Society and Health
Sociology for Health Professionals

Society and Health
Sociology for Health Professionals

Richard K. Thomas, Ph.D.

Kluwer Academic / Plenum Publishers
New York   Boston   Dordrecht   London   Moscow

Library of Congress Cataloging-in-Publication Data

Thomas, Richard K.
  Society and health: sociology for health professionals/Richard K. Thomas.
    p. cm.
  Includes bibliographical references and index.
  ISBN 0-306-47746-7
    I. Social medicine. 2. Sociology. 3. Medical personnel. I. Title.

  RA418.T535 2003
  362.1—dc21
                                                                    2003050643

ISBN: 0-306-47746-7

© 2003 Kluwer Academic / Plenum Publishers, New York
233 Spring Street, New York, New York 10013

http://www.wkap.nl/

10 9 8 7 6 5 4 3 2 1

A C.I.P. record for this book is available from the Library of Congress

Permissions for books published in Europe: *permissions@wkap.nl*
Permissions for books published in the United States of America: *permissions@wkap.com*

Printed in the United States of America

Preface

The publication of *Society and Health: Sociology for Health Professionals* represents the results of an information-gathering process that has extended over a 30-year career as a health professional. It reflects a determination to frame medical sociology as a multidisciplinary endeavor that must, of necessity, draw information from a wide range of fields. While sociologists themselves have certainly contributed their share to the development of the field of medical sociology, representatives of many other fields have also made important contributions. Many of these did not initially approach their subject matter from a sociological perspective, only to find that there was indeed an important social dimension to their research. This book owes a great deal to those representing epidemiology, public health, social psychology, psychiatry, demography, biostatistics, and related fields that have contributed so much to our knowledge concerning the social aspects of health and healthcare.

In *Society and Health* I have tried to step back from my respective roles as academician and practitioner in order to transcend any disciplinary or occupational constraints, in order to view the body of knowledge presented here in the most open-minded manner possible. The intent has been to reflect the breadth and depth of the study of the social aspects of health and healthcare and, in so doing, serve to bear witness to the various influences that have converged to bring this combination of materials together.

Nearly thirty years ago, it was argued that a new perspective on the medical model was required, one that combined the biological, psychological, and social perspectives. This new paradigm, it was felt, would provide the framework for analysis of the healthcare system for a long time to come. This volume is intended to reflect that perspective and, indeed, expand on that approach to offer the most inclusive perspective on health and healthcare possible. Its intent is to demonstrate the extent to which healthcare cannot be considered apart from the influence of social, cultural, economic, and political factors, among others. Hopefully, the notion of health and healthcare as integral parts of social life—and not as topics to be singled out for separate consideration—is reflected in this book.

RICHARD K. THOMAS

Contents

Chapter 1

Introduction to the Sociology of Health and Illness

THE FIELD OF SOCIOLOGY

Sociology is the scientific study of human social activity. Any type of human activity that involves social circumstances—and that is virtually everything—is appropriate for sociological analysis. Certainly any form of social interaction is amenable to sociological study, and an individual's solitary behavior and even his thoughts are influenced to a great extent by social factors.

Sociology is distinguished from other sciences by its use of the "sociological perspective." The sociological perspective involves a search for patterns that exist in observed human behavior. Virtually nothing happens randomly when it comes to human behavior, and patterns can be found in all human activity. Even accidents do not occur randomly in society, but are more likely to affect individuals with certain characteristics. Doctors do not act randomly, nor do patients. Like everyone else in society they act in accordance with societally established guidelines that are appropriate for the roles they perform.

Like proponents of the natural sciences, early sociologists set out to identify "laws" of social behavior. They believed that behavior was not random or governed by external forces but involved identifiable patterns that could be linked to social characteristics. To the extent that these patterns become embedded into the fabric of society, they could be considered analogous to the laws of natural science.

Although well established as an academic discipline today, sociology faced a difficult challenge in becoming accepted in U.S. society. The American ethos places inordinate emphasis on individualism and touts the American's ability to think for himself and transcend group constraints. Although the U.S. is certainly less individualistic than it was 50 years ago, as a society we still tend to hold individuals accountable for their actions and expect individuals to work toward their own best interests in most cases, rather than the best interests of their social group. Thus, a brilliant physician is likely to be praised for his individual efforts, while a patient who fails to follow doctor's orders or pay his medical bill on time—the "bad" patient—is blamed as an individual for his actions. Yet, neither one of these individuals acts the way he does because of his individual traits. They are both to a great extent products of the "system"—that is, the social system in which they function. The fact that we are all creatures of our society and our social environment rather than some more deterministic factor explains why Americans behave differently from the French or the Chinese and, further, why rich Americans behave differently from poor ones.

Over time, Americans have come to realize that, as a society, we are not nearly as individualistic as we perceive ourselves. True, Americans emphasize self-actualization to the point of appearing narcissistic, but this is tempered by the same type of "herd instinct" that characterizes all types of human groups. Like all people everywhere, Americans are influenced by the larger society in which they live. While the mantra of the 1960s—society made them do it—may represent an extreme view of deviant behavior, it is difficult to find any pattern of behavior—from our hairstyles to our housing choices to our selection of healthcare provider—that is not influenced by our sociocultural background and the social groups with which we interact.

The society's institutions continuously guide our behavior as we develop as society members, and they reinforce that behavior once we are socialized into the society. Like members of other societies, Americans are influenced by the groups in society with which they interact. Fraternities, political parties, and professional associations all influence our thoughts and actions, and we are influenced to a considerable extent by our immediate group surroundings—by our families, friends, and business associates. These social influences act simultaneously to shape the beliefs, values and behavior of the individual.

BASIC TENETS OF SOCIOLOGY

Sociologists posit several important notions related to the nature of society. First, sociologists contend that the human being comes into the world as a "blank slate", ready and eager to be inscribed upon by its social group. There is little about human behavior that is innate and, indeed, this perspective would disdain the notion of "instincts" within human beings. While some aspects of our being may be conveyed through genetic matter, our social "being" is a product of our social environment. The recent spate of international adoptions by Americans has clearly proven this point. Everywhere we turn in the U.S. today, there are children from China, Romania and Colombia, who are as American as George Washington. For those adopted as infants, they have known only one social environment and that environment has filled up their "slate."

This means that we are not born knowing how to follow healthy lifestyles or pursue healthy diets. And we are certainly not born knowing how to act like patients. These behavior patterns are imprinted through the socialization process on an essentially blank slate and it is up to the sociologist to describe and analyze these processes.

Second, sociologists would argue that society—or any social group, for that matter—represents more than just the sum of its parts. A nation of ten millions residents is, thus, more than just the characteristics of the ten million residents added together. By being part of a social group, something new and different arises that transcends any characteristics of individuals. Rules, preferences, and expectations evolve from the interaction of individuals that would not occur to individuals left to their own volition. Studies have found that individuals will do things as part of a group that never would have even occurred to them as individuals. The classic case is probably the lynch mob, in which no individual would have taken it upon himself to personally deal out "justice" to the victim of the mob. The mob takes on characteristics that transcend those of any individual. Would an adult male ever agree to wear a necktie if a rule had not evolved from the group that mandated it? Would any reasonable person embark on a potentially dangerous crash diet if it weren't for the influence of the social group?

This leads to a third point. Once a society or social group is established, it takes on a life of its own. That is, individual society members have limited ability to influence the nature of society and, in fact, must generally bend to society's will. In effect, we are all born into a game that is already underway and have limited influence over the rules. True, there is the occasional revolutionary—the Karl Marx or Martin Luther King, Jr.—who comes along and makes a major impact on society. But the work of revolutionaries often takes decades before it makes an impact on the deep-seated characteristics of the society. Indeed, decades after the assassination of Martin Luther King, Jr., America as a society is still trying to work out the details of racial integration. And, long after observers reported a "crisis" in healthcare, reformers are still trying to overcome deeply ingrained physician practice patterns and insurance practices in order to create a more efficient delivery system.

WHY A SOCIOLOGY OF HEALTH AND ILLNESS?

Why do we need a sociology of health and illness? Why not leave healthcare to the doctors? Indeed, what is *social* about health and healthcare? First we need to consider what is social about anything. In the final analysis, individual human behavior is social behavior and this means that "health behavior" is social behavior, influenced by the societal factors that influence all behavior, as well as the particular behavior patterns engendered by the healthcare institution. Sick people do not act randomly, but follow certain "rules". In fact, if they don't follow the rules, they may be criticized by their social group and the healthcare system and even "thrown out" of the sick role.

Since healthcare is an endeavor that is highly technical and characterized by strict rules of conduct, how can we say that social factors play a role in health behavior? These rules that guide clinical trials, doctor-patient relationships or surgical protocols arise out of a social situation and are established by social beings. In fact, a rigorous endeavor like medical science is rampant with examples of how social factors influence supposedly strict clinical protocols. Why did male physicians and the medical power structure oppose the training of female doctors for so many decades? Why do male physicians tell women undergoing menopause that their symptoms are "all in their head"? Why do African-American patients receive different treatment than white patients who have the same symptoms? Why are physicians eager to "write off" elderly patients rather than aggressively pursuing improved health?

These situations all reflect the variation that exists in health behavior even among professionals who have sworn to uphold rigorous standards, variations reflecting the influence of social factors on health professionals. Indeed, it has been found that the best predictor of a psychiatric diagnosis for a patient is often the demographic characteristics of the patient and the psychiatrist—not the patient's symptoms.

There are many additional arguments for health behavior as social behavior. Indeed, the defining condition of the system—sickness—is a social construct. As will be seen later, individuals may develop symptoms of illness, and these may be identified through clinical tests. However, the individual is not "officially" sick until someone—that is, a physician or someone in the individual's social group—concedes he is in fact sick.

The fact that sickness is a social condition is supported by the differential assessments of symptoms by those within the respective social groups. In some social circles, premenstrual syndrome is considered a condition that requires rest and medical attention, while in others it is normal state that one takes in stride—and certainly not a medical issue. Among some groups in U.S. society, pregnancy is considered similar to a sickness and requires extensive medical intervention, while to others pregnancy is a natural process that will take care of itself. Among some groups minor aberrations in emotional state are considered anxiety disorders and require clinical intervention, while to others these represent normal variations in human emotions and are, therefore, odd or eccentric at best. Among some social groups, the disorientation accompanying aging is seen as a symptom of advancing Alzheimer's disease and requires medical intervention; to others, it's a normal part of the aging process and is something that will run its unfortunate course.

Not only do social considerations determine what one considers a sickness, but we attribute social meaning to health conditions. We only have to consider the social stigma attached to conditions like sexually transmitted diseases, AIDS and schizophrenia. These conditions are attributed meaning above and beyond their medical consequences, and the affected parties are now seen in a different light as people. In fact, even individuals with a "routine" illness—something that can happen to anyone—may also be seen in a negative light. Sickness in U.S. society is associated with inferiority and the condition implies that sick persons are not as capable as well ones. Our compassion for the infirm is tempered by a concern that the individual is not pulling his or her weight as a society member. In the U.S., a particular stigma is associated with those who live off of disability payments, and those who linger in the sick role for too long are likely to be viewed in a negative light.

The social significance of sickness is seen in the impact it has on social relationships. Even beyond extreme examples such as AIDS and mental illness, a disruption of social relationships is an inherent component of sickness. The affected individual may be unable to carry out social obligations in terms of work, school or church and unable to function in terms of interpersonal relationships. Not only does the person's role of "employee" suffer, but he may be unable to perform the role of "husband", "father", or "friend." The sick person is seen in a different light by those in his social group and, indeed, he comes to see himself differently, not only in physical terms but in social terms as well.

An additional argument for the salience of sociology to modern healthcare is the fact that social factors have come to play such an important role in the prevalence and distribution of health conditions within the U.S. population. Indeed, much of this text is devoted to that issue. As acute conditions have given way to chronic conditions as the leading health problems and causes of death, we have found that biological factors are playing a diminished role in the etiology of disease. In fact, some estimates suggest that biological factors account for only 10% of the health problems in contemporary U.S. society, and this only increases to 20% when heredity is thrown in. What then is to blame?

While the environment is certainly a factor in the etiology of disease— and this to a great extent reflects social considerations—lifestyle has come to be the major contributor to and predictor of health problems in U.S. society. While we are all cognizant of the influence of lifestyle on such conditions as cancer and heart disease, even minor conditions are often correlated with social factors and lifestyle-related behaviors. An individual's sociocultural background and social group influences determine to a great extent the type and severity of the physical and mental illnesses that occur. Indeed, many of the greatest threats to an individual's health and physical well-being today can be attributed to unhealthy lifestyles and high-risk behavior. Healthy lifestyles and the avoidance of high-risk behavior advance the individual's potential for a longer and healthier life, while unhealthy lifestyles and high-risk behavior are primary contributors to the burden of illnesses in U.S. society.

While the common cold occurs relatively randomly within a population, the likelihood of that cold progressing to bronchitis or even to pneumonia is a function of the demographic and social characteristics of the individuals involved. Thus, the facts that one is African American rather than white, male rather than female, or affluent rather than poor are major determinants with regard to the risk of health problems.

The social dimension of the health/illness process is further indicated by the importance of social support. Individuals who do not have adequate social support tend to be more likely to experience the onset of health problems, develop more severe problems, experience conditions of longer duration, and experience progression to more serious phases. The availability of social support depends to a certain extent on the sociocultural characteristics of the individual.

In the final analysis, health behavior is social behavior. In fact, early social analysts even argued that health was not a medical problem but a social problem. And that assertion appears to have even more validity as more research findings on health behavior are generated. Whether we are talking about the actions of physicians, patients, hospital administrators, nurses, or managed care executives, their behavior is primarily determined by social considerations. Participation in the healthcare system does not insulate us from the forces that pervade society. Indeed, the healthcare system serves in many ways as a microcosm for the study of the larger society.

SOCIAL ROOTS OF HEALTHCARE

Just as health behavior is a function of the social forces that impinge upon members of society, any healthcare system is ultimately a product of the society in which it exists and the cultural traits characterizing that society. The healthcare system can only be understood within its sociocultural context. No two healthcare systems are exactly alike, and the differences that are found between healthcare systems are primarily a function of the contexts in which they exist. The social structure of the society, along with its cultural values, defines the system. The form the system takes and the functions it performs reflect the form and functions of the society in which it resides. Much of the focus of this book will be on the influence of social factors on the health status and health behavior of individual society members and on the system in which this behavior occurs.

Social factors influence the manner in which societies organize their resources to respond to sickness and to deliver care to their members. Individuals and societies tend to respond to health problems in a manner consistent with the prescriptions (and proscriptions) of their culture. Social and political values influence the policies established, the institutions formed, and the types of programs that are funded. It is no accident that the United States has the form of healthcare delivery it does and that other nations have their particular forms. The development of a system of healthcare is therefore not simply a matter of responding to biological threats, but involves a number of factors that are social, cultural, political, and economic in nature. Thus, those who would understand the U.S. system of healthcare must understand society.

THE HISTORY OF THE SOCIOLOGY OF HEALTH AND ILLNESS

As sociology emerged as a discipline in the late nineteenth century, it founders ignored the healthcare institution in their analysis of society. Unlike frequently studied institutions such as the family, the political system and religion, healthcare was neglected because it had yet to emerge as a full-blown social institution. For this reason, medical sociology as an accepted field did not emerge until after World War II, nor did it achieve any significant development until the 1960s. Consequently, medical sociology matured in an intellectual climate far different from nineteenth- and early twentieth-century environment that spawned early social thought.

The use of the term "medical sociology" has been noted as early as 1894 in an article by Charles McIntire on the importance of social factors in health. Medical sociology was established as a specialized field within sociology in the United States during the 1940s and 1950s. The emergence of this subdiscipline was given impetus by virtue of the interest in social medicine that surfaced in the 1920s and 30s and the emergence of the field of social epidemiology in the 1940s and 1950s. These two movements bolstered the belief that social science had something to contribute to medical research. As a result, the first applications of this new subdiscipline within sociology were in the medical schools. Even so, because of the apparent success of the medical model in dealing with sickness and its domination of medical thought for a century, the significance of non-clinical factors for the health and illness equation was essentially ignored. In fact, it was only in the last third of the twentieth century that the contribution of the sociological perspective to the study of health and healthcare came to be appreciated.

Recognition of the complex relationships between social factors and the level of health characteristic of various groups has made the sociology of health and illness an important substantive area within the general field of sociology. Just as sociology is concerned with the social causes and consequences of human behavior, the sociology of health is concerned with the social causes and consequences of health and illness. The sociology of health brings sociological perspectives, theories, and methods to the study of health and healthcare.

Medical sociology emerged at a time when government agencies and medical funding sources had little interest in purely theoretical sociology. Thus, the pressure has always been on medical sociology to produce work that could be applied to medical practice and the formulation of health policy. In the United States, where medical sociology has reached its most extensive development, the development of the field has paralleled government investment in health-related research. Funding from federal and private organizations helped stimulate cooperation between sociologists and physicians with regard to research on health problems. As a result, the early focus of medical sociology in the United States was on applied or practical problem solving rather than on the development of theory.

The direction taken by medical sociology early in its development is best summarized by Robert Straus (1957). Straus suggested that medical sociology had become divided into two separate but closely interrelated areas: a sociology *of* medicine and a sociology *in* medicine. The sociology of medicine deals with such factors as the organization, role relationships, norms, values and beliefs of medical practice as a form of human behavior. Thus, the initial work in medical sociology was from the point of view of medicine rather than sociology. The emphasis was on the social processes that occur in the medical setting and how these contribute to our understanding of medical behavior in particular and our understanding of social life in general. The sociology of medicine shares the same goals as all other areas of sociology and is characterized as research and analysis of the medical environment from a sociological perspective.

The sociologist in medicine is a sociologist who collaborates directly with physicians and other health personnel in the study of the social factors that are relevant to a particular phenomenon in the healthcare arena. The work of the sociologist in medicine is intended to be directly applicable to patient care or to the solving of a public health problem. (The various perspectives on the role of the sociologist of health and illness are described below.) These analyses are made available to health practitioners, health planners and policy setters to assist them in addressing health problems and problems in the delivery of care. Thus, sociology in medicine can be characterized as "applied research and analysis primarily motivated by a medical problem" rather than a sociological problem (Cockerham, 2001).

While sociology itself had its origins in Europe, medical sociology has evolved as a particularly American perspective. The first university programs for the training of medical sociologists in the U.S. were instituted in the 1940s and a section of the American Sociological Association dedicated to medical sociology was formed in 1959. At present, medical sociologists constitute the largest and one of the most active groups of professionals doing sociological work in the United States and Western Europe. Not only have the numbers of medical sociologists continually increased, but the scope of matters pertinent to medical sociology has clearly broadened as our conception of health and illness have broadened and issues of health, illness, and medicine have become a forum through which larger issues of society may be addressed.

THE NATURE OF THE SOCIOLOGY OF HEALTH AND ILLNESS

As the title of this book indicates, the term "medical sociology" is not the label of choice for this field for this author. While the term "medical sociology" is still in common usage, there has been a definite trend toward use of the term "sociology of health and healthcare" or the "sociology of health and illness." This shift in nomenclature reflects the paradigm shift (discussed in a later section) that characterized the U.S. healthcare system in the closing years of the twentieth century. Without belaboring issues to be discussed later, suffice it to say that, for many, "medical" is much too narrow a term, especially in light of the expansion of the boundaries of what is to be considered under the heading of "health", "illness" and "healthcare". As will be seen, this broadening of the boundaries of health and healthcare has led to a concomitant broadening of the perspective of medical sociology. (We will continue, however, to use the term "medical sociology" as a convenience.)

The sociology of health and illness is a far-ranging discipline and its scope is difficult to define in a few words. Medical sociologists approach the field from a variety of perspectives and typically emphasize one or more aspects of the discipline. Some focus on *social epidemiology* and study the distribution of illness within a population, how social characteristics contribute to its etiology and distribution, and the correlations between sociodemographic characteristics and health status. Others focus on *socio-culturally determined responses* to illness and study the manner in which individuals react (or don't react) to the onset of symptoms and how the values we hold influence our reaction to illness.

Some medical sociologists focus on the *interactional aspects* of health-care and study, for example, doctor-patient relationships or doctor-nurse interaction. Others emphasize the *organizational aspects* of healthcare and focus on the organization of the hospital or the structure of medical educa-tion. Some medical sociologists focus on patterns of *health services utilization* and study variations in utilization in different communities and the social correlates of the use of health services. Others may emphasize the soci-ology of *health occupations* and study the characteristics of physicians and nurses or social stratification within the health professions. Medical so-ciologists may focus on the study of *mental health and illness*, examining the distribution of mental disorders within the society or professional and lay perceptions of mental patients. Still others may focus on the *"political" aspects* of healthcare and study the power structure of healthcare, the role of the American Medical Association, or trends in the "medicalization" of society. Finally, some medical sociologists may focus on *health policy issues* and study the manner in which U.S. health policy is formulated and the role of various parties in establishing health policy.

The evolution of medical sociology owes a debt to several other dis-ciplines whose concepts, methods and data have contributed to the devel-opment of the field. Research on the sociology of health and illness relies heavily on methods and data from *demography* and, indeed, the emerging field of health demography is becoming increasingly important. Any un-derstanding of the social correlates of health status and health behavior requires an appreciation of the demographic characteristics of the popu-lation under study and skills in demographic analysis on the part of the researcher. The medical specialty of *epidemiology* has contributed much of the methodology that underlies sociomedical research, and social epidemi-ology has become a major field in its own right. Other medical specialties that have contributed to the development of the field include *public health* and *psychiatry*. The former has provided a perspective that emphasizes the "public" aspects of healthcare and reminds us that health should be a community concern as well as an individual issue. Psychiatry has provided insights into the nature of mental health and illness and contributed to our understanding of the social correlates of mental disorder. Some key perspectives within the sociology of mental illness have been contributed by psychiatrists.

The sociology of health and illness also owes a debt to other social sciences. *Medical anthropology* has been in the forefront of theoretical perspectives that have become incorporated into medical sociology. Anthropologists have led the way in the examination of cross-cultural differences in perceptions of and responses to health conditions and have sensitized the field to the significance of ethnic and subcultural factors in health status and health behavior in the U.S. Anthropologists have also led us to understand that symptoms may be interpreted quite differently in various societies and introduced us to the salient attributes of traditional medical systems. *Medical geographers* have offered insights into the spatial distribution of health-related phenomena and provided the foundation for examining geographical variations in health conditions and health services utilization. *Medical economists* have provided a perspective that reminds us that we are "economic man" as well as "social man", that economics drives the U.S. system, and that the U.S. healthcare "market" is indeed unique.

Although the intent of this text is to be as comprehensive as possible, not every conceivable topic of interest to medical sociology can be covered. Here, as always, the author must focus on the topics that are considered most salient and the content that is essential to an understanding of the sociology of health and illness. Although most of the following topics are addressed at least in passing, they are typically given limited coverage.

The text does not deal extensively with the regulation of healthcare, although the implications of the laws and regulations originating from various agencies and organizations are significant. Similarly, legal issues related to the operation of the healthcare system are not addressed in detail. The financing of healthcare is provided limited coverage and is a topic of enough complexity to require its own venue. The implications of the physical environment for health are generally not addressed, although the social environment is dealt with in great detail. Ethical issues are provided limited coverage, although the controversy surrounding issues such as euthanasia, cloning, genetic engineering, and abortion are major considerations in today's healthcare environment. Health policy issues are not addressed, primarily due to the fact that the United States does not have a formal health policy in any real sense. Finally, the sociology of health and illness is not examined in cross-cultural perspective. Occasional references will be made to research from other countries or comparisons between the U.S. and other societies, but this is a significant enough topic as to require separate attention.

PURPOSE OF THE BOOK

The idea for this book came about in response to a perceived void in the resources available to sociologists interested in healthcare and particularly to those in the health professions who require an understanding of the sociology of health and illness. While there are several medical sociology textbooks available, they are typically geared toward students who know a lot about sociology but very little about healthcare. The growing market for this material, however, is among those in the health professions who are coming to appreciate the importance of social factors for health and healthcare and require a resource that is appropriate for students and professionals who know a great deal about healthcare but little about sociology. The challenge was to develop a resource for students approaching the convergence of sociology and healthcare from either perspective.

The interest in the sociological aspects of health and healthcare has never been higher. The significance of non-biological factors for health status and health behavior is now conceded by even the most "clinical" of medical professionals. Every day new information relating social factors to health characteristics is reported, and we are clearly beginning to operate under a new paradigm that involves a biopsychosocial view of health and healthcare. Most health training programs now offer a course on this topic and the interest continues to grow. Within sociology itself, medical sociology remains one of the largest subdisciplines and no well-trained sociologist can neglect this area of study.

A major motivation for this book has been the realization on the part of the author—after thirty years spent in applying medical sociology to concrete health problems—of how little of this knowledge has been made available to clinicians or healthcare administrators. Neither the people who run health facilities nor the physicians and others who provide care have been privy to much of the knowledge that has been generated by medical sociologists and other researchers on the topics dealt with in this text. Information on the causes of health problems, on lay perceptions of these problems, on the approaches that people use to address these problems, and on what patients think of the healthcare system—none of these have been widely disseminated among the professionals responsible for the operation of the system. This book attempts to provide this information in a context that will not only instill in sociologists an appreciation of the application of concepts from sociology to the healthcare arena but, at the same time, arm health professionals with the knowledge they need to manage the system and deal effectively with patients.

ORGANIZATION OF THE BOOK

The organization of this book is fairly straightforward. Chapters 1–5 provide basic information on the nature of sociology and basic definitions and concepts from healthcare, indicating the extent to which they interface. These first chapters also provide information on the history of healthcare in general and particularly for the United States. The social and cultural factors influencing the development of the healthcare system are emphasized here.

Chapters 6 and 7 describe aspects of sociology that have particular relevance for healthcare—social groups and occupations and professions. Chapter 8 provides an overview of social epidemiology and sets the stage for much of the remaining discussion of the interface of social factors and healthcare.

Chapters 9 and 10 offer what some would consider the core material of the book. These chapters examine the social correlates of health status and sickness behavior. These chapters build on the voluminous research on these topics that has been accumulated over the past three decades.

Chapters 11 and 12 deal with the particularly sociological concepts of social stratification and deviance. The extent to which social class plays a role in health status and health behavior cannot be overemphasized and the relevance of social stratification to the operation of the healthcare system is highlighted. Chapter 11 also addresses the role sex, race and age play in social stratification. The topic of deviance is of particular importance in that sickness represents a form of deviance that all persons experience at one time or another.

Chapter 13 deals with the important topic of the sociology of mental illness, presenting the core concepts and looking at the field from the unique sociological perspective. Chapter 14 presents the sociological perspective on social change and technology and relates the concepts therein to healthcare. Likely future developments in healthcare and their implications for the sociology of health and illness are also discussed in this chapter.

Chapters generally begin by presenting a basic introduction to the sociological or healthcare concept under study and proceed from there to apply it to a concrete setting. Each chapter includes sidebars to illustrate concepts noted in the text, along with tables and graphs where appropriate. In addition to references for each chapter, a section on additional resources includes other readings and materials relevant to the topic. Each chapter also includes a list of Internet sites that might be useful. An index and a glossary of relevant terms are included at the end of text.

REFERENCES

Cockerham, William C. (2001). *Medical Sociology*. Upper Saddle River, NJ: Prentice Hall.
Straus, Robert (1957). "The nature and status of medical sociology." *American Sociological Review*, 22:200–204.

ADDITIONAL RESOURCES

Bird, Chloe E., Peter Conrad, and Allen M. Fremont (eds.) (2000). *Handbook of Medical Sociology*: 5th edition. Upper Saddle Creek, NJ: Prentice Hall.
Brown, Phil (1996). *Perspectives in Medical Sociology*, 2nd ed. Prospect Heights, IL: Waveland Press.
Pescosolido, Bernice A., and Jennie J. Kronenfield (1995). "Health, illness, and healing in an uncertain era: Challenges from and for medical sociology. *Journal of Health and Social Behavior*, extra issue: 5–35.
Sullivan, Thomas J. (1998). *Applied Sociology: Research and Critical Thinking*. Boston: Allyn and Bacon.

INTERNET LINKS

The American Sociological Association homepage: www.asanet.org
The American Sociological Association Medical Sociology Section homepage: www.kent. edu/sociology/asamedsoc
The Society for Applied Sociology homepage: www.appliedsoc.org
SocioSite: Sociology of Health: www.pscw.uva.nl/sociosite/TOPICS/ Health.html

Chapter 2

The Language of Healthcare

DEFINITIONS IN HEALTHCARE

Defining the concepts is the first step in the establishment of any science. However, in the evolution of both medical sociology and the U.S. healthcare system, little attention has been paid to the formulation of some key concepts. At the outset, the concepts of health and healthcare need to be defined, and this is no simple matter. In fact, most books on medical sociology or healthcare make no attempt to define either concept. Despite the fact that Americans are obsessed with their "health", there is no consensus on a definition for this concept among either professionals or laypersons. In the final analysis, what constitutes health–and its counterparts sickness and disease–depends on one's frame of reference. Medical sociologists and others studying the meanings of these terms have had to settle for several definitions, each linked to a different explanatory model.

The concepts used to define and organize any system of healthcare reflect the social organization and culture of the society in which it exists. The health-related concepts that are familiar to Americans are a function of the unique worldview characterizing U.S. society. Many of the health-related concepts that are so familiar to members of U.S. society today did not exist in premodern societies. Notions of "health," "sickness," and "disease," although taken for granted in contemporary Western societies, are recent social constructs; they have no counterparts in earlier social systems. For most premodern societies, these health states were an inherent part of the nature of things and could not be separately objectified.

DEFINING HEALTH

"Health" is perhaps one of the most difficult of healthcare terms to define. Not only is it a difficult concept to define in absolute terms, its meaning has been changing over time. A variety of definitions have been proffered representing different perspectives and none can be considered clearly right or wrong. As will be seen, the acceptable definition depends on one's perspective.

The very notion of health is a social ideal and its conceptualization varies widely from culture to culture and from one historical period to another. For example, in the nineteenth century the ideal upper-class woman was pale, frail, and delicate. A woman with robust health was considered to be lacking in refinement (Ehrenreich and English, 1978). In other periods, cultures, or subcultures, the ideal of health might be identified with traits such as strength, fertility, righteousness, fatness, thinness, or youthfulness. The ideal of health, thus, embodies a particular culture's notions of well-being and desired human qualities.

The Medical Model

There are at least three commonly used paradigms for dealing with the concepts of health and illness (Wolinsky 1988). The historically dominant model in U.S. society is referred to as the *medical model*. The medical model had its genesis in the establishment of germ theory as the basis for modern scientific medicine. This perspective emphasizes the existence of clearly identifiable clinical symptoms, reflecting the conviction that illness represents the presence of biological pathology. Thus, illness is a state involving the presence of distinct symptoms; health is the negative, residual state reflecting an absence of symptoms.

Health and illness are conceptualized under the medical model in terms of biological "normality" and "abnormality." While many would argue for a more meaningful definition of these concepts, this view of health and illness continues to be widely accepted, since it is the view supported by medical practitioners. The manner in which most health problems are conceptualized and managed reflects this orientation. Both medical education and the organization of care reinforce this perspective. Health insurance constitutes an excellent example in that no treatment is covered without a physician's (i.e., a medical-model orientation) diagnosis based on the presence of symptoms.

As Freund and McGuire (1999) note, the medical model assumes a clear dichotomy between the mind and the body, and physical diseases are presumed to be located within the body. The philosophical foundations for this mind/body dichotomy may go back to Descartes' division of the person into mind and body. The practical foundations, however, probably lie in medicine's shift to an emphasis on clinical observation toward the end of the eighteenth century and pathological anatomy beginning in the nineteenth century. This notion implies that the body can be understood and treated in isolation from other aspects of the person inhabiting it (Hahn and Kleinman, 1983).

This medical perspective sees the body as docile—something physicians could observe, manipulate, transform, and improve. Diseases are conceptualized in terms of alterations of tissues that are visible upon opening the body, such as during autopsy. This mode of conceptualizing disease had a profound effect in splitting body from mind in the practice of clinical medicine. In fact, health came to be seen as a residual state involving the *absence* of pathology.

The medical model also assumes that illness can be reduced to disordered bodily (biochemical or neurophysiological) functions. This physical reductionism excludes social, psychological, and behavioral dimensions of illness (Engle, 1977). The result of this reductionism, together with medicine's mind-body dualism, is that disease is localized in the individual body. Such conceptions prevent the medical model from considering external factors such as the way in which aspects of the individual's social or emotional life might impinge upon physical health.

A related assumption of this biomedical model is the belief that each disease is caused by a specific, potentially identifiable agent. This assumption emerged from the nineteenth century work of Pasteur and Koch, who demonstrated that the introduction of specific virulent microorganisms (germs) into the body produced specific agents with a causal link to specific diseases. This doctrine of specific etiology was later extended beyond infectious diseases and applied to other diseases less amenable to this explanation.

Dubos (1959) noted that while the doctrine of specific etiology has led to important theoretical and practical achievements, it has rarely provided a complete account of the causation of disease. Why, for example, do only some people get sick some of the time? Accordingly, an adequate understanding of an illness etiology must include broader factors, such as nutrition, stress, and metabolic states, that affect the individual's susceptibility to infection. The search for specific illness-producing agents worked relatively well in dealing with infectious diseases but is too simplistic to explain the causes of complex, chronic illnesses.

A variation of the medical model compares the body to a machine. From this perspective, disease represents the malfunctioning of some constituent mechanism and disease represents a "breakdown" of some organ. Modern medicine has not only retained the metaphor of the machine but also extended it by developing specializations along the lines of machine parts, emphasizing individual systems or organs to the exclusion of an image of the totality of the body. The machine metaphor further encouraged an instrumentalist approach to the body; the physician could "repair" one part of the body in isolation from the rest (Berliner, 1975).

The medical model has been widely accepted because of its scientific basis and its usefulness in addressing certain types of disorders. It has been criticized, however, for its focus on acute rather than chronic conditions, its inability to account for nonphysical and/or asymptomatic conditions, and its reliance on professional "consensus" on what is considered normal and abnormal (Wolinsky 1988). The fact that the medical model was becoming less and less effective in dealing with contemporary health problems has contributed to a significant paradigm shift in healthcare.

The Functional Model

A second context for defining health and illness is referred to as the *functional model*. This model contends that health and illness reflect the level of *social* normality rather than physical normality characterizing an individual (Parsons 1972). This approach de-emphasizes the biologically based medical model in favor of a model based on social role performance. This view reasons that an individual with clinically identifiable symptoms, but who is adequately performing his or her social functions, should be considered "well." Conversely, if an individual has no clinically identifiable symptoms but is unable to function, it may be appropriate to classify this individual as "sick."

The functional model is rooted in lay conceptualizations of health and illness rather than professional ones. From this perspective, the "diagnosis" is made by the social group based on societally based criteria rather than clinical ones. "Treatment" is geared toward restoring the affected individual to social normality rather than biological normality. The individual is seen as "cured" when he or she can resume social functioning, not when the clinical signs have disappeared.

Examples of the tension between the medical model and the functional model would include the alcoholic who, for years, is able to perform his job and maintain an adequate family relationship. This person would be considered sick under the medical model but not under the functional model. Conversely, an individual complaining of chronic back pain would be considered sick under the functional model (assuming that the symptoms interfered with his or her social role performance), even if physicians could not identify any underlying pathological disorder. Another example would involve individuals with disabilities; an amputee may be considered sick from the medical-model perspective but actually be capable of performing all required social roles.

The Psychological Model

Although the medical and functional models are considered the dominant paradigms, the *psychological model* should also be introduced (Antonovsky 1979). Alternately referred to as the "stress model," this is by far the most subjective of the three approaches. This model relies solely on self evaluation by the individual for the determination of health and illness. If the individual feels well, he or she is well; if the same individual feels sick, he or she is sick. This approach focuses on the importance of stress in the production of sickness and argues that much of physical illness is a reaction to stress on the part of the individual. This perspective has gained some respect, now that the mind/body connection has been rediscovered and increasing emphasis is being placed on psychosomatic conditions.

The Legal Model

One final model that should be noted primarily applies to mental illness. This is the *legal model*, and it is applied in situations where the legal "health" or competence of the individual is in question. A legal definition comes into play in cases where competence must be determined for involuntary hospital admission, guardianship, or custody decisions, and in cases where the individual's ability to manage his or her affairs is in question. Although a physician is generally required to certify the individual's competence, it is ultimately the courts that decide based on criteria established by the legal system.

To summarize the definitions of health and illness from these various perspectives, the following might be considered: From the medical-model perspective, health is a biological state characterized by the absence of disease and disability. Under the functional model, health is a condition characterized by optimal performance of social roles, regardless of the individual's physical state. From the psychological perspective, health is a state of well-being identified by the individual and, as such, is not amenable to easy description. From the legal perspective, health—or, more appropriately, illness—is a state defined by the legal system that may or may not have any relation to other definitions of health and illness.

One other definition of health that might be noted is the one formulated in the 1960s by the World Health Organization (WHO), the health arm

---

Box 2-1

The Discovery of a New Disease: The Case of Menopause

A variety of factors may contribute to the discovery of a "new" disease. This may involve the identification of a here-to-fore unknown condition (e.g., Legionnaire's disease or AIDS) and the subsequent classification and naming of it. It may involve the discovery of a syndrome involving a set of symptoms not previously connected before. Or it may involved the redefinition of an existing condition as a health problem (e.g., alcoholism).

The last means of disease discovery is relevant to menopause which was added to the list of diseases in the *International Classification of Diseases* in the 1980s. Although menopause is considered to be a normal biological process, it has become increasingly "medicalized" over the past 50 years. During this period, the condition has been transformed from symptoms that were essentially "all in the head" of affected women to a clinical condition involving estrogen deficiency or ovarian dysfunction.

Despite the universality of menopause among women regardless of the society, there are remarkable differences in the biophysical, social and emotional dimensions of the condition from culture to culture. The various social connotations and expectations associated with menopause are ignored by modern Western medicine. The condition is reduced to a set of biochemical processes presumed to characterize all female bodies, regardless of the social or cultural context. The notion of menopause as a pathological condition originated with a specific body of research but, once the condition was isolated, the "disease" took on a life of its own, unaffected by subsequent research. Early research, for example, was based on women who had experienced surgically induced menopause or who suffered from extreme conditions that involved unusual physical side effects. The findings drawn from an abnormal

---

of the United Nations. Health is defined by WHO as a state of complete physical, psychological, social, and spiritual well-being and not merely the absence of disease and infirmity (World Health Organization 1999). While this rather idealistic definition has generally been rejected as unworkable in today's healthcare environment, it is ironic that the U.S. healthcare system has come to be seen by the public as serving to meet the disparate needs encompassed by this definition. American society has come to expect the scope of healthcare to extend far beyond the treatment of physical problems and into the management of psychological, social, and spiritual problems.

Ultimately, there is no *one* definition of "health". In fact, the definitions posed by health professionals may be quite different from lay definitions. (See Box 2-1 for a discussion of lay definitions of health and illness.) Each of the examples above may be appropriate for certain purposes under certain

population were extrapolated to the general population, and the notion of menopause as a disease became firmly entrenched.

Recent research utilizing more normal populations for subjects has found no evidence of pathology or medical problems. Not only did most women not experience abnormal symptoms but, among those few who did, there were typically other health problems accompanying the onset of menopause. Thus, it could be argued that other health problems contribute to problem menopause and not the other way around. Researchers have subsequently argued that physicians have been too eager to attribute various problems to the menopausal state of the patient.

To a great extent, the identification of menopause as a pathological condition was a result of a "campaign" by a handful of sex endocrinologists who were proponents of menopause as a hormonal disorder during the 1930s and 40s. Other physicians were willing to accept this notion because if fit well with their medical model concept of disease. As is often the case, the identification of menopause as a disease was facilitated by the availability of inexpensive drug therapy. Not only could a pathological state be identified, but a medical treatment (estrogen replacement therapy) had become available for its management. Thus, despite the fact that 15 percent or less of American women experienced a problem menopause, in 1975 it was found that 51 percent of women had taken estrogen replacement drugs at some point.

Despite the risks now known to be associated with estrogen replacement therapy, the medical community continues to debate the existence of menopause as a disease. The fact that there are proponents on both sides of the issue reminds us that the formal identification of a disease is often a function of the perspectives of the health professionals involved. It could be argued, in fact, that there are very few diseases in an absolute sense, with the identification of disease being as much a social process as a clinical one.

circumstances. Each has its advantages and disadvantages. As will be seen, the medical model has lost much of its salience as the epidemiological transition has shifted the burden of disease from acute conditions to chronic conditions.

DEFINING NON-HEALTH: ILLNESS, SICKNESS, AND DISEASE

Defining Non-Health

The condition of "non-health" could be considered the converse of the state of health described above, although, as will be seen, this greatly oversimplifies the situation. Like "health," non-health can be defined in different ways depending on one's perspective. According to the medical model, illness involves the presence of clinically identifiable biological pathology. In fact, from this perspective, "health" only exists as a residual category—that is, the absence of symptoms. The focus of medical education and practice is on the presence of pathology—that is, biological abnormality—with little attention given to what constitutes a state of health and no concern for the non-biological factors involved in ill-health. This perspective underlies most of the operation of the healthcare system which expends it efforts eliminating these pathological conditions.

According to the functional model, ill-health involves a state of social "abnormality". Individuals who do not or cannot comply with social norms related to role performance would be considered "ill" under this model. While the intent under the medical model is to return the affected individual to biological normality, the actions within the functional model attempt to restore social normality by allowing the affected individual to reassume appropriate social roles (regardless of his or her biological condition).

According to the psychological or stress model, the individual is considered in ill-health if the individual so defines himself. An individual who feels "disordered", out of sync with his social environment, or otherwise emotionally in disequilibrium would be considered ill under this model. This condition may manifest itself in physical or social abnormalities although the root cause is some internally based condition.

The legal definition of health is typically applied only to ill-health. Thus, in the case of involuntary commitment to a mental institution, a psychiatrist must determine the extent to which the individual is a threat to himself—or others—and the extent to which he is competent to properly take care of himself. The "judge" is not generally capable of making a judgment of "competence" but only "incompetence", with competence reflecting a lack of evidence of incompetence. Although a psychiatrist performs the examination, the courts determine competence or incompetence in the final analysis. The situations in which the legal definition might be applied to physical illnesses would be in the case of certain "reportable" diseases or conditions requiring quarantine. A test for a sexually transmitted disease that comes back positive defines the affected person as legally ill and allows public health authorities to take action to bring about treatment and/or limit the spread of the disease.

Illness and Sickness

To sociologists, the characterization of non-health is more complex than presented above. In a basic sense, a state of illness or sickness constitutes "ill health" and is the converse of a state of "health." However, the subjective nature of conditions of health and illness has led medical sociologists to formulate a more complicated depiction of these concepts (Wolinsky, 1988).

A major distinction in this regard is made between illness and sickness. *Illness* refers to the individual, private, and usually biological aspect of the state of ill health. The term illness relates to the set of symptoms known only to the individual, and in this sense is private as opposed to public. It is argued that illness (but not sickness) is a state shared by human beings with all other animals; that is, it is a state of biological dysfunction known only to the individual organism. Under this definition, it could be contended that the actual level of illness is similar from society to society, reflecting the primarily biological nature of illness.

Sickness refers to the public or social component of ill health. Illness is transformed into sickness when the condition becomes publicly known through announcement by the affected party, observation by significant others, or professional diagnosis. Thus, while illness is primarily a biological state, sickness is a social state. Sickness is social not only because it is recognized beyond the bounds of the individual per se, but also because it has implications for social role performance and interpersonal interaction.

Some simple examples may help clarify the distinction between illness and sickness. An individual who feels bad (e.g., headache and nausea) is clearly ill. However, if the individual never discloses his or her symptoms to others (or they go unobserved by others) and continues to perform social roles adequately, he or she, although "ill", would not be considered "sick". Conversely, if an individual is unable to perform social roles due to some generalized condition, although clinically identifiable symptoms cannot be found, this individual would be considered "sick."

Unlike illness, the amount of sickness varies widely from society to society and within the same society at different time periods. The amount of sickness reflects the perceptions of society at that point in time. This means that the level of sickness is much more "elastic" than the level of illness. Examples of the elasticity of sickness can be found during wartime when military physicians at induction centers adopt a quite different standard of what constitutes disability than in peacetime.

U.S. society today, in fact, reflects this notion of elasticity in that a larger proportion of the population is under medical management than at any time in the past. However, it could be argued that the population as a whole is healthier than it has ever been. In this situation, there is a relatively low level of illness but a relatively high level of sickness. Thus, there is little relationship between the level of illness in society and the amount of healthcare consumed.

Defining Disease

The concept of disease is one of the most problematic within healthcare. Like all of the concepts being discussed here, it is modern in its origin.

Originally referring to a state of "dis-ease," the term has come to be used in a variety of ways. The most significant one involves the identification of a medically recognized pathological condition. Technically, this means a syndrome involving clinically identifiable and measurable signs and symptoms reflecting underlying biological pathology. This view of disease clearly reflects an orientation derived from a healthcare environment dominated by infectious illnesses. This conceptualization continues to be important, since it underlies the medical model perspective on health and illness and is the definition instilled in health professionals. (See Box 2-1 for a description of the process of identifying a "new" disease.)

In medical sociology, a disease is considered an adverse physical state consisting of a physiological dysfunction within an individual, as compared to illness or sickness. In actual practice, the term disease is applied rather liberally to a wide variety of conditions that do not precisely fit the definition. One of the more controversial areas relates to mental illness. It could be argued that many, if not most, mental disorders would not be considered diseases under the definition above. The same could be said of other conditions that have been identified as "diseases" at various times. Examples include certain sexual deviations, alcoholism, and drug abuse. These conditions do not necessarily have the requisite clear-cut symptomatology and underlying biological pathology. They are nevertheless frequently treated as if they were diseases. One explanation for this is clear: In order for a condition to be treated by the healthcare system, it must be identified as a disease. Therefore, there is a tendency toward an overly broad conceptualization of disease.

Obviously, the general public is not attuned to the academic definitions of health, sickness and disease described above. "Folk" conceptualizations of health, sickness and disease are common, with wide variation in perspectives on these concepts found among various subpopulations. Subgroups based on sociodemographic attributes (e.g., ethnic groups) are likely to maintain distinct conceptualizations of health, sickness and disease, conceptualizations that may vary significantly from the formal definitions of these concepts. (See Box 2–2 for a discussion of lay perceptions of health and illness.)

A Biopsychosocial Model of Health and Illness

The modern view that many factors interact to produce disease may be attributed to the seminal work of George L. Engel, who put forward the biopsychosocial model of disease (Engel, 1977). The purpose of the biopsychosocial model is to take a broad view, to assert that simply looking at biological factors alone—which had been the prevailing view of disease at the time Engel was writing—is not sufficient to explain health and illness.

According to Engel's model, biological, psychological and social factors are all involved in the causes, manifestation, course, and outcome of health and disease, including mental disorders. Few people with a condition such as heart disease or diabetes, for instance, would dispute the role of stress in aggravating their condition. Research bears this out and reveals many other relationships between stress and disease.

Engel's model ultimately seeks to resolve the definitional dilemma by eliminating the either/or contention. It is not a matter of ill-health being caused by biological factor *or* social factors *or* psychological factors but a combination of the above is typically involved. Everyone, it could be argued is exposed to disease organisms in the environment; this is a necessary but not sufficient factor in the onset of many diseases. Other factors—social and/or emotional—come into play to trigger the disease episode. It is almost always the case with chronic conditions, in fact, that the condition results *only* through a combination of these three factors. Many people carry the indicator for rheumatoid arthritis in their blood, but only a small proportion are affected. Those affected have typically had some social or psychological factors come into play that serve to activate the disease.

DEFINING HEALTHCARE

The concept "healthcare" is as difficult to define as health and illness. Although hospital-based medical services involving advanced technology automatically come to mind when the issue is raised, the provision of this intensive level of care is more the exception than the rule. In the United States today, only a fraction of the activities of the healthcare system is directed toward the management of life-threatening conditions involving intensive services.

Even if healthcare were to be defined simply in terms of a description of its existing structure, this also represents a challenge. The difficulty of such an approach is exacerbated in the United States by the system's size, complexity, and technological emphasis, as well as by its diversity of functioning units, its various levels of "control," its combination of public, quasi-public, and private interests, and its mixture of for-profit and not-for-profit entities.

In the final analysis, healthcare is what society defines as healthcare. In the contemporary United States, healthcare has come to include formal, institutionalized care, along with "alternative" therapies, self-care and any other activities designed to prevent the onset of disease, treat illness, improve the quality of life, and/or preserve health.

--- *Box 2-2* ---

Lay Perceptions of Health and Illness

It has been well documented that lay perceptions of health and illness frequently vary—often significantly—from those held by health professionals. Long before any outside help (medical or otherwise) is sought, individuals interpret their own condition. Underlying all such evaluations is a set of ideas about health and illness. These notions of health and illness are not those of science or medicine, although they may be borrowed, accurately or inaccurately, from those formal systems of knowledge. They are the perceptions held by ordinary people whose experiences, cultural background, and social networks shape and continually modify their notions of health and illness.

Researchers have found that laymen's perceptions of health and illness vary widely from group to group. Many people think of health as simply the absence of illness. Others describe health in terms of an absence of illness, equilibrium in daily life, and a capacity to work. While both working-class and middle-class persons share the notion that health means the absence of illness, working-class people tend to emphasize what is essential for their everyday lives—the ability to carry out their tasks, especially job and family duties. Middle-class persons are more likely to mention broader, positive conceptions of health that include such factors as energy, positive attitudes, and the ability to cope well and to be in control of one's life.

The sense of being in control is particularly important to the middle class for it meshes with their experiences of making decisions and having a degree of control in their work and daily life. By contrast, because working-class persons have control over far fewer areas of their lives, this value may be remote or inconceivable to them. Thus, American middle-class values have expanded the notion of health to something that must be actively achieved and proven.

There are important differences in lay conceptions of health and illness within various subcultures as well. Americans raised in different ethnic subcultures typically incorporate their group's ideas about health and illness, including perceptions of the nature of health, the causes of illness, and appropriate responses in the face of symptoms. Religious subcultures likewise influence not only their members' responses to illness but also their very definitions of health and illness. From a fundamentalist Christian perspective "health" and "wholeness" are words that reflect "salvation". A healthy person would be one that is whole in spirit, soul, mind, and body.

Just as lay notions of health are shaped by individuals' social and cultural backgrounds, so are the ways people understand their illnesses. People seek to comprehend what is wrong within a context that makes sense to them. Individual belief systems about illness are typically drawn from larger cultural belief systems, which give shape to the illness experience, help the individual to interpret what is happening, and offer a number of choices about how to respond.

Lay images of various diseases reveal why certain responses "make sense." A study of middle-class New Yorkers found that people regularly refer to disease and diseased body parts as "its"—as objects separate from the person. The image allows ill persons to distance themselves from their problems. The concept of disease as an "it" also meshed with notions that the problem had its source in some external agent that invaded the body. Because lay images of illness reflect people's diverse experiences, they vary by such factors as social class, gender, ethnicity, and religion. Thus, the causal categories used by laypersons to explain illness onset may not be correct in bioscientific terms but are generally rational and based upon the kinds of empirical evidence available to laypersons.

Lay understandings of illness typically address the broader issues of meaning and addresses questions like: Why me? Why now? What did I do to deserve this? Indeed, in much lay thinking cause and meaning are not separate interpretative categories. Serious illnesses in particular evoke broader causal interpretations that are often used in combination with medical interpretations.

In addition to these underlying ideas about health and illness, a number of other social factors influence whether an individual will perceive a particular disturbance and come to define it as distressing enough to warrant further attention. People react to the meaning of a symptom, not merely the symptom itself. The significance of symptoms is not self-evident; the person must actively give attention and interpretation to them. A person with a gaping and painful wound that is bleeding profusely is not likely to ignore the bodily disturbance. Other disturbances, however, are more open to varying interpretations, including those that make the person less likely even to recognize them. It has been suggested that the usual response to such disturbances involves testing hypotheses by observing the situation over time, taking a wait-and-see stance on the assumption that many conditions are self-limiting.

Ultimately, individuals develop notions of health and illness that are consistent with the worldviews of their respective cultural milieus. People rely on their social group to provide an understanding of illness, its causation, and acceptable reactions, not only because individuals may not have access to a "professional" framework for analyzing the situation but also because, even if they did, the professional perspective would not answer questions that are important to the affected individual but outside the scope of the clinician.

Source: Peter E.S. Freund and Meredith B. McGuire (1999). *Health, Illness, and the Social Body*, 3rd ed. Englewood Cliffs, NJ: Prentice Hall.

The behavioral definition of healthcare is "medicinal and preventive measures taken by the self or others to maintain functional health status". The institutional definition is "a society's cultural and organizational arrangements directed at maintenance of the health status of its population" (Cockerham and Richey, 1997). An even more appropriate definition for our purposes may be: *Any* action taken with the intent of restoring, maintaining or enhancing health status." (See Box 2-3 for a discussion of what activities should be considered under the heading of "healthcare".)

PHYSICAL ILLNESS AND MENTAL ILLNESS

The U.S. healthcare system clearly distinguishes between physical illness and mental illness. This distinction is well established today, but it was only in the twentieth century that it became widely applied in healthcare. Traditional societies viewed all illnesses under the same umbrella. Whatever the form of the malady, it was thought to be a function of disequilibrium on the part of the individual, the intervention of some supernatural force, or some other nonscientific phenomenon. Differential diagnosis (i.e., the precise classification of disease) was not emphasized, and the etiology (cause) of the problem was the main consideration in evaluating a symptomatic individual.

Modern Western thinking led to a clear distinction between the physical and the mental domains. This perspective was reinforced by the deep entrenchment of germ theory in the medical model paradigm. This model's emphasis on biological causes led to the separation of conditions that demonstrated clear biological pathology (physical illnesses) from those that did not (mental disorders). This distinction is reflected in what is essentially a separate sector within the healthcare system for the treatment of mental disorders, with distinct facilities and practitioners. A clear distinction is maintained today between mental hospitals and general hospitals and, in medical science, between psychiatrists and other physicians.

Mental illness and physical illness do differ from each other in a number of ways. Physical illness is generally characterized by clear-cut, clinically identifiable symptoms, while mental illness is not. The symptoms of physical illness reflect biological pathology while those of mental illness reflect disorders of mood, behavior, and thought patterns. Clearly, the diagnosis of most mental disorders is more subjective than that of physical disorders because of the lack of clinical diagnostic tests. Although a small portion of mental disorders can be attributed to some underlying biological pathology (e.g., nervous system damage), most mental conditions are thought to reflect either internal psychological pathology or the influence of external stressors. Neither of these lends themselves to traditional medical diagnostic techniques.

Note that the definitions of mental health and illness reflect the same models or perspectives associated with physical health and illness. The medical model remains important, primarily due to the pivotal role of the psychiatrist. However, the functional model is particularly relevant in that mental pathology is more likely to be identified based on some functional impairment rather than a biological impairment. Ironically, the psychological model probably has the least salience in that it assumes the individual making an assessment of healthiness is in his or her "right mind." It should also be remembered that mental health or illness is sometimes defined from a legal perspective.

Mental illness also differs from physical illness in that most mental disorders are considered to be both chronic and incurable. The basic goal of medicine is the treatment and cure of disease, yet most mental disorders are considered to be permanent and, thus, cannot be cured, only managed. This makes the medical model of limited usefulness as a framework for viewing mental illness. Mental illness is also perceived much differently by the general public than is physical illness. Mental illness carries more of a stigma than do most physical illnesses: one can recover from the latter, but not the former. At the same time, the unpredictability of the behavior of the mentally ill tends to make the "normal" person uncomfortable in the face of psychiatric symptoms.

One final distinction relates to the treatment of physical and mental illnesses by medical science. In general, mental disorders do not lend themselves to treatment by the modalities derived from the medical model. In some cases, drug therapy is utilized for mental disorders; in rare cases, surgery is as well. However, most mental disorders are treated by counseling and psychotherapy. "Talking" therapies (rather than the standard armamentarium of the medical scientist) are commonly utilized, further reinforcing the conceptual gap between physical and mental illness. (See Chapter 8 on the sociology of mental illness for more detail on these issues.)

One additional model that relates specifically to mental illness is the *societal reaction model*. Proponents of this perspective contend that there is no such thing as mental illness in a scientific sense. Mental illness is a concept constructed by society as a means of controlling residual deviant behavior—i.e., behavior that doesn't fit nicely into the sin or crime categories but is nevertheless found to be objectionable. Thus, the behaviors or attributes that society (or powerful interests in society) reacts negatively to become labeled as mental illness. It is no surprise that those who are typically labeled as mentally ill are those who are on the margins of society and relatively powerless. The societal reaction approach argus that certain behaviors of certain categories of people are selectively chosen for labeling as mental illness. For example, middle-class therapists may label certain "normal" behaviors of lower-class patients as symptoms of mental disorder although they are common to all members of this category. Further,

---

Box 2-3

What Should Be Legitimately Considered as "Healthcare"?

With the expansion of the scope of U.S. healthcare since the 1960s, questions have increasingly been raised concerning what should appropriately be considered under the umbrella of care. The question has been raised for a variety of reasons. Consumers have asked this because of their concern over what conditions it is appropriate to seek treatment for. Insurance plans and federally subsidized health programs have been concerned over what should legitimately be covered as a medically necessary procedure. Policy setters and critics of healthcare have expressed concern over what is the legitimate role of medicine in society.

In a simpler time, one might have concluded that the treatment of life-threatening conditions was raison d'etre for the healthcare system. Yet, relatively little of the activity of the U.S. healthcare system today deals with life-threatening conditions. In fact, a growing proportion of the resources are dedicated to the "treatment" of well persons rather than sick person. As the institution expanded its scope, it took "ownership" of more and more conditions, conditions that historically had been deemed to be outside the realm of medicine. "Conditions" such as pregnancy, aging, adolescent adjustment problems, and eating disorders were brought under the wing of healthcare and "new" conditions were constantly being identified. The inclusion of these new conditions under the aegis of healthcare has led more and more parties to question what constitutes the legitimate role of healthcare in U.S. society.

This issue might be examined by identifying some categories of conditions that are managed by health professionals. There are the aforementioned life-threatening conditions that are unquestionably appropriate for medical care. (Although the question could be raised about the appropriateness of continued care once the case has been declared terminal.) These are joined by a category that includes illnesses that medical practitioners (and insurers) would consider "medically necessary." That is, there is an accepted diagnosis that requires medical treatment. These medically necessary therapies are distinguished from "elective" procedures that, arguably, are not medically necessary. Thus, tennis elbow is considered an elective surgery. The patient could benefit from the procedure, but it is not considered medically necessary.

There is another category of conditions that could arguably benefit from medical intervention, although the patient could probably get along fine without the care. These include conditions like premenstrual syndrome, pregnancy, menopause, and many emotional disorders. Some would consider these to be "natural" conditions for which medical care is unnecessary.

There are other conditions that require medical involvement where it could be argued that medical care is inappropriately provided. Procedures such as abortion on demand, facelifts and various other forms of cosmetic surgery are carried out by medical doctors. Many question whether these are appropriate uses of the healthcare system.

Many other conditions that were not historically considered appropriate for medical intervention are now routinely managed by clinicians. These include hyperactivity in children, alcoholism, drug abuse, child abuse, eating disorders and a wide range of emotional problems. Critics argue that, by redefining these conditions as medical problems, more people are brought under medical management and the institution acquires more power and more revenue. This expansionism has made the healthcare system the source of care for more than traditional medical conditions, but as a source of care for social and emotional problems a well.

With the growing appreciation of the contribution of non-biological factors to health and illness, the healthcare system is now offering family planning, nutritional counseling, fitness and lifestyle counseling and other non-clinical services. While it could be argued that these do not fall within the purview of the healthcare system, it could also be argued that they might make more of a contribution to improved health status than the clinical procedures that are often performed.

Taking this argument one step further, it might be argued that the best way to reduce morbidity and improve health status would be to invest not in medical facilities but in a safe environment, adequate housing, and crime reduction. Healthcare dollars spent in this manner would serve the ends of the institution much more effectively.

Clearly, as a society we have developed a confused notion of what the appropriate role of the healthcare system should be. There is obviously no correct answer and what is considered the appropriate role for healthcare will be a function of one's perspective. If one feels that sick people should be the only concern of the healthcare system, the approach is quite different than an approach that focuses on well people (i.e., keeping them well). If one feels that only clinical tools should be used to improve health status, little emphasis will be placed on cleaning up the environment. If one believes that health status is improved by treating one person at a time, the approach will be different from one that feels like the community should be the "patient" if you really want to improve health status.

As the future of the U.S. healthcare system continues to be debated, questions like these must be asked if policy makers are going to have an appreciation of the implications of the decisions they make.

Table 2-1.　Health and Sickness from Various Perspectives

	Medical model	Functional model	Psychological model	Legal model	Societal reaction model
Definition: Health	Absence of pathology	Ability to function	Self-assessed well-being	State of competency (mental); absence of communicable disease (physical)	Absence of societally recognized symptoms
Definition: Sickness	Presence of pathology	Inability to function	Self-assessed lack of well-being	State of incompetency (mental); presence of communicable disease	Presence of societally recognized symptoms
Source of Definition:	Medical scientists	Social group	Affected individual	Criminal justice system; public health agencies	Powerful social groups
"Certifying" Agent:	Physician	Significant other	Affected individual	Criminal justice system; public health system	Agencies controlled by powerful social groups
Therapeutic Objective:	Remove pathology	Restore functioning	Restore well-being	Protect individual, society	Control deviance

the fact that most of the behavior patterns of symptomatic individuals are normal in no way detracts from the mental illness label. Once the label is applied, the affected individual is seen in a new light by society and by himself. The individual begins to act in keeping with the label—i.e., in response to societal expectations. Permanent stigmatization may result and continue to be attached to the individual regardless of the outcome of the episode. (See Table 2-1 for a perception of health of illness from various theoretical perspectives.)

REFERENCES

Antonovsky, Aaron (1979). *Health, Stress and Coping*. San Francisco: Jossey-Bass.

Berliner, Howard S. (1975). "A larger perspective on the Flexner Report," *International Journal of Health Services* 5:573–592.

Cockerham, William C., and Ferris J. Richey (1997). *The Dictionary of Medical Sociology*. Westport, CT: Greenwood.

Dubos, Rene (1959). *Mirage of Health*. New York: Harper and Row.

Ehrenreich, Barbara, and Deirdre English (1978). *For Her Own Good: 150 of the Experts' Advice to Women*. Garden City, NY: Doubleday.

Engle, George L. (1977). "The need for a new medical model: A challenge for biomedicine," *Science* 196:129–135.

Freund, Peter E.S., and Meredith B. McGuire (1999). *Health, Illness and the Social Body*, 3rd ed. Englewood Cliffs, NJ: Prentice Hall.

Hahn, Robert A., and Arthur Kleinman (1983). "Biomedical practice and anthropological theory: Frameworks and directions," *American Review of Anthropology* 12:305–333.

Parsons, Talcott (1972). "Definitions of health and illness in the light of American values and social structure," pp. 107–127 in E.G. Jaco, ed., *Patients, Physicians, and Illness*. New York: McMillan.

World Health Organization (1999). Website, URL: www.who.int/aboutwho/en/definition.html.

Wolinsky, Frederic D. (1988). *The Sociology of Health: Principles, Professions, and Issues*, 2nd ed. Belmont, CA: Wadsworth.

ADDITIONAL RESOURCES

Haubrich, William S. (1984). *Medical Meanings: A Glossary of Word Origins*. New York: Harcourt, Brace, Jovanovich.

INTERNET LINKS

http://www.medicinenet.com. On-line medical dictionary.

The Societal Context of Healthcare

THE INSTITUTIONAL FRAMEWORK

The healthcare system of any society can only be understood within the sociocultural context of that society. No two healthcare delivery systems are exactly alike, with the differences primarily a function of the contexts within which they exist. The social structure of a society, along with its cultural values, defines the healthcare system. Thus, the form and function of the healthcare system reflect the form and function of the society in which it resides.

A common way of looking at society by sociologists is in terms of a "system". A system is an assemblage of parts combined in a complex whole. Each of the parts is interconnected either directly or indirectly and, thus, all are interdependent with the others. These parts working in concert create a dynamic, self-sustaining system that maintains a state of equilibrium. The various parts perform their respective functions, and each component must work in synchronization with the others if the system is to function efficiently and, indeed, survive as a system. Anything that happens to

35

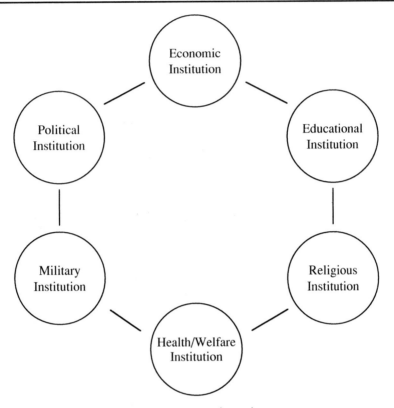

Figure 3–1. Diagram of social system

one part (e.g., damage) has repercussions throughout the system, and the system must act to address this "dysfunction" or the entire system could be impacted.

Every society (and, indeed, every social group) can be viewed in this manner. Society, like any system then, is composed of various components. Unlike a mechanical system (such as a machine) the components of a social system are not "things" in the material sense, but they are processes. Sociologists refer to these major components of a social system as "institutions" that, rather than being tangible things, constitute patterns of behavior. These are not undirected patterns of behavior but patterns established to accomplish some societal goal. (A diagram of a stylized social system is presented in Figure 3–1.)

These goals emerge in response to the needs that face every social system. These societal needs, sometimes referred to as "functional requisites", are the tasks that every society (or every social group for that matter) must perform in order to survive. These functions include: reproducing new society members, socializing the new members, distributing resources, maintaining internal order, providing for defense, dealing with the supernatural, and, importantly, providing for the health and well-being of the population. Organizational structures (i.e., institutions) evolve to meet each of these needs. Thus, some form of family evolves to manage reproduction, some form of educational system to deal with socialization, some form of economic system to deal with the allocation of resources, and so forth. A healthcare/social services system of some type evolves to assure the health and welfare of the population. (Note that this conceptualization of society is not the only one formulated by sociologists. See Box 3-1 for an introduction to other perspectives on the nature of society.)

In any society these social institutions "evolve" over a period of time. They are not created overnight but are gradually established through the repeated behavior of individuals attempting to address personal needs within the context of the institutional framework. Some institutions, like healthcare, are dependent upon a certain level of knowledge and even technology to be able to fully develop. Thus, healthcare was one of the slowest of U.S. institutions to be formally established, with many tracing its origins as a modern institution only to the post-World War II period.

The form that a particular institution takes varies from society to society. A society's cultural history, its environment, its relationships with other societies, and its demographic characteristics all contribute to the shaping of its various institutions. These are numerous forms that can be taken by the family, the political institution, and economic institutions, with the particular form being uniquely tailored to the situation of that society. Similarly, there are a variety of forms the healthcare institution can take.

Thus, one might speak in terms of "traditional" healthcare systems (e.g., shamanism among American Indians), more complex traditional systems such as holistic Asian systems (e.g., Aryuvedic healthcare), capitalistic systems (e.g., for-profit healthcare in the United States), socialized systems (e.g., the National Health Service in Great Britain), and communistic systems such as that that once existed in the Soviet Union and is found today perhaps only in Cuba.

From a sociological perspective, no one system is intrinsically better or worse than any other; each has evolved in response to social, cultural, and environmental considerations, and each is uniquely suited to its particular society. Indeed, if the system is not suited to the society, it must transform itself to be responsive to societal needs or risk extinction. The traditional healthcare systems of many native American societies could not successfully adapt to the challenges presented by the introduction of European diseases, resulting in not only the collapse of the indigenous healthcare system but the ultimate extinction of many of these societies.

Box 3-1

Differing Paradigms for Understanding Society

The *structural-functional paradigm* represents a convenient framework for examining the healthcare system, and that is the approach taken throughout this book. The structural-functional paradigm is a framework for building theory that sees society as a complex system whose parts work together to promote solidarity and stability. As its name suggests, this paradigm emphasiees social structure involving relatively stable patterns of social behavior. Social structure gives our lives shape, whether it be in families, the workplace, or the college classroom. Second, this paradigm looks for a structure's social function, or the consequences of any social pattern for the operation of society as a whole. All social patterns—from a simple handshake to complex religious rituals—function to keep society going, at least in its present form. The structural-functional paradigm depicts culture as a complex strategy for meeting human needs. Cultural values, in other words, give meaning to life and bind people together.

The strength of structural-functional analysis is in its depiction of the ways in which culture operates to meet human needs. From this perspective, the healthcare institution is viewed as society's strategy for keeping its members healthy. In this scheme, illness is dysfunctional because it reduces people's ability to perform their roles. Society responds to illness by providing a sick role, patterns of behavior defined as appropriate for those who are ill. Yet, by emphasizing a society's dominant cultural patterns, this approach directs less attention to cultural diversity.

Moreover, because this approach emphasizes cultural stability, it downplays the importance of change. In short, cultural systems are not as stable or as much a matter of consensus as structural-functional analysis leads us to believe. For example, not everyone agrees on what is beneficial and what is harmful. What is functional for one category of people (say, hospital administrators, health insurance compar.ies) may well be dysfunctional for another category of people (say, physicians or health plan enrollees).

The chief characteristic of the structural-functional paradigm is its vision of society as orderly, stable, and comprehensible. While most sociologists historically favored this approach, in recent decades its influence has declined. By focusing attention on social stability and unity, critics point out, structural-functionalism tends to ignore inequalities of social class, race, ethnicity, and sex, which can generate considerable tension and conflict. Its focus on stability at the expense of conflict and change makes this paradigm somewhat conservative. Such an approach calls for support of the status quo as a means of preserving the institutions of society and inherently discourages radical social change. Needless to say, the "haves" of society are more likely to ascribe to this approach that the "have nots", making it a frequent target for those with a more social activist bent.

The advantage of macro-level forms of analysis like structural-functionalism, however, is that this approach shows how social and economic conditions beyond the direct influence or control of the average person can create stressful circumstances that force people to respond to them. For vulnerable people, the stressful circumstances may promote ill health.

While this is a useful approach for examining the healthcare system, there are other sociological paradigms that could have been utilized. A second approach, the *social-conflict paradigm*, points out the connection between health and social inequality and ties health to capitalism. Researchers have focused on three main issues: access to medical care, the effects of the profit motive, and the politics of medicine.

Health is important to everyone. But by making health a commodity, capitalist societies allow health to follow wealth. The access problem is more serious in the United States than in most other industrial societies because our country has no universal healthcare system.

Conflict theorists concede that capitalism provides excellent healthcare for the rich but not for the rest of the population. Most of the 42 million people who lack healthcare coverage at present have low incomes.

Some social-conflict analysts go further, arguing that the real problem is not access to medical care but the character of capitalist medicine itself. The profit motive turns physicians, hospitals, and the pharmaceutical industry into multibillion-dollar corporations. The quest for higher profits encourages unnecessary tests and surgery and an overreliance on drugs (Kaplan et al. 1985).

Of some 25 million surgical operations performed in the United States each year, three-fourths are "elective", intended to promote long-term health and are not prompted by medical necessity. And, of course, any medical procedure or use of drugs is risky and harms between 5 and 10% of patients. Therefore, social-conflict theorists contend that most surgery reflects the financial interests of surgeons and hospitals as much as the medical needs of patients. Physicians often have a direct financial interest in the tests and procedures they order for their patients.

Although science declares itself to be politically neutral, scientific medicine frequently takes sides on significant social issues. For example, the medical establishment, opposed to increased government regulation of fees and services, has always strongly resisted proposals for national healthcare programs. Moreover, the history of medicine shows that racial and sexual discrimination have been supported by "scientific" opinions (Leavitt, 1984).

Even today, according to conflict theory, scientific medicine explains illness in terms of bacteria and viruses, ignoring the damaging effects of social inequality. In other words, scientific medicine depoliticizes health in the United States by reducing social issues to simple biology.

Social-conflict analysis provides still another view of the relationships among health, medicine, and society. According to this paradigm, social

(*continued*)

inequality is the reason some people have better health than others. However, the most common objection to the conflict approach is that it minimizes the advances in U.S. health supported by scientific medicine and higher living standards. Though there is plenty of room for improvement, health indicators for our population as a whole rose steadily over the course of the twentieth century, and we compare well with other industrial societies.

The social-conflict paradigm is a framework for building theory that sees society as an arena of inequality that generates conflict and change. Unlike the structural-functional emphasis on solidarity, this approach highlights inequality—disorder rather than order, dysfunction rather than function, conflict rather than cooperation. Guided by this paradigm, sociologists investigate how factors such as race, ethnicity, sex, and age are linked to the unequal distribution of various goods in society (including healthcare). A conflict analysis rejects the idea that social structure promotes the functioning of society as a whole, focusing instead on how any social pattern benefits some people while depriving others.

Sociologists using the social-conflict paradigm look at ongoing conflict between dominant and disadvantaged categories of people—the rich in relation to the poor, white people in relation to people of color, men in relation to women, or doctors in relation to patients. Typically, people on top strive to protect their privileges, while the disadvantaged try to gain more for themselves.

A conflict analysis of the health care system would consider such issues as: the way that access to healthcare is determined by socioeconomic status, the ways in which the elite operate the system to their own benefit, the ways in which powerful medical interests influence policy setting, and the ways in which healthcare might be used for social control.

The social-conflict paradigm draws attention to the link between culture and inequality. Any cultural trait, from this point of view, benefits some members of society at the expense of others. Social-conflict analysis ties American competitive values to our society's capitalist economy, which serves the interests of the nation's wealthy elite. The culture of capitalism further teaches us to think that rich and powerful people have more energy and talent than others, and therefore deserve their wealth and privilege. Viewing capitalism as somehow "natural" also discourages efforts to lessen economic disparity in the United States.

Eventually, however, the strains of inequality erupt into movements for social change. Two examples in the United States are the civil rights movement and the women's movement. Both sought greater equality and both, too, encountered opposition from defenders of the status quo. The social-conflict paradigm suggests that cultural systems do not address human needs equally, allowing some people to dominate others. This inequality, in turn, generates pressure toward change. Yet by stressing the divisiveness of culture, this paradigm understates ways in which cultural patterns integrate members of a society. Thus, we should consider both social-conflict and structural-functional insights for a fuller understanding of culture.

Both the structural-functional and social-conflict paradigms share a macro-level orientation, or a concern with broad patterns that shape society as a whole. Macro-level sociology takes in the big picture, rather like observing a city from a helicopter and seeing how highways help people move from place to place or how housing differs in rich and poor neighborhoods. Yet sociology also has a micro-level orientation, a focus on small-scale patterns of social interaction in specific settings. This involves analyzing society at "street level", perhaps watching how physicians and nurses interact within a hospital or how physicians and patients communicate with each other. A third model, the *symbolic-interaction paradigm*, offers a framework for building theory that sees society as the product of the everyday interactions of individuals.

Society "emerges" from the on-going experiences of tens of millions of people in that society and is a product of the reality that people construct based on their everyday experiences. Human beings are creatures who live in a world of symbols, attaching meaning to virtually everything. "Reality" is a reflection of how we define our surroundings, our own identities, and our relationships with others. As individual players in society, we observe how people respond to us and develop a picture of reality based on this, not based on our relationship to large-scale organizations. Thus, a physically disabled individual is likely to develop a picture of society from his or her particular perspective, based on the reaction of people around him.

The symbolic-interaction perspective views the individual in society as a creative, thinking organism who is able to choose his or her behavior, instead of reacting more or less mechanically to the influence of social processes. It assumes that all behavior is self-directed on the basis of symbolic meanings that are shared, communicated, and manipulated by interacting human beings in social situations.

Without denying the existence of macro-level social structures such as the family and social class, the symbolic-interaction paradigm reminds us that society basically amounts to people interacting. That is, micro-level sociology tries to convey how individuals actually experience society. But the other side of the coin is that, by emphasizing what is unique in each social scene, this approach risks overlooking the widespread effects of culture, class, sex and race. According to the symbolic-interaction paradigm, society is less a grand system than a series of complex and changing realities. Health and medical care, therefore, are socially constructed within everyday interaction. If we socially construct both health and illness, it follows that people in a poor society may view malnutrition as normal. Similarly, members of U.S. society give little thought to the harmful effects of a rich diet.

To ensure that the situation is defined as impersonal and professional, the medical staff wear uniforms and furnish the examining room with

(continued)

nothing but medical equipment. The doctor's manner is designed to make the patient feel that, to him, the examination of the genital area is no different from treating any other part of the body. A female nurse is usually present during the examination, not only to assist the physician but to dispel any impression that a man and woman are "alone together in a room".

The symbolic-interaction paradigm reveals that what people view as healthful or harmful depends on a host of factors that are not, strictly speaking, medical. This approach also shows that, in the course of any medical procedure, both patient and medical staff engages in a subtle process of reality construction. Critics fault this approach for implying that there are no objective standards of well-being. Certain physical conditions do indeed cause specific changes in people, whatever we may think about it. People who lack sufficient nutrition and safe water, for example, suffer from their unhealthy environment whether they define their surroundings as normal or not.

The following table summarizes the features of these three paradigmatic approaches to the understanding of society.

Theoretical Paradigm	Orientation	Image of Society	Health-Specific Issues
Structural-function	Macro-level	A system of inter-related parts each serving a function and contributing to the stability of society	What are the component parts of the system? What is the function of health-care within the system and how does it relate to other institutions?
Social-conflict	Macro-level	Society as a context for	How does social inequality

Obviously, not all societies are populous enough or complex enough to support fully developed institutions of each of these types. In cases where this situation exists, a single institution may perform the functions of two or more institutions. For example, the family within a traditional society may perform the functions of the educational institution, the economic institution, and others as well. An absence of emphasis on rationality and a dependence on the supernatural as an explanatory factor in the existence of health, illness, and death in premodern societies precluded the development of a distinct healthcare system.

		on-going conflict between those seeking to further their own interests resulting in constant change and reorganization	contribute to disparities in health status among different groups in society and how is healthcare used as a means of social control?
Symbolic-interaction	Micro-level	The "reality" of society is constructed through the interaction of society members as they perform their everyday activities	How do the symbols (e.g., uniforms) worn by various healthcare workers contribute to the patient's construction of reality? How does doctor-patient communication serve to construct the patient's view of society?

In these cases, functions usually reserved for the healthcare system in modern societies were typically performed by the family or the religious institution.

Once established, institutions take on a certain permanence and, in fact, develop mechanisms for preserving themselves and enhancing their influence. Institutions establish rules that govern the behavior of individuals vis-à-vis those institutions and develop the ability to enforce those rules through both positive and negative sanctions. This is perhaps nowhere more clear-cut than with regard to the religious institution that, regardless of the religion, typically lays out strict rules to be followed by its believers. In most religions, the reward for following the rules is eternal life; the punishment for not following the rules is eternal damnation.

The rules established by the healthcare institution may not be quite so dramatic and clear-cut. However, there are guidelines that are put forth that say, in effect, if you follow these rules, you will live a long, healthy life. If you don't follow these rules, you risk sickness and death. These guidelines are often formalized in the form of "doctor's orders." Since individuals in a free society cannot be forced to live a healthy lifestyle, the institution invokes various legal and regulatory contrivances to enforce its requirements. Thus, all individuals are required to obtain certain childhood immunizations, addicts are forced to enter rehabilitation, and patients with contagious diseases are isolated from the rest of the population.

On another level, we find that some healthcare providers will not accept patients without insurance, that health maintenance organizations require annual checkups in order to maintain a low premium, or that insurance plans charge high premiums for individuals involved in risky activities. While it cannot be argued that society deliberately sets out to create a system that controls the patterns of behavior that support the healthcare system, it can be seen that various parties, appearing to act in their own self interest, are actually working toward the goals of the healthcare institution through the promulgation of such rules.

Despite the "permanence" that institutions take on in society, they must also have the flexibility to adjust to changing conditions. Throughout time, the institutions of most societies changed little over the centuries and most individuals who have ever lived have experienced little or no institutional change in their lifetimes. But change does eventually occur as the environment changes, as contact is made with other societies, as discoveries occur. Thus, each institution must have the flexibility to adapt and change in keeping with the new situation. Institutions that are too rigid to adapt may eventually contribute to the destruction of their society.

The history of institutional change in the United States points out the adaptability of institutional structures. The economic system of postindustrial America is much different from that of industrial America or agrarian America. It could be argued, however, that these different economic systems do not represent a radical transformation of the economy but evolutionary changes, involving adaptation to new situations while still retaining the basic characteristics of the institution. The U.S. educational system, its religious institution, its political system, its military, and its arts and entertainment institution have all undergone tremendous change over the past century. Even the family institution changed dramatically during the last half of the twentieth century.

While many observers may decry these changes and attribute them to the deterioration of society, from a sociological perspective these modern institutions are no better or worse than their historical antecedents. They are, in fact, the systems that are appropriate under the circumstances. While the extended family may have certain nostalgic value for many, it was not a suitable family form for industrial society. The nuclear family became the norm in view of the demands of urbanized, industrialized society.

As we will see later, no other institution has undergone the dramatic change that healthcare experienced in the twentieth century. At the start of that century, healthcare was a very rudimentary institution with limited visibility and credibility in society. Hospitals were places that people went to die, and doctors were to be avoided at all costs. Indeed, there was little the doctor could do for the patient anyway. There was no agreement on the nature of health and illness, and only the beginnings of scientific evidence for the effectiveness of medical care were emerging. Healthcare was not even on the national radar screen for the first half of the twentieth century and accounted for a negligible amount of the gross national product.

Contrast that to the healthcare institution at the end of the twentieth century. Not only has the institution become well established in the United States but it has come to play a dominant role in American society. The importance of the institution has become such that sociologists often refer to the "medicalization" of American society. Indeed, there are few members of contemporary U.S. society that are not under some type of medical management. In the last half of the twentieth century, the institution came to be accorded high prestige and began to exert a major influence over other institutions. The healthcare institution at the beginning of the twenty-first century can claim 15 percent of the gross national product and 10 percent of the nation's workforce.

The significance placed on a particular institution differs from society to society. While all societies must address the same basic needs, the importance of various needs and the significance of the associated institution vary from system to system and from time period to time period. The importance of a particular institution will be determined by the conditions facing that society and by the values (discussed below) that characterize that society. In the Islamic world today, the religious institution holds inordinate significance, especially compared to the role of the religious institution in the United States (and the rest of the Western world, for that matter). Yet three hundred years ago, religion was one of the dominant institutions in the lives of the European settlers in what would become the United States. In most of the world's societies the family is a more important institution than it is in the United States today. Yet, at one time the family was arguably the most important institution in a fledging America.

American society today is dominated by the economic and educational institutions and, increasingly, by the healthcare institution. Economic success is a driving motivation for the behavior of Americans, and we spend an inordinate amount of time earning money, spending money, and planning how to invest our money. Indeed, much of our activities in other institutions serve to support the goal of economic success. Thus, the education system is seen not so much as a virtue in its own right but as a means to improves one's position vis-à-vis the economic system. As a society, the U.S. is obsessed with education. We value credentials, and a significant portion of the population is involved in some type of education or training at any given time. Education is one of the nation's major employers and often the subject of the largest line item in the budgets of state and local governments. No other society comes close to the U.S. in terms of its emphasis on these two institutions.

The rise of these institutions in the twentieth century was given impetus by the growing dependence on formal organizations of all types. The industrialization and urbanization occurring in the United States involved a transformation from a traditional, agrarian society to a complex, modern society in which change, not tradition, is the central theme. In such a society, formal responses to societal needs take precedence over informal responses.

Healthcare provides possibly the best example of this emergent dependence on formal solutions, since it is an institution whose very development was a result of this transformation. Our great-grandparents would have considered formal healthcare as the last resort in the face of sickness and disability. Few of them ever entered a hospital, and not many more regularly utilized physicians. Today, in contrast, the healthcare system is often seen as the "first resort" when health problems arise, rather than a necessary evil. Traditional, informal responses to health problems gave way to complex, institutionalized responses. "High-touch" home remedies could not compete in an environment that valued high-tech (and subsequently high status) responses to health problems. In fact, the system's influence is such that Americans turn to it not only for clear-cut medical problems, but also for a broad range of psychological, social, interpersonal, and spiritual problems.

Industrialization and urbanization clearly influenced the direction of the development for the healthcare system, as the traditional managers of sickness and death—the family and church—gave way to more complex responses to health problems. The "management" of health became a responsibility partly of the economic, educational, and political systems and, eventually, of a fully developed and powerful healthcare system.

There are several ways in which we might gauge the importance of an institution within a society. One measure might be the proportion of societal resources that are devoted to that institution. A large share of the gross national product is related to production functions of the economy, education takes another large share, and healthcare now accounts for a significant 15 percent of the GNP. Other institutions such as the political institution, the military, and the arts receive comparatively fewer resources.

Another measure would be the extent to which the institution impinges on our daily lives and the amount of influence the institution exerts on our personal behavior. As noted above, most Americans spend most of their waking hours involved in some activity related to the economic institution. We also express inordinate concern over educational issues, with constant pressure being exerted to upgrade our degrees, enhance our skills, and acquire continuing education certification. At the same time, we have become increasingly obsessed with our health as a society. On public opinion polls, respondents frequently site "health" as among their most pressing personal concerns and "healthcare" as a leading national concern. On the other hand, more traditional institutions such as the family and religion make comparatively fewer demands on our time and exert less influence on the behavior of most Americans today.

Yet another measure that might be applied is the influence that an institution has over other institutions in the society. Certainly in medieval Europe and in contemporary Islamic societies, the religious institution is associated with inordinate control over other institutions. In contemporary America, however, the influence of religion is limited and, in fact, there are clear prohibitions against church involvement with the state and vice versa. On the other hand, the economic institution in the United States exerts extraordinary influence over other institutions. The political institution is heavily influenced by lobbyists and contributions from economic interests, and it has been argued that our educational system was designed to support the needs of America's economic functions. Indeed, the fact that the United States has the world's only for-profit healthcare system reflects the power of the economic institution to influence other institutions.

Healthcare's significance can be viewed in a similar light. The size of the institution has attracted substantial resources from other industrial sectors, healthcare is an unavoidable issue in political contests (and the AMA and AHA are among the major lobbying groups), and much of our educational system is devoted to the training of health personnel. The fact that the federal government now is responsible for 60 percent of personal healthcare expenditures indicates the influence of healthcare on the central government.

Perhaps more telling has been the extent to which the healthcare institution has been successful in the medicalization of everyday life. During the "golden age" of medicine in the 1960s and 1970s, the success of medicine resulted in an expansion of the scope of the field and led it to encompass various conditions that heretofore had not been considered medical matters. Thus, "conditions" like drug and alcohol abuse, homosexuality, child abuse, hyperactivity in children, and obesity came to be defined as medical problems. These developments served to increase the breadth of influence of the healthcare institution, enhance the prestige accorded to the institution, and garner grant funds and other sources of wealth for the institution's representatives.

In the late twentieth century Americans increasingly turned to healthcare as the solution for a wide range of social, psychological, and even spiritual issues, and physicians came to be regarded as experts in regard to virtually any human problem. This expansion of scope is evidenced by the fact that less than half of the people in a general practitioner's waiting room suffer from a clear-cut medical problem. They are there because of emotional disorders, sexual dysfunction, social adjustment issues, nutritional problems, or some other non-clinical threat to their well-being. Despite the fact that physicians are generally not trained to deal with these conditions, the healthcare system is seen as an appropriate place to seek solutions for these and other maladies.

A fourth measure, in an age of media overkill, might be the amount of "air time" allocated to various aspects of the society. Certainly, Americans continue to be deluged by advertisements for all manner of consumer goods. To a lesser degree, promotionals for various educational programs are increasingly common in the media. Coverage of religion by the media or expressed through promotionals is relatively rare. The most obvious change over the past decade or two is the explosion of advertisements and paid programming related to health, beauty and fitness. A tally of television advertisements would indicate the extent to which health products and services have come to dominate the advertising channels. Paid programming featuring fitness programs and cable television channels devoted solely to healthcare indicate the extent to which the healthcare institution has gained ascendancy.

All things considered, healthcare was the up-and-coming institution of the second half of the twentieth century. The growing significance of health for our personal lives and healthcare's growing role in the public arena cannot be denied. Indeed, many corporations have indicated that health benefits are one of their single largest costs. The increasing involvement of U.S. citizens in the use of health services and our annual per capita expenditures on health services set the U.S. apart from other countries. Subsequent sections will address the factors involved in healthcare's ascendancy in American life.

Society at the Micro-Level

The discussion to this point has focused on the macro-level aspect of society—the "big picture"—so to speak. While we have addressed the overall structure of society, we have not considered the individual and his or her place in the system. Indeed, how can a society member relate to something as overwhelming as the social structure? The individual cannot do this directly nor as an individual per se. The individual can only relate to the macro-level through intermediary structures and through the occupation of various positions within the system.

The link between the social system and the individual involves a number of steps. In effect, there is a "step-down" process from the macro-level to the micro-level. Each institution can be thought of as a subsystem within the larger social system. As a subsystem, the institution is broken down into its component parts—that is, the parts that come together to allow the subsystem to function. Within the healthcare institution, components of the subsystem would include hospital systems, the medical education component, employers who provide health insurance, medical research institutes, the pharmaceutical industry, and the federal agencies that administer Medicare and Medicaid, among others. These components must work together in order for the institution to function and achieve its goal of providing for the health and well-being of the U.S. population.

Each of these subsystems is further broken down into other subsystems. Thus, medical education would be subdivided into medical schools, dental schools, allied health schools, and nursing schools. These could also be divided into public state-sponsored educational programs and private for-profit technical training schools. Other components would include the residency programs sponsored by hospitals, the research programs associated with the professional schools, and the agencies that accredit training programs. All of these subsystems within the medical education component operate in concert to carry out the goal of educating individuals for healthcare occupations.

These subsystems are further broken down into their component parts, with a medical school involving administrators, researchers, medical students, and faculty, with the latter broken down into the various departments each with its own organizational structure. As we approach the micro-level, the subgroups are becoming smaller and more specialized. In fact, these formal groupings eventually give way to informal groupings of small numbers of individuals. Within school medical departments, cliques of colleagues are likely to develop involving a subgroup of the department faculty, and certain students are likely to cluster together in study groups or friendship groups that exclude other students.

As will be seen in the chapter on social groups, the establishment of these small groups is essential to the effective functioning of individuals within that setting. As human beings, we cannot relate very well to large formal structures. We need to bring this down to a more human scale. Small informal groups serve as a buffer between the individual and the larger society. Group members can help to interpret the rules of the formal organization and provide the social support that all society members require.

In this example, the interface of faculty and medical students may be seen as the context for discussing the micro-level of society. Sociologists do not think in terms of individuals with all of their idiosyncracies, but they see the lowest unit of the social system as the social statuses that individuals occupy. A "social status" is a recognized position within the social structure occupied by an individual that exists only in relation to other statuses. (Sociologists do not use the term "status" in its everyday meaning of "prestige", as when a neurosurgeon has more "status" than a family practitioner. Sociologically, both "neurosurgeon" and "family practitioner" are statuses or positions within the healthcare institution.) The pivotal statuses in healthcare are often thought to be those of "doctor" and "patient". These statuses are social positions that only exist each in relation to the other. Thus, if there are no "patients" there can be no "doctors"; if there are no "doctors" there can be no "patients".

In all societies, but particularly in modern industrialized societies, society members occupy many statuses at once. Thus, sociologists use the term status set to refer to the statuses a person holds at a particular time. A female medical student may be a daughter to her parents, a sister to her brother, a friend to others in her social circle, a student in anatomy class, and a volunteer at a nursing home. A person's statuses change over a lifetime, so that a child turns into a parent, a medical student becomes a doctor, and single people become husbands or wives. Joining an organization or finding a job enlarges our status set; retirement or withdrawing from activities makes it smaller. Thus, over a lifetime, an individual gains and loses many different statuses.

Some statuses matter more than others to the individual and may be singled out as a master status, or a position that carries exceptional importance and may dominate other statuses. For most Americans, their occupation represents a master status because one's occupation conveys a great deal of information about their social background, socioeconomic status, and lifestyle. At the same time, a serious disease can also operate as a master status. Cancer patients or people with AIDS may be avoided by friends as a result of this status.

Social statuses are both reciprocal and complementary. One or more reciprocal statuses must exist for a particular status to exist, and these statuses complement each other in terms of the tasks they perform. These tasks are referred to as "roles" and each status carries a particular role with it. The role is that set of rights and obligations that characterize a particular status. The rights indicate what the status incumbent may do, and the obligations indicate what the incumbent must do. In the case of the medical school faculty and students, the status of professor involves a certain role that the individual occupying the role of professor is expected to perform. Similarly, the status of student involves a set of expectations and behaviors constituting the student's role.

The roles of professor and student are complementary and it takes the two working together to accomplish their portion of the goal of the institution—that is, providing medical education. Thus, the two roles working in concert accomplish the task of transmitting medical knowledge. If either status incumbent fails to carry out his obligations, the system breaks down. Thus, if the professor does not convey the correct information or the student does not incorporate the knowledge because of a neglect of his studies, this component of the healthcare institution is deficient.

Because we occupy many statuses at once, everyday life involves multiple roles. Thus, every society member has a role set involving the various roles that correspond to the individual's status set. Most people in industrial societies juggle a variety of responsibilities dictated by their various statuses. Sociologists thus identify role conflict as the inevitable consequence of incompatibility among roles corresponding to two or more statuses.

Even roles associated with a single status can make competing demands onerous. Role strain refers to incompatibility among the roles corresponding to a single status. Doctors are ethically constrained from treating members of their own families due to the role strain that is likely to be involved. Thus, performing the roles of even a single status can involve something of a balancing act.

Having described the micro-level of society, how, then, can we link the micro-level of the social system back to the macro-level, especially with so many interceding levels? It should be recalled that an institution is a pattern of behavior for accomplishing a certain societal goal—in this case, assuring the health and well-being of society members. But where do these patterns of behavior reside? They reside in the role performance of individuals occupying the various statuses within the healthcare institution. Thus, there are doctors interfacing with patients, medical school faculty interfacing with students, researchers interfacing with clinical trial subjects, doctors interfacing with nurses, insurance clerks interfacing with hospital billing clerks, and so forth. The interactions of millions of persons occupying thousands of statuses and performing their respective roles become the "patterns of behavior" that constitute the institution. All of these statuses performing all of the associated roles ultimately carry out the work of the institution.

The Functions of the Healthcare Institution

As noted earlier, the primary objective of the healthcare institution is to provide for the health and well-being of the population it serves. However, this is not the only function of the healthcare institution and, in a society as complex as the United States, this institution serves a number of other purposes as well. Even in more traditional societies, the healthcare institution may carry out other functions that, indeed, given the limited efficacy of pre-modern systems, may be more important than curing sickness.

The U.S. healthcare institution attempts to achieve its goal through curing sickness and, secondarily, through prevention and health maintenance. Implicit in this function is the staving off of death and the prolonging of life. These are certainly overt functions of the healthcare institution but do not nearly complete the list. Other direct functions of the healthcare system include the promotion of public health and safety. Thus, assuring that society members have safe drinking water and clean air to breath, along with the myriad other functions carried out by public health agencies and government organizations such as the Environmental Protection Agency, is a significant but often overlooked function of the healthcare institution. Indeed, without the successful operation of this function, treatment and cure would face an uphill battle in maintaining the health status of the population.

The U.S. healthcare institution performs many other functions that indirectly contribute to the goals of the institution. Healthcare organizations—often the same ones involved inpatient care—provide training for health professionals and participate in research toward the furtherance of our understanding of the nature of health and illness. At the same time, these organizations typically perform humanitarian and community service functions, through the provision of free or discounted care, community education programs, and the sponsorship of community events. Further, many healthcare organizations serve as conduits for the transmission of religious tenets.

The healthcare institution also performs an important economic function in U.S. society. As a $1.3 trillion a year industry, healthcare contributes to the creation of wealth in the society and provides jobs for 10 percent of the workforce. For-profit healthcare organizations are expected to return a profit to their owners. In many small communities, the local hospital may be the largest employer in the area.

These are all generally recognized functions of the healthcare institution in the United States and, to a lesser degree, in other developed countries. There are some also not-so-overt functions of healthcare systems that are found in varying forms in most societies. One of these functions is resource management. In centrally planned healthcare systems (e.g., the British National Health Service), the major goal of the system may be the efficient management of government resources. Curing disease is an important, albeit secondary, function.

The healthcare system also provides an answer for the "why" of sickness and death. Whether the explanatory system is based on supernaturalism or the rationality of the medical model, the system helps explain why people get sick and why they die. It doesn't change the reality of sickness and death, but human beings seem to have at least some explanation for the events that befall them.

The healthcare institution also contributes to the overall operation and stability of the society in which it resides. As will be discussed later, the healthcare system serves as a method of social control. Remembering that sickness represents a form of deviance in society and is therefore dysfunctional, some means of controlling deviance and restoring functionality must be maintained. By identifying the biologically abnormal, the institution can isolate them and provide them the care that will restore them to normality and, at the same time, protect the rest of society from the potentially harmful effects of deviants within its midst.

One other function of the healthcare system identified by anthropologists is the integrative role it performs. The operation of the system in the face of sickness serves to bring the community together in a common effort and reaffirms the belief system of the society. By rallying around the sick person and participating in shared rituals, the community is brought together and its integration reinforced.

ADDITIONAL RESOURCES

Cassell, Eric J. (1976). "Disease as an 'it': Concepts of disease revealed by patients' presentation of symptoms," *Social Science and Medicine* 10:143–146.

Cassell, Eric J. (1986). "Ideas in conflict: The rise and fall (and rise and fall) of new views of disease," *Daedalus: Journal of the American Academy of Arts and Sciences* 115(2):19–41.

Comaroff, Jean (1978). "Medicine and culture: Some anthropological perspectives," *Social Science and Medicine* 12B:247–254.

Cockerham, William C., and Ferris J. Richey (1997). *The Dictionary of Medical Sociology*. Westport, CT: Greenwood.

Murdock, George Peter (1965 [1949]). *Social Structure*. New York: Free Press.

Parsons, Talcott (1951). *The Social System*. New York: The Free Press.

Chapter 4

The Cultural Dimension of Healthcare

THE NATURE OF CULTURE

The social structure of a society is difficult to observe with the naked eye, since institutions, being patterns of behavior, do not take tangible form. It is true that the structural evidence of these institutions can be seen in the form of factories, churches, schools and hospitals, but this is not the same as seeing the social structure. What is actually being observed is the outward manifestation of the social structure or the cultural traits of that social system. The factory is a bricks-and-mortar representation of the economic institution, the cathedral of the religious institution, and the hospital of the healthcare institution. Indeed, when we visit a foreign country, what we observe is not the social system but differences in clothing, food, language and architecture. All of these are representations of the social system of that particular culture. Culture establishes the "flavor" of a society and, when we compare Americans to Frenchmen to Chinese, we do this in terms of cultural differences.

"Culture" can be defined as the way of life characterizing a particular society. Culture includes the values, ideas, techniques for dealing with the environment that are shared among contemporaries and passed on from generation to generation. Social structure and culture are two sides of the same coin, with the social structure providing the underlying framework and culture being the outward manifestation. Culture represents the pattern of living characterizing the members of a society, and it includes both the nonmaterial aspects of social life and the products created as people follow their daily activities.

Anthropologists point out that there are two dimensions of culture— the material and the non-material. Material culture refers to the tangible, man-made artifacts that are developed for use by that culture. These "things" would include clothing, tools, art forms and other tangible products of the culture. While sociologists do not overly emphasize material aspects of culture, they are important to our understanding of the non-material aspects of culture and ultimately the social structure. Objects are seldom solely utilitarian, but have attributes that provide clues into the lifestyles, values and beliefs of those who produced them. It is for this reason that archaeologists can reconstruct the social life and, hence, the social structure of long extinct societies from the few representatives of tangible culture they can retrieve.

The healthcare institution is certainly not short of examples of material culture. We associate all types of biomedical equipment, hospital furniture, surgical instruments, and uniforms with healthcare. The hospital is the concrete symbol of the healthcare system and the stethoscope symbolizes the expertise and authority of the physician. From the country doctor's black bag to the magnetic resonance imaging machine, we associate healthcare with its material components.

Sociologists are generally more interested in the non-material culture that characterizes a society than in the material. This includes the ideas, beliefs, values and rules that characterize the society and provide clues to the patterns of behavior that sociologists seek to identify. Non-material culture in a sense represents the "ideals" of that culture—the beliefs one should hold, the values one should strive after, the norms one should comply with. Non-material culture is couched in a symbol system that, beginning with language, reflects a systematic and logical framework for understanding and dealing with the world. Non-material culture may be either conscious or unconscious, spoken or unspoken. There are some rules that we "just know" (actually because they were instilled in us at an early age) and others that are constantly articulated.

These non-material traits of a culture give a society its ethos and are reflected in the behavior of society members. Indeed, these traits serve to guide the behavior of society members. Thus, when Americans are depicted as avaricious, Englishmen as reserved, or Germans as methodical, these are not necessarily stereotypes but reflect underlying aspects of the non-material culture of the respective societies.

LANGUAGE: THE FOUNDATION FOR CULTURE

Language forms the foundation for any culture. Not only does it allow members of the same culture to communicate with each other but it serves many other purposes as well. To the extent that culture is transferred from generation to generation, this is carried out either orally or through written documents using language. By learning a particular language—our society's language—we are predisposed to see the world in a certain way. Thus, until relatively modern times, most languages did not have a term for "health" in the sense that we use it today. Without this concept embedded in the language, it is difficult to conceive of a healthcare system in a formal sense.

Language represents a sort of training program for new society members. They are introduced to the tenets of that society by learning the concepts embodied in the language. At the same time, the individual is *not* exposed to the concepts of other cultures by being excluded from their language, with his language thereby serving as a filtering device. Indeed, those who have tried to translate documents from one language to another are often stumped by the fact that a concept in one language may not have a counterpart in another.

Language has other less obvious but no less important functions as well. Language serves to construct reality for the individual and make sense out of an otherwise chaotic world. The fact that there is no word for "secular" in Arabic establishes a framework for religion within that culture. Languages of traditional societies that have no word for "mental illness" develop a different view of health and illness than those in cultures that speak English. The English term "self-actualization" represents a concept unlikely to be found in most languages and, thus, not a part of their culture's ethos.

Not only does language help the society member interpret the world but it gives meaning to the objects in one's environment. The words "man" and "woman" don't simply denote different sexes, but the words used for the two sexes in any language are pregnant with meaning. Various behaviors are explained by saying, "He's a man" or "She's a woman". This is supposed to explain it all due to the meanings associated with those terms. The English language usually treats whatever has greater value or significance as masculine. For example, the adjective "virtuous" meaning "morally worthy" or "excellent," is derived from the Latin word "vir," meaning "man". In contrast, the disparaging adjective "hysterical", meaning uncontrollable emotion, comes from the Greek word "hyster", meaning uterus. Thus, hysterectomies were historically thought to remove the hysteria from women. Language both mirrors social perceptions and helps to perpetuate them.

Even such basic notions as "time" are embodied in a culture's language. The English language emphasizes tenses utilizing, unlike some other languages, past, present and future tenses. This linguistic structure serves to help establish a view of history and reality. Thus, we tend to view history as a linear progression of events from one period to the next, each connected in some manner. This is contrary to the views posed by virtue of other languages. This linguistic context causes Westerners in general and English speakers in particular to think in terms of cause and effect. Any event, it is held, must have some precedent event that "caused" the second event. This notion is the basis for the scientific method and for the diagnostic process underlying allopathic medicine. Thus, we speak of the "progression" of a disease. While this notion seems logical to those who have grown up speaking English, the notion may not be accepted by those who speak other languages.

Healthcare—and the medical profession in particular—epitomizes the use of language as more than a means of communication. Medicine, for example, understandably has its own unique terminology for use in the management of ill-health, allowing practitioners to speak with precision in a common jargon. The use of "myocardial infarction" for a heart attack provides precision and differentiates this type of "heart attack" from other types. The fact that patients "expire" rather than "die" reflects the underlying explanatory system for understanding health and illness.

At the same time, however, language is often used by physicians as a means of establishing their superiority vis-à-vis patients, exerting power in the doctor-patient relationship, and/or maintaining control over social interaction. Language is thus used to reinforce the asymmetrical power relationships between doctor and patient and to limit the amount of information that is provided the patient. The use of language in healthcare will be noted throughout this text.

THE COMPONENTS OF NON-MATERIAL CULTURE

The sociologist is particularly interested in the non-material aspects of culture. Beyond language, the major components of non-material culture are beliefs, values and norms. Each of these components of culture plays an important role in the management of society and in the achievement of societal goals.

Beliefs

For sociologists, beliefs are notions held by society members for which no socially acceptable means of proof exists. These include notions about man, the world, the universe, and God. Examples of these would be beliefs in one god rather than many gods or none at all, or the belief that human beings are intrinsically "good" or "evil". With regard to the healthcare institution in our society, Americans *believe* that it is appropriate to intercede medically in the face of illness, a belief, incidentally, not held by all societies. We *believe* that every human life is worth saving, another belief not universally held.

The beliefs held by members of a society fit together to form a belief system, and this system becomes the foundation for the ideas, values, and behavior patterns that characterize the culture. Because they fit together in a system, it is difficult to modify one aspect of a belief system without modifying other components. Missionaries who converted the "heathen" to Christianity often contributed to the demise of the society by virtue of tampering with one component of the belief system while neglecting others.

Beliefs are often unspoken and simply "understood", or they may be constantly reaffirmed as through the religious institution. Particularly in modern, industrialized societies, we are often not very cognizant of the beliefs that contribute to our worldview. These beliefs are often nebulous and may be hidden in the cultural background but, nevertheless, exert an influence on our thoughts and behavior.

Values

The second component of non-material culture is values. Values represent ideas, preferences, and objects—tangible and intangible—we consider of worth. They also include desirable ends that we would like to attain. Values might be considered as statements, from the standpoint of culture, of what "ought" to be. These values mesh into a value system and typically reflect the underlying belief system.

Values are more directly relevant to society members than are beliefs in the sense that they guide the behavior of individuals. Members of any society behave in accordance with the values that they incorporate through the socialization process, a process that teaches us the values our society considers important for the attainment of societal goals. Thus, Americans learn to value competitiveness over cooperation, the individual over the group, and youthfulness over old age. A society's values serve to create its national character. Americans display certain attitudes and preferences not because of any individual traits but because of the values promulgated by the society.

What then are the dominant American values? These can be identified for American culture (or any culture) by determining what society members consider important. The American values that immediately come to mind include economic success, educational achievement, freedom and equality, individuality, scientific advancement and technology. We also value human life to an extent not found in other societies and place emphasis on humanitarianism. American contributions to charity and involvement in humanitarian efforts are unparalleled anywhere. While family life and religion may be given some value, it is hard to argue that they constitute major values in contemporary America. Some have suggested that American values fit together in cultural themes that would involve groupings like: freedom/democracy/equality; economic success/free enterprise; and progress/scientific advancement/technology.

Since World War II "health" has been added to the list of personal values held by Americans and, its institutional counterpart "healthcare" to the list of societal values. In fact, up until the 1960s health was not singled out as a distinct value to be pursued, and healthcare was not seen as a component of the national agenda. During the last third of the twentieth century, however, Americans came to be obsessed with health as a value and with the importance of institutional solutions to health problems.

There are other American values that might not appear too obvious on the surface. One of these is an orientation toward the future. Americans place a great deal of emphasis on the future and typically demonstrate a willingness to sacrifice in the present for gains at some future date. As a society, we encourage investing in education for future career benefits, participating in retirement plans, and purchasing insurance against possible future events. With some important exceptions, Americans tend to keep their eyes on the horizon, seldom looking nostalgically back at the past or dwelling on the issues of the present time.

One other important value characterizing American culture is "activism." Americans are not the type of people to passively let things happen to them. American culture emphasizes aggressive action and the controlling of one's destiny. Americans seek to control their environment and, relative to many other societies, appear almost frantic in their attempts to manage their situation. This is in stark contrast to societies where such activism would be considered inappropriate. In those societies, "passivism" is emphasized as a cultural value, and it is considered inappropriate to attempt to control one's fate. More than that, it may even be considered blasphemous to question the master plan of that culture's particular deity. (Box 4-1 illustrates the implications of one cultural value for healthcare.)

The values that a society emphasizes may change over time, with change more likely to occur in rapidly developing societies as opposed to traditional societies. In fact, it could be argued that "change" itself has become a value in American culture. The society's emphasis on "progress" and technological advancement make a certain amount of change inevitable. This is perhaps epitomized by the hawker's common phrase: New and Improved! The rate at which Americans change jobs, residences and even lifestyles suggests that change has become a national value. In healthcare there is always the prospect of the breakthrough drug or procedure that will revolutionize medical care. (This emphasis on change as it relates to healthcare runs counter to the basically conservative nature of the institution, in which the benefits of any new approach must be scientifically demonstrated before its application.)

It should be noted that some values contradict others. For example, the controversy over abortion pits the value we place on human life against the value we place on freedom of choice for individuals. Similarly, the issue of physician-assisted suicide juxtaposes the value of human life with the value we place on quality of life. The strain created for healthcare organizations as they try to balance their humanitarian missions with the need to show a profit is another example. Such value conflicts often lead to awkward balancing acts in our convictions. Individuals may decide that one value is more important than another; in other cases, they simply learn to live with inconsistencies. Thus, while access to abortion services has been established as a legal right for American women, many physicians still refuse to perform abortions. Physicians may quietly allow terminal patients to die, without actively practicing euthanasia.

An appreciation of societal values is important for an understanding the nature of the U.S. healthcare system or any system for that matter. When one examines the values that are dominant in U.S. society, much of the nature of the healthcare system is explained. First and foremost is the value our society places on health and human life. Both of these values have led to excessive use of health services by some segments of the population and a willingness to expend whatever resources are necessary to save a single human life. Supporting these values is the emphasis Americans place on activism. If our healthcare system is anything, it is proactive in its approach to sickness and death. The system aggressively pursues the treatment of health conditions, and individual society members proactively utilize clinical services and are quick to respond to potential health threats.

At the same time, the emphasis placed by American society on scientific advancement encourages the use of innovative technology in healthcare, making the U.S. system the most high-tech in the world. Our emphasis on educational achievement has led us to establish credentialing procedures for all manner of health workers and has made the training of health personnel a major "industry". Our emphasis on economic success and the free enterprise system has encouraged the development of the world's only for-profit healthcare system, and the value we place on freedom of

---

Box 4-1

The Health Implications of Our Obsession with Youth

Because America is a young country, American society has always placed an emphasis on youth. This is in contrast to older societies where age may be valued over youthfulness. It took the developments of the second half of the 20th century, however, to elevate "youth" to the status of a societal value. In the last half of that century, U.S. society became almost obsessed with the notion of youthfulness, and the personal goals of many Americans included maintaining their youthful looks and vigor. The emergence of youth as a value was given particular impetus by the Baby Boom generation. This generation had always had things pretty much its way and was used to being in good physical condition and having all parts in working order. This generation was not about to submit to the ravishes of aging and has pushed the envelope in terms of mechanisms for remaining youthful.

The implications for society of an emphasis on youth can be seen everywhere. Instead of young people emulating their elders, we witness elders emulating their children. Consumer goods are designed to appeal to young people but are subsequently purchased by older people. Youth drive the movies, television shows and music that the rest of the population adopts. Despite the fact that older Americans far outnumber youth, disproportionate amount of market research focuses on what youth are interested in, and a subsequent disproportionate amount of marketing dollars are devoted to this relatively small segment of the consumer population.

While youth-oriented fashions may be widely promoted, the implications of fashion for society are relatively superficial. However, the implications of the value placed on youth are particularly significant for healthcare. When combined with the emphasis placed on "health" as a value, this youth/health orientation drives much of the activity of the healthcare system. This aspect of healthcare is now being given particular impetus by 70 million aging Baby Boomers. Not only is there growing emphasis on maintaining high health status, but there has been a dramatic growth in interest in procedures and products designed to retard aging.

Americans have long been obsessed with dieting, and this may be the most ubiquitous evidence of our obsession with youthfulness. Youth is associated with a svelte figure and a firm body (despite growing evidence that few Americans fit this picture). Billions of dollars are spent, mostly by

---

choice has become a rallying cry for physicians who fear loss of control, if patients cannot freely choose their physician. On the other hand, as noted above, the emphasis we place on humanitarianism results in a value conflict vis-à-vis the profit motive characterizing many healthcare organizations.

The conceptualization of "health" as a value described earlier represented a major development in the emergence of the healthcare institution.

women, trying to live up to a virtually unattainable image of the youthful figure. And, as with many other aspects of society, weight management has come to be defined as a medical concern. Whether or not some measure of success can be achieved by these dieters, positive results have been produced for promoters of diet programs (and the clinicians that support them) and negative results have been achieved for the health of many individuals who pursue such diets.

The emphasis Americans are placing on youthfulness is nowhere more obvious than in the area of cosmetic surgery. Cosmetic surgery is arguably the fastest growing component of the healthcare system. The determination of Americans to remain youthful has led to a surge in interest in tummy tucks, facelifts, hair replacement and treatments for aging skin. While these procedures have been long endured by older American women, statistics indicate that men are equally as interested in procedures that change their image. In fact, the average age for first exposure to cosmetic surgery has dropped from the mid-50s to the mid-40s. Besides cosmetic surgery, another area of significant growth among medical practitioners is skin care.

Perhaps more obvious to the typical American than the burgeoning cosmetic surgery industry is the plethora of products that are being offered to promote youth and beauty. Even a casual glance at newspaper and magazine advertising or television commercials indicates the extent to which youth-preserving products are being offered. Products that promise to restore youthful skin, regrow hair, increase energy levels or improve sexual vigor are promoted through every possible medium. As the Baby Boom cohort continues to age, the number of products of this type can only increase.

This emphasis on youth has some far-reaching implications for the healthcare industry. Besides elevating the visibility of cosmetic surgeons and dermatologists, it also influences preferences for specialty training. Despite the rapidly growing elderly population in the U.S., few medical students are interested in geriatric medicine. In fact, there are essentially no more geriatricians in the U.S. than there were two decades ago. The number of pediatricians trained far exceeds the number of geriatricians, despite a growing number of older Americans and a relatively smaller number of children. There are other reasons, of course, for choosing pediatrics over geriatrics, but the reality is that, regardless of the specialty, future physicians are going to be constantly faced with demands from their patients for preservation of their youthfulness.

Prior to World War II health was not perceived as a distinct value in its own right but was vaguely tied in with other notions of well-being. Public opinion polls prior to WWII never indicated that personal health was an issue with the population, nor was healthcare delivery considered a societal issue. By the 1960s, personal health had climbed to the top of the public opinion polls as an issue and concerns surrounding the healthcare system were beginning to make healthcare a top societal issue in the mind of the American public.

Once health became established as a value, it was a short step to establishing a formal healthcare system as the institutional means for achieving that value. With the ascendancy of "health" as a value, an environment was created that encouraged the emergence of a powerful institution that supported many basic values of American culture. Some of them, like the value placed on human life, were considered immutable. The emerging scientific, technological and research communities contributed to the growth of the healthcare industry. Support from the economic, political and educational institutions assured the ascendancy of this new institutional form.

Norms

The third component of non-material culture is norms. Norms represent the rules and regulations society establishes to guide behavior. The term "norm" is used in two different senses. On the one hand, sociologists use the term to refer to the behavior expected of society members—that is, what is appropriate and what is inappropriate. In this sense, the norms represent the dos and don'ts of behavior in society. Conceding that many society members cannot or do not abide by all of the rules of society, the term also refers to what behavior is actually performed—in other words, the "average" behavior. While the speed limit (the formal norm) may be set at 40 miles per hour, it can be observed that motorists "normally" drive five miles over the speed limit.

Compared to beliefs and values, norms are relatively specific and impact the behavior of individual society members much more directly. In fact, we often comply with norms without being consciously aware of it and frequently do not even understand the reason for the rule that is being followed. The more effective the socialization process is, the better society members internalize the rules. The more "automatically" society members comply with the norms without the need for positive or negative sanctions, the more smoothly the society operates.

Norms are important above and beyond their role in encouraging society members to act appropriately. They provide a basis for inducing the level of conformity needed for the orderly operation of social transactions and for smooth social interaction. Importantly, norms make human behavior predictable, and this predictability is necessary for the efficient operation of the social system. Indeed, one of the traits that makes us uncomfortable with the mentally ill is their unpredictability. We worry less about their more radical behavior than we do the fact that we cannot predict what they are going to do or say.

The ultimate function of norms is their contribution to the institutional goals of society. If institutions represent patterns of behavior geared toward the achievement of some societal goal, where do those patterns come from? They are created through the operation of individuals complying with the norms of society. Thus, there are norms that govern the operation of the economic system, the educational system, and the healthcare system. The rules that govern doctor-patient relationships, beyond serving to facilitate orderly transactions between the two parties, also serve to accomplish the goal of the healthcare institution—that is, assuring the health and well-being of the population. Thus, without society members ever being aware of the ulterior purpose of their behavior, they are contributing to the goals of various institutions through their everyday actions.

There are four categories of norms that sociologists generally recognize—customs, mores, laws, and fads. "Customs" involve those rules that guide the everyday behavior of society members. Also referred to as folkways in deference to the fact that they emerge from the grassroots of society, customs include rules of hygiene, dress, conversation and social interaction. Much of what we think of as manners amounts to customs (sometimes codified as rules of etiquette). Rules that guide everyday interactions between males and females, between young and old, and between peers involve customs. Clothing styles, dietary habits and work schedules reflect "customary" behavior. It's customary for Americans to begin the workday around 8 or 9 in the morning, while it's customary for Japanese workers to begin the workday at sunrise. In the classroom, students customarily do certain things—e.g., take notes, ask questions, and address the instructor with respect. In taking notes, students in American classes use pens and pencils (and increasingly computers) for note taking, while different customs might guide the behavior of students in other cultures. At the same time, instructors follow certain customs with regard to preparing lectures, making assignments, and encouraging discussion.

In healthcare, it is customary for various health professions to wear different uniforms and insignia, and the methods of address among health professionals and between clinicians and patients are based on custom. It is even customary for certain segments of the population to resort to folk medicine prior to or as an alternative to the use of conventional medicine. In everyday life, there are certain health-related customs that we observe, such as washing our hands before meals, eating chicken soup when sick with a cold, and purchasing over-the-counter drugs when faced with minor symptoms. While we take these behaviors for granted, there are plenty of societies in which these behaviors are not customary.

Customs tend to be relatively informal types of norms and are typically not written down (except in the case of etiquette books or, say, a school's policy manual). They are also informal in the sense that they are typically not "legislated"—that is, no one makes them up. They arise out of the everyday transactions of individuals and evolve over time. In this sense, they are the most "traditional" of the various types of norms. Quite often, customs originated for some practical purpose as in the case of cuffs on men's pants or buttons on the sleeves of men's sports coats. Long after the reason for the rule has been forgotten, customs remain strong factors in the control of everyday behavior.

Customs are also informal in the sense that they are not precisely defined. They serve as general guidelines and therefore are open to some interpretation. It is customary for children to obey their parents, but anyone who has ever had children will concede that this custom can be broadly interpreted. At the same time, there is no clear-cut reaction to violations of customs. Unlike some other types of norms, we don't have rules that prescribe the punishment for talking back to parents or not taking all of the pills prescribed by the physician. The reaction—and punishment, if any— typically depends on the situation and who observes the violation. Parents, teachers, employers and other authority figures are perhaps more likely to note and react to violations of norms than, say, peer group members. Indeed, the fact that no one is formally assigned to police customs violators further reflects the informality of this type of norm.

A second category of norm involves "mores" (always used in the plural). Mores are like customs in many ways but tend to deal with more serious issues. Like customs, mores are relatively informal in the sense that they evolve through social interaction rather than being legislated, they are not stated very precisely, they do not carry a specific punishment for violation, and no one is specifically assigned to monitor their compliance. Like customs, they have the objectives of assuring conformity and predictability in behavior and furthering the achievement of the goals of society.

Mores differ from customs, as noted in that they deal with much more serious issues. While customs serve to regulate manners, styles, and taste, mores deal with such issues as sexual relationships, religious observances, and professional ethics. Issues of premarital and extramarital sex, sinful behavior, and doctor-patient confidentiality are the subjects of societal mores, as the term's kinship with "morality" suggests. Violations of customs may create a temporarily awkward situation, but violations of mores potentially threaten the basis of social order. Bad manners is not likely to topple the society, but rampant illicit sexual behavior—read sexual behavior considered inappropriate by that society—certainly has the potential to damage the family institution as well as other institutions.

Some societies carry the enforcement of mores virtually to the point of becoming a legal issue, and the punishment is swift and sure. However, in the United States and most societies, mores are not precisely defined and the response to violations of mores is likely to be situational and, again, depend on who observes the violation. Premarital sex between consenting teenagers may violate accepted societal mores but is likely to be interpreted in the light of the situation. If the situation involves an older man and an underage girl, then the reaction is likely to be much more severe.

In healthcare there are numerous examples of mores as they relate to professional ethics. These mores in healthcare cover everything from referral relationships between colleagues to euthanasia. In recent years, physicians have faced the dilemma of whether to advertise their services or not. Professional ethics have historically prohibited advertising on the part of physicians, although such actions have not been illegal. Clinicians may also face situations in which a relationship between the practitioner and the patient may be developing, and such a relationship would clearly violate the mores governing practitioner-patient relationships.

Similarly, the confidentiality of doctor-patient interaction is sacrosanct and would involve a serious violation of societal mores as well as professional ethics if such confidences were betrayed. However, the latitude involved in the interpretation of mores sometimes is evidenced by, say, a situation in which a psychiatrist has the choice of violating doctor-patient privilege in order to save the life of the patient or someone else. Everyday, physicians face the question of allowing terminal patients to die even though they could be kept alive indefinitely on life-support systems. Professional ethics call for preserving life at all costs but, increasingly, the profession and the public are conceding that quality-of-life issues may represent mitigating circumstances.

A third type of norm involves "laws". Laws are different in many ways from customs and mores and are the most formal of the norms to be discussed. Interestingly, for most of the societies that ever inhabited the Earth, customs and mores have been sufficient to maintain social order and further the goals of the society. However, as societies grow larger and more complex, informal means of social control begin to lose their power and more formal means are required. While laws typically reflect the same values that spawned the customs and mores of the society, they are qualitatively different. Indeed, the laws of society may actually run counter to majority public sentiment in some cases.

Laws are formal in the sense that they are legislated and enacted in a deliberate manner and do not evolve over time as do customs and mores. They are formal in the sense that they are clearly stated for all to see and much more precise than customs and mores. They are formal in the sense that there are clear-cut penalties for violations of laws. Finally, they are formal in the sense that there are entities that are formally charged with the enforcement of these norms and the identification, apprehension and punishment of the violators. There is a lot less latitude for interpretation than with customs and mores, and we often speak of "the letter of the law". In addition, customs and mores are considered situational and may be applied differently in different situations. Laws, on the other hand, are universal and, theoretically at least, applied uniformly across the board. Thus, in the United States, all are considered equal before the law.

In healthcare, laws have been enacted to cover a variety of aspects of the field. Most clinical practice is governed by the laws of the state in which the practice takes place, and to practice medicine without a license, for example, is a legal offense. Laws govern billing practices, price fixing, fee-splitting and other activities that health professionals and organizations may be involved in. A whole set of laws governs the prescription of controlled substances to patients. Federal law governs what drugs can be sold to the public and what claims can be made for these drugs. Recent cases involving Medicare and Medicaid fraud, false product advertising, and illegal sale of pharmaceuticals via the Internet indicate the extent to which state and federal laws impact healthcare.

A final type of norm that should be mentioned is the "fad". A fad is more like a custom than any of the other types of norms in terms of its informality, its lack of precision, lack of specific punishment, and so forth. A fad differs from a custom in that it does not typically reflect traditional behavior patterns, and it does not have a very long existence. A fad is thus a standard of behavior that arises precipitously (and may, in fact, be "manufactured") and has a sometimes dramatic but short-lived impact. Clothing styles, hairstyles, trendy foods and entertainment activities are likely to be faddish. Unlike other norms, fads are likely to affect only a portion of the society and not become engrained in the societal ethos.

Why consider fads in the context of healthcare? Interestingly, we find that some health-related behaviors—on the part of both patients and practitioners—take on many of the characteristics of fads. We are used to hearing the term "fad diet", but the same notion could be applied to activities such as exercise, health food consumption, and therapeutic bracelets.

Table 4–1.   Health-Related Social Norms

Customs	Laws
Uniforms/insignia	Prescription restrictions
Methods of address	Medical licensure
Folk medicine	Blood-handling regulations
Mores	*Fads*
Doctor-patient confidentiality	Tonsillectomies
Professional ethics	Ear tubes
Nurse in examination room	Cosmetic surgery

Of a more serious nature are some of the "fads" that have affected clinical practice. We now know that the traditional removal of tonsils of children was more of a fad than it was a medically necessary procedure, and now that fad has been replaced by the trends toward indiscriminate insertion of ear tubes into children and prescription of drugs for misbehaving children. Many of the therapeutic modalities introduced by mental health clinicians over the years are now viewed as fads that had no clinical underpinning. Indeed, given the fact that only 20 percent of medical procedures are known to reflect evidence-based research findings, one could argue that many common medical procedures border on being faddish within the profession. (See Table 4-1 for examples of healthcare-related norms.)

CULTURAL COMPLEXITY IN THE UNITED STATES

Any discussion of the components of culture assumes that society members hold a consensus with regard to the beliefs, values and norms that constitute the culture's ethos. And this is the case for most societies that have ever existed. However, the size and diversity of the U.S. population challenges the validity of this assumption. Do Americans, in fact, all ascribe to the same beliefs, pursue the same values, and adhere to the same norms?

The complexity of contemporary American society mitigates against any type of consensus with regard to beliefs, values and norms. The diversity of racial and ethnic groups, religious communities, immigrants of virtually every nationality, regional differences, and extreme variations in lifestyle result in multiple sets of beliefs, values and norms. This was most clearly demonstrated during the debate in the 1970s as to what constitutes pornography. The non-decision by the court threw that determination back on the local community, on the assumption that standards with regard to pornography would vary from community to community.

The existence of numerous subcultures within the society further contributes to variations in perceptions. In some cases, these varying interpretations of the tenets of the culture result in conflict between ethnic groups or subcultures and the larger society. While the society allows great latitude with regard to religious beliefs and childrearing approaches, the interests of the larger society intercede in the case of child deaths caused by faith healing practices. While one cannot help be impressed with the diversity of beliefs, values and norms held by a society as diverse as the United States, we see that certain basic principles surface at times of crisis such as the terrorist attacks of September, 2001. Americans of all persuasions rallied in support of what were thought to be basic American values.

Even within healthcare, an endeavor presumably guided by rigorous scientific principles, we find considerable variation in values and norms. There are practitioners who wholeheartedly support the rights of physicians to perform abortions or euthanasia and others who consider these criminal acts. There is tremendous variation in the rate of hospitalization and the numbers and types of procedures performed from community to community. This phenomenon has less to do with differences in health problems than with standards of practice that vary from community to community.

THE INTERFACE OF THE SOCIAL SYSTEM AND CULTURE

In the previous chapter, the "social structure" was discussed and in this one its counterpart "culture" was described. How is it that these two sides of the same coin interface? As noted earlier, the main components of the social system, institutions, represent patterns of behavior for accomplishing goals that society considers important. One of the things that determine what is important are the values emphasized by the culture. Thus, if the culture values economic success, educational achievement, and military dominance, these values will be reflected in the importance of the economic, educational and military institutions. On the other hand, if the culture values religiosity and family relations, then the religious and family institutions will be more important.

The relationship between social structure and culture, of course, is a two-way street. Once the institutions are in place they institute methods for maintaining and enhancing the values that encouraged their development in the first place. Thus, the values of culture influence the nature of its institutions and, in turn, these institutions reinforce the important values of the culture.

Since Americans have come to value health, a large and powerful healthcare institution has emerged. Once established, the healthcare institution has introduced formal and informal means of reinforcing the value of health within the culture. While health insurance was offered as a benefit to the insured, the influence of the healthcare institution can be seen in the fact that employees often *must* participate in the health insurance plan and taxpayers *must* contribute to the Medicare program. Similarly, while at some point society determined that it would be beneficial to immunize children against certain diseases, the institution today mandates that all school children have immunizations before registering. While society may have determined that having "asylums" available to shelter and care for the severely mentally ill was socially beneficial, the institution has used the legal system to enact laws that allow for the involuntary incarceration of certain categories of the mentally ill.

Looked at differently, the culture's values can also be seen as the "goals" that culture establishes for its members. Americans are encouraged to have successful careers, improve their education, and follow healthy lifestyles. These individual goals can be seen as contributing to the societal goals posed by the various institutions. By striving after personal ends, well-socialized society members are serving the ends of the system.

If values can be viewed as "ends," then the norms that guide behavior in pursuit of these goals can be seen as the "means." Thus, the rules that society members internalize related to career pursuit, educational advancement, and health maintenance serve to advance the ends mandated by cultural values. By complying with the customs, mores and laws associated with the various institutions, society members contribute to the furtherance of societal goals and the efficient operation of the system. Individuals who brush their teeth twice a day (custom), follow their doctor's orders and avoid risky sexual behavior (mores), and make their federally mandated Medicare contributions (law) are participating in the actions that constitute the patterns of behavior that constitute the healthcare system. Thus, we, as individuals obeying the rules while striving after goals, are actually performing the work of society's institutions.

CULTURES AND SUBCULTURES

Subcultures are specific groupings within a culture that follow their own distinctive ways of behavior. Subcultures exist within the framework of the larger culture and, by definition, maintain considerable overlap with the dominant culture. Members of subcultures for the most part speak the language of the dominant society and participate at some level in its various institutions.

At the same time, subcultures are likely to differ from the dominant culture in some important ways. They may hold different beliefs and values from the dominant culture, or at least foster modifications of the accepted values. They are likely to have different sets of norms than the rest of society and, in fact, for most people this is what sets subcultures apart. The lifestyles of members of subcultures are often different or even deviant, and "unusual" lifestyles are often spawned by subcultural groups.

Subcultures, like any cultural unit, are characterized by internally homogeneous sociocultural characteristics. These shared characteristics are taught to new subculture members and passed from generation to

---

Box 4-2

Corporate Culture and Healthcare

One aspect of culture that has come to the public's attention in recent years is referred to as "corporate culture". It is not that this is a new development within American organizations, but only in recent years has it been given a label. Many health professionals have observed that each healthcare organizations creates its own environment, an environment that might differ widely from organization to organization. The importance of this phenomenon has been noted because of its ability to create a unique environment and to influence the behavior of participants in that environment.

Corporate culture refers to that set of values, norms and understandings shared by members of an organization. In some ways, a corporate culture is similar to the cultural milieus that evolve within subcultural groups and set them apart from the rest of society in terms of beliefs, values, and norms. The primary difference, however, is that corporate culture is associated with a formal organization or legal entity, while a subculture is more informal and may grow or decline depending on various internal and external social factors.

The concept of corporate culture was originally identified in corporations outside of healthcare but its application to healthcare organizations was soon realized. Perhaps the development that most brought attention to corporate cultures in healthcare to the fore was the corporatization of healthcare that began in the 1980s and introduced a range of new players into the field. Healthcare had been dominated by clinicians for most of 20th century but by the 1980s power was being usurped by businessmen, accountants, lawyers and a range of other individuals who not only were not clinicians but often had no experience with healthcare. In extreme cases, a culture that valued service over profits came face to face with a culture that valued profits over any other goal.

While the corporate culture may become embodied in policies and procedures, for the most part the culture is unwritten and unspoken. Corporate employees adopt the worldview proffered by the corporation and, often unbeknownst to them, incorporate the values and norms that support that culture. The aspects of the culture that emerge from the social interaction that takes place within the organization are often subtle but sometimes uncomfortably palpable so that even an outsider can sense it.

At one level the corporate culture may be embodied in the standards that are established—such as the orientation toward customer service or worker productivity. But the corporate culture may also be seen in the manner in

---

generation. Subcultures establish rules and the means for enforcing these rules. Members of a subculture are expected to display similar attitudes, and the subcultures establish protocols for dealing with the larger society.

which rewards (and punishments) are meted out or in the informal dress codes that are established. The physical space of the organization may reflect and support the culture as in the case of frequent religious reminders in religion-sponsored hospitals or in the Spartan furnishings of hospitals run by certain religious orders.

Quite often, the corporate culture is established—either implicitly or explicitly—by the leadership of the corporation. Often a charismatic leader will be brought into the corporation and create a different culture. Or a new management team may be brought in with a different approach to running the corporation. In fact, health professionals often complain of the problems associated with adjusting to differing corporate cultures as rapid administrative turnover occurs.

Sometimes the culture emerges over a period of time and cannot be attributed to any particular individuals. The cultures associated with public "charity" hospitals or pubic health clinics have often been cited for their particular traits. The mission to provide free care to patients coupled with a rigid bureaucratic structure often results in a corporate culture that demonstrate a lack of concern for the cost of care or efficiencies of operation. Such cultures are likely to be resistant to change and fail to appreciate innovations that will save labor or improve efficiency. Indeed, any change in the operation may be thought to threaten bureaucratically assured employment of the workforce.

While the existence of different corporate cultures has been frequently noted in healthcare, the extent of the problem was highlighted as a result of the consolidation that took place in healthcare in the 1990s. As healthcare providers, health plans and other healthcare organizations merged or were acquired, considerable problems were encountered as a result of existing corporate cultures. Attempts at merging operations or portions of the workforce ran into resistance and/or failed as a result of clashing corporate cultures, and even the ability to communicate via information technology ran aground due to contrasting cultures. It was not unusual to hear during the rush of mergers in the 1990s that a planned merger to two hospitals or health systems was called off because of incompatible corporate cultures.

As healthcare organizations increasingly adopt the business philosophies and practices of organizations outside healthcare, the issue of corporate culture is likely to become more important. Longstanding cultures are likely to face significant change fostered by these outside influences, and anyone seeking to understand the nature of U.S. healthcare in the future must be sensitive to the extent to which corporate cultures can shape philosophies and behaviors.

The values and norms of the subculture would be considered appropriate by subculture members and may even be considered superior to those of the larger society.

Subcultures arise in a variety of ways in a society as complex as the United States. They may arise "naturally" from the interactions of individuals with similar ethnic, nationality, or religious backgrounds. Immigrants may attempt to transplant much of their native culture—at least temporarily—to America. Subcultures also arise as a result of repeated interaction of individuals with common interests. Thus, people may be involved in a singles-bar subculture, a pop music subculture, or a gay subculture. Some of these lifestyle-based subcultures are tolerated by the larger society as insignificant or ephemeral. Others are considered to be "deviant" subcultures and their lifestyles criticized and even persecuted by the larger society. Some subcultures may be inadvertently created by the larger society through the operation of its sanctions. This was certainly true of gay and lesbian subcultures some years ago when the disapproval of the larger society drove such individuals "underground" and unwittingly encouraged them to form deviant subcultures.

The existence of subcultures in U.S. society has numerous implications for health and healthcare. Some subcultures contribute directly to the existence of health problems, as in the case of gay or drug subcultures. Other subcultures may emphasize drinking and smoking and other risky health behavior. The persistent "welfare" subculture found in the U.S. not only promotes unhealthy behavior, it also fosters certain attitudes with regard to the healthcare system and the use of its services. Subcultures based on ethnicity may also hold differing perceptions of the healthcare system and even encourage the use of non-conventional therapists. (Box 4-2 describes how an organization can develop its own culture.)

ADDITIONAL RESOURCES

Collis, Harry, and Joe Kohl (1999). *101 American Customs: Understanding Language and Culture Through Common Practices*. Columbus, OH: McGraw-Hill/Contemporary Books.

Hall, John R., and Mary Jo Neitz (1993). *Culture: Sociological Perspectives*. Englewood Cliffs, NJ: Prentice Hall.

Harrison, Lawrence E., and Samuel P. Huntington (editors) (2001). *Culture Matters: How Values Shape Human Progress*. New York: Basic Books.

Sumner, William Graham (1959 [1906]). *Folkways*. New York: Dover.

Wardbaugh, Ronald (2001). *An Introduction to Sociolinguistics*. Malden, MA: Blackwell Publishers.

Chapter 5

The U.S. Healthcare Institution

THE EVOLUTION OF MODERN HEALTHCARE

A minimal understanding of the history of the development of healthcare is essential as background for the examination of the contemporary U.S. healthcare system. Such an understanding contributes to an appreciation of the evolution of the present healthcare system from past iterations. And it underscores the importance of non-medical factors in this evolutionary process. The healthcare system that exists today in the U.S. (actually in every country) represents in significant ways an extension of healthcare systems of the past. At the same time, however, contemporary healthcare systems have characteristics that set them qualitatively apart from earlier systems.

The sections below summarize the historical development of healthcare and then focus on the emergence of the U.S. healthcare system. It should be noted that the emphasis is on "healthcare" and not "medicine". The former term is clearly broader than the latter which, in common usage, is restricted to organized medical practice. In this context we are interested in much more than the direct provision of care, especially when many of the factors contributing to the nature and operation of healthcare delivery systems exist outside the medical arena.

The presentation of a brief overview of the history of healthcare is somewhat problematic. Most attempts at this result in a tedious list of time periods, each with its notable events, a laundry list of inventions, discoveries, and breakthroughs, or a list of people who have made significant contributions to the field. These approaches may be useful when discussing the history of *medicine*, but are not very beneficial for explicating the history of *healthcare*.

These traditional approaches tend to be misleading in many ways, in fact. First, they imply a steady progression of events culminating in the present form of healthcare. Second, they place undue emphasis on specific people and events rather than ideas. Third, they fail to emphasize the intellectual atmosphere that made such advances possible. That is, they ignore the sociocultural context that allows a particular breakthrough to occur.

The challenge here is to present historical development in a manner that is both meaningful and adequate in detail—and in a way that focuses on our primary concern here: the relationship between a society and its system of care. As one prominent medical historian has noted: "... [T]he medical behavior of a period can be regarded as a kind of projective test of the total culture of that period. We know much more about a society when we know how it treated its sick and what it thought a disease to be" (Ackerknecht, 1955).

Advances in the theory and practice of medical science have often depended more on the existence of a hospitable cultural environment than on the skills and creativity of medical scientists and practitioners. The historical record is full of medical and scientific breakthroughs that were before their time. Unless we can appreciate the intellectual climate of a particular time and place, we cannot hope to understand the stages in the development of contemporary healthcare.

THE PARADIGMATIC APPROACH

One approach to examining the history of healthcare involves the utilization of the concept of "paradigm". A paradigm constitutes a theoretical framework within which the universe and its component parts can be understood. This concept has been most clearly explicated by Thomas Kuhn (1970) as a result of his analysis of scientific "revolutions". Revolutions in scientific thought, he points out, are not the result of some dramatic event; breakthroughs and discoveries simply verify existing beliefs. (E.g., each new "wonder drug" did not represent a revolution but confirmation of the efficacy of the germ theory.) Revolutions take place through the development of new organizing principles that order the objects of the universe in a different way. A dominant paradigm will continue to be accepted although anomalies are discovered that do not fit that framework. Eventually, enough anomalies will accumulate that the existing paradigm is called into question. Ultimately, the existing paradigm gives way, albeit grudgingly, to a new one that can accommodate the factors that were not compatible with the old paradigm.

Kuhn's notion of paradigm has much in common with the concept of world-view developed by anthropologists. Every culture develops a unique world-view involving a systematic and integrated set of beliefs, assumptions and understandings. This world-view is shared by members of that particular society and serves as the primary organizing factor of the individual's perceptions and actions. The character of the society's institutions is shaped by the particular world-view, and all behavior takes meaning within this context. The world-view of a society determines the prevailing intellectual atmosphere, and this atmosphere influences the nature of the healthcare system.

The stages (that is, paradigms) in the development of healthcare for our purposes are: primitive healthcare, pre-scientific healthcare, early scientific healthcare, early technological healthcare, and late technological healthcare. One final stage will be discussed that reflects the current transformation occurring in healthcare in the U.S. It should be noted that not all stages evolve from the stages temporally preceding them; in fact, many discontinuities are found in this developmental process. Indeed, some of the earliest approaches to healthcare persist in certain parts of the world today and some of these, we might add, are actually finding acceptance within the framework of modern healthcare.

Regardless of the dominant paradigm, the *healthcare system* in any society can be separated into two components: the disease theory system and the service delivery system. The disease theory system involves the underlying explanatory framework that provides meaning to the system. This component is unique to each society and reflects that society's world-view. It addresses such issues as the nature of health and illness, the meaning of life and death, the appropriateness of intervening in the face of sickness, and the prolongation of life for the terminally ill. In effect, the prevailing paradigm encompasses the assumptions that underlie the system and provides the basis for the creation of healthcare delivery mechanisms.

The second component, the healthcare delivery system itself, is the mechanism through which society discharges its responsibility for providing for the health and welfare of its members. As such, it involves both structural aspects (such as facilities, organizational arrangements, and role relationships) and functional aspects (such as treatment, research, and education). It is the component of the system that we as healthcare consumers come face to face with, while the disease theory system remains in the background. Unless some type of crisis or public debate develops,

participants in the delivery system are not likely to give much consideration to the underlying disease theory system. Nevertheless, changes in the
nature of the disease theory system will have major implications for any
healthcare delivery system.

THE STAGES OF HEALTHCARE DEVELOPMENT

Primitive Healthcare

For most of the societies that have ever existed some form of primitive
healthcare has been utilized to meet society's responsibility for the health
and well-being of the population. The term "primitive" should not be
equated with crudeness, as many of the explanatory frameworks and techniques utilized in such systems are mind-boggling in their complexity.
These systems are clearly primitive with regard to their technology (a major criterion for us). Very little was utilized in the way of equipment, tools
and instruments, creating a system that was much more person centered
than technology centered. (It may be more politically correct today to refer
to them as "traditional" systems.)

Primitive healthcare is usually divided into the components of "folk
medicine" and "primitive medicine". *Folk medicine* (literally the healthcare
of the people) involves the treatments, remedies and actions known by
all members of society. Everyone in traditional societies was familiar with
certain herbs and other substances with medicinal effects that were specific
for various health problems. And everyone typically knew how to bandage
a wound or splint a broken bone. The term "nostrum", in fact, which we use
to refer to a folk remedy originally referred to a cure particular to a certain
family. Thus, the family with its knowledge of basic treatment represented
the first line of treatment for the individual. (We also see here where the
family institution overlaps with the healthcare institution.)

Primitive medicine was turned to for more serious problems, especially
if the supernatural was thought to play a role in their etiology or causation.
The practitioner of primitive medicine was typically an ordinary member
of society who was thought to have some special talents for curing health
problems and/or someone who had apprenticed with another practitioner.
Sometimes a separate status of "shaman" or "curer" developed. The term
"magician-priest" may, in fact, be a better term since it reflects the importance of religion in the management of sickness. More likely, however, the
primitive practitioner was indistinguishable from other society members
unless some serious health problem arose and his services were needed.

Supernaturalism provided the explanatory paradigm in primitive
healthcare systems. Most health problems (beyond the minor, routine problems) were explained by reference to intervention by some supernatural
being or by utilization of supernatural powers by some other member of

society. Members of such societies were not so naïve as to ignore natural causes of health problems and every society identified many of these. Many traditional societies were familiar with the practices of quarantine, cauterization of wounds, and amputation. In fact, there is now evidence that as long as 20,000 years ago, some groups were practicing a form of brain surgery called trepanning.

But many episodes of injury and disease were not easily explained within a naturalistic framework and, besides, a supernatural explanation helped answer the "why?" of ill fortune. Since most such systems emphasized a oneness with the universe and all other objects of nature, primitive healthcare systems emphasized a balance between the individual and nature as well as the individual and his social group. The notion of equilibrium pervades the lore of primitive societies, and the first function of diagnosis was to determine the extent of imbalance characterizing the situation. The failure to observe societally-mandated ceremonies or the infraction of societal mores were often causes of imbalance and subsequent illness or injury. Similarly, the malicious actions of one society member toward another could result in illness.

The diagnosis of a health problem involved the identification of the cause of the disequilibrium that was believed to exist. Consequently, the examination by the practitioner deemphasized physical symptoms and signs and concentrated on social psychological factors. The diagnostician required information on the nature of the patient's social relationships and his recent interactions with other society members. The social history thus took on more importance than the medical history.

Just as causation was relegated to the realm of the supernatural, treatment involved a comparable framework. The therapeutic techniques available to the primitive practitioner would be considered nonscientific, although certain drugs and surgical techniques were known even though the practitioner was not likely to have understood the reason for their efficacy. In most societies, medical activities were indistinguishable from religious activities. (In fact, the words "healthy" and "holy" have the same etymological root.) Ceremony and ritual supplant science and technology in the primitive healthcare system, and these responses to health problems were seen as appropriate for the patient's needs. Curing activities were geared toward restoring equilibrium between the patient and his world. The restoration of balance was attempted by appeasement of the offended or mischievous spirits or by redressing the wrong done to some other member of society. If the patient had been cursed by someone, then counter-magic was in order.

The approach to primitive healthcare was holistic in that the individual was not only seen as a total entity (as opposed to a collection of tissue, organs, etc.), but was viewed as inextricably tied into a social network. Diagnosis could only be made with reference to the patient's social milieu

---

Box 5-1

Can We Learn Anything from Traditional Healers?

For over a century, Western medicine has been distancing itself from the practices that have characterized healers in traditional societies for time immemorial. Scientific medicine is thought to have little in common with the "primitive" techniques utilized by the shaman, the witch-doctor or the tribal herbalist. And, certainly, there is little that modern practitioners can learn from these traditional healers. Or is there?

As the U.S. healthcare system has begun evolving from a system emphasizing medical care to one emphasizing healthcare, a variety of "innovative" techniques are being introduced. Many of these techniques, however, are not new and, in fact, have been around for thousands of years. The following traits associated with traditional healers are increasingly of interest to modern medical practitioners.

- The traditional healer diagnoses the health problem within the patient's sociocultural and environmental context.
- The traditional healer takes into consideration all aspects of the patient's existence (including non-biological factors).
- The traditional healer is holistic in his orientation, taking the whole of the person into consideration.
- The traditional healer views health and ill health as the end-points of a continuum rather than as the two components of a dichotomy.
- The traditional healer emphasizes a high touch/low tech approach to diagnosis and treatment.
- The traditional healer does not label the affected individual as a "patient", thereby avoiding the stigma associated with the patient status.
- The traditional healer has an appreciation of the relationship between the mind and body and their effect upon one another.
- The traditional healer involves the patient (and his significant others) in diagnosis and therapy processes.
- The traditional healer relies upon natural remedies and the body's ability to heal itself rather than "heroic measures".
- The traditional healer places a great deal of responsibility on the "patient" for his own cure.
- The traditional healer ultimately views the welfare of the community as more important than the welfare of any individual.

Ironically, the paradigmatic shift from an emphasis on medical care to one on healthcare embodies many of the attributes attributed to primitive health systems. In fact, as one describes the healthcare system that is emerging in the United States, many of these attributes are featured. The holistic health movement embodies most of these precepts, and they represent attributes that are increasingly being requested by U.S. healthcare consumers.

and treatment almost always involved other members of society. It was believed that treatment should only occur within the individual's familiar surroundings and isolation of the patient was rare. Recovery, in fact, required the marshalling of all available social and emotional support, with family and friends usually participating in the therapy. (See Box 5-1 for a discussion of the value of traditional therapies.)

Prescientific Healthcare

Prescientific healthcare can be traced to the early civilizations of the Middle East some 10–12,000 years ago. Arising out of, and often coexisting with, the supernaturalistic paradigm, the development of this natural-medical view of health and illness represented an important step in the direction of scientific healthcare. During this period, the first steps were taken toward rationalizing man's view of disease and introducing the empirical study and scientific treatment of health problems.

The oldest records available on these fledging attempts to systematize the management of health problems survive the Babylonians. Many historians, in fact, trace the roots of modern medicine to this culture. The Egyptians, near contemporaries of the Babylonians, pioneered the use of drugs and herbs, both of which played an important role in the religion of that culture. The Egyptians were the first to organize the healthcare system, and their society offered care on three levels. During this same period, civilizations on the Indian subcontinent had produced medical textbooks that described in detail surgical procedures for cataract removal, hernia repair, the performance of Caesarean sections, and plastic surgery. These texts identified thousands of instruments used in the provision of care and over 700 medicinal herbs.

These early attempts at more formal medical care were halting due to the recurring belief in the supernatural. Most of the members of society adhered to nonscientific notions of health and illness and the acceptance of any new therapy was undoubtedly limited. While advances were made in selected areas of healthcare, the dominance of the older supernaturalistic paradigm made scientific innovations spotty and limited in their acceptance.

As the early civilizations waned and Greek culture became dominant around 2,000 B.C., the evolution of modern healthcare received a boost in the form of the medical system developed and administered by the Greeks. Greek philosophers and medical practitioners made the first systematic attempt to separate science from supernaturalism and thus develop a paradigm based on naturalism. The development of a new paradigm in this case did not result from research breakthroughs or new insights into the nature of disease as much as it did from a new philosophical orientation based on rationalism. This philosophy encouraged the systematic study of disease and the detailed observation of the course of illness, a radical innovation for the time. This rationalism was reflected in the formalization of medical education and in the nascent idea of social causation of disease.

Hippocrates urged the development of a scientific medicine based on a rational and systematic approach. He pushed for the elimination of the supernatural as a cause of disease and injury and encouraged formal training for physicians. Treatment involved many natural therapies (diet, rest, exercise, fresh air) and encouraged the involvement of the patient. Hippocrates was also responsible for the development of a code of ethics for medical practitioners.

Even at this point, it should be noted, these early attempts at a rational view of health and illness represent a minority viewpoint. Although many Greek physicians and some members of the upper classes welcomed this new paradigm, supernaturalistic views still pervaded the rest of society. In fact, other competing paradigms existed side by side with the supernaturalistic and naturalistic. A variety of practitioners made claims as to the efficacy of their particular view of health and disease with theories on causation being numerous. The simultaneous existence of competing views was possible—indeed, inevitable—due to the lack of an empirically-testable paradigm.

The Greek period was superceded by Roman domination of the known world. The Romans "inherited" much of the medical knowledge developed by the Greeks although they contributed little of their own. They were not original thinkers but good organizers and did bring some order to both the body of medical knowledge and the organization of care. The Romans were credited with developing the first public health systems and introduced sanitary measures. They provided free public baths and free "medical care" for the public. They also developed the concept of the "hospital", not surprisingly as a result of their battlefront need for medical care.

The Roman Empire eventually deteriorated and the Middle Ages (700–1500 A.D.) ensued. This period is alternatively referred to as the "Dark Ages" because of the subsequent loss of much existing knowledge—although scholars still debate just how "dark" the Dark Ages were. It certainly represented the Dark Ages for medicine and healthcare as most of the knowledge of previous centuries and earlier civilizations disappeared. What knowledge remained was retained by the Catholic Church and by Arab cultures that were not affected by these developments in Europe.

The European continent during this period was faced with tremendous health problems and widespread social chaos. There was essentially no central government in operation anywhere and no organized response to the health threats that were rampant. The fragmented societies that comprised the continent fell back on the remaining institution that had any stability, the Catholic Church. This involved a reversion to an otherworldly orientation that removed the focus from practical health matters. Previous advances in sanitation were lost, and there was no public hygiene and no organized healthcare.

Medical practice in its prescientific guise, however, did not entirely disappear and some curers in isolated pockets continued to pursue the teachings of Classical medical practitioners. Overall, however, the Church became the main provider of healthcare during this period. It was successful at preserving some medical knowledge and even sponsored the establishment of hospitals (although these were more akin to what we refer to today as "hospices", or places where people go to die). There was virtually nothing in the way of what we would consider medical care today. Priests and nuns served as the healers, although their purposes could be considered more religious and social than medical.

During the Renaissance period in Europe (14th–17th centuries), the continent witnessed the first incipient movement toward the establishment of scientific medicine. The knowledge preserved by the Catholic Church was recovered, and the medical lore of the Arab world rediscovered. This period witnessed advances in many aspects of healthcare. Some of the Classical approaches to health and illness were revived and sanitary methods were reinstated. The first known dissections were preformed and principles of anatomy were established. The major development was a new emphasis on empiricism and rationality, and the first attempts at separating medicine from philosophy appeared.

The structure of society became more formalized, and this period witnessed the rise of powerful nation-states. The diminished power of the Catholic Church opened the door for increased control by secular forces, and much authority was transferred from the Church to the State. This control extended to healthcare as governments took over the responsibility for public sanitation and the management of the few hospitals that existed.

Early Scientific Healthcare

The eighteenth century was truly a revolutionary time in Western social development. The American and French Revolutions questioned the validity of existing institutions. Capitalism as an economic system replaced the feudal system and other agrarian systems in Europe and the United States, and Europe was experiencing the beginnings of the Industrial Revolution.

Sometimes referred to as the age of "humanistic medicine", this period witnessed a renewed interest in the social aspects of health and illness. Many, in fact, trace the public health movement to this period. The period actually witnessed the eradication of many epidemic diseases not through medical care, which was still in its infancy, but through social reforms.

The concept of "social medicine" was developed and a population-based approach to healthcare was formulated. While doctors were still not able to provide much in the way of a cure, the use of the microscope led to an understanding of microorganisms and the importance of immunization came to be understood. The first scientific classification of diseases was introduced, a necessary first step in the development of diagnostic processes.

Early Technological Healthcare

The nineteenth century is generally recognized as the beginning point for modern Western medicine. As in every case described above, the new era was ushered in by social changes. Indeed, historians would consider this the period in Europe and the United States in which the transition from a "traditional" orientation to a "modern" orientation was taking place.

Medicine came to be seen as a social science in Europe and reached its highest state of development in Germany during this period. The maintenance of health came to be recognized as an obligation of the state. The population rather than the individual came to be seen as the patient, and community health was thought of as more effective than one-on-one treatment. The importance of lifestyle, environment, and socioeconomic conditions for the health status of the population was recognized.

Despite these developments, medicine was still essentially ineffective in the face of most health problems. "Heroic" measures such as blistering, purging, vomiting, and bleeding were practiced. Physical examinations were uncommon, and medicine remained an art based on personal interaction. There was still very little in the physician's "black bag".

In actuality, there was no *one* medicine during this period. There were numerous competing paradigms and, particularly in the young United States with its emphasis on egalitarianism, no one approach was considered superior to others. In fact there was no scientific basis for evaluating any of the healing systems. Thus, there were herbalists, mesmerizers, and practitioners of botanic, magnetic, electrical, and homeopathic approaches. While those who practiced allopathic medicine were considered "regulars" and the others "irregulars", there was really little difference in the results that the various practitioners produced at this time.

The Rise of Western Medicine

The rise of modern "Western" medicine required the establishment of certain conditions. At a minimum, allopathic medicine as practiced by the regulars required some empirical basis for its claims of being the "true" solution to sickness and death. It needed some basis for differentiating this system of treatment from the numerous others that made comparable claims of efficacy. And, the regulars needed a "political" breakthrough, independent of any proofs of efficacy, that would provide legitimacy for this system of care over other claimants.

The breakthrough in terms of empirical evidence occurred in the late nineteenth with the recognition of the connection between microorganisms and ill health. Once this connection was made, it was possible to develop a theoretical framework for explaining the etiology of many forms of illness. The "germ theory" that emerged based on these revelations not only provided an explanation as to the causes of illness, but pointed toward an appropriate response. Illness could be prevented, it was thus argued, by limiting exposure to harmful microorganisms, and cure could be obtained, if illness did occur, by counteracting these organisms. Given the fact that most of the health problems of the day were communicable, infectious and parasitic diseases caused by microorganisms, this did indeed represent a breakthrough in our understanding of the illness process.

For the first time an approach to treatment could offer scientific proof of its efficacy. As the twentieth century dawned, the medical regulars made their case to the powers that be and to the public for the legitimacy of their modality. The scientific method could be applied in the assessment of the efficacy of treatments provided by allopathic practitioners and the findings used to confirm the soundness of the germ theory and its concomitant therapeutic approach. This new cadre of medical scientists petitioned the government (that is of the states) to certify the allopathic practitioner as *the* official medical practitioner, thereby providing them legitimacy before the law. The regulars were granted this request and licensing processes were established by the various states.

The political victory did not end there, as these newly legitimized physicians went on to insist that no other type of practitioner be recognized as legitimate. Thus, physicians lobbied governmental agencies against the granting of any type of license for non-allopathic physicians, making it a criminal act to practice medicine without a license. The success of this approach served to eliminate most of the competing practitioners from the field and the rest were driven underground. The victory for medical regulars was so complete that it would be decades before any competing practitioners gained licensure approval.

The granting of sole licensure was accompanied by demands that physicians be allowed to practice undisturbed by outside interference. Arguing that the subject matter of medicine was too arcane to be understood by laypersons, physicians argued successfully for the right to maintain their own standards and to police their own. The American Medical Association emerged as a powerful force for physician interests and would play a major role in healthcare policy setting throughout the twentieth century.

THE EMERGENCE OF THE U.S. HEALTHCARE SYSTEM

Despite the emergence of an acceptable framework for understanding sickness and directing treatment, healthcare remained an institutional infant for the first half of the century. True, physicians were able to explain more in the way of sickness, utilize immunizations against many health threats, and actually cure some patients. Yet, until World War II medicine was not fully accepted as a solution to health problems, and hospitals were still considered places to go to die. In fact, we know now that much of the success in fighting disease claimed by medical practitioners should really be attributed to improved diets, living conditions, and public sanitation.

It is not appropriate to speak of a modern healthcare system in the United States until after World War II. Prior to that time, healthcare as an institution was poorly developed and accounted for a negligible proportion of societal resources. It remained an institutional non-entity until the period following World War II when it began a rapid rise to become a major U.S. institution. The development of the healthcare system following World War II can be divided into six stages, roughly equating with the six decades of the last half of the twentieth century and the beginning of the twenty-first. Each of these stages will be briefly discussed in turn. (See Table 5–1 for an overview of the stages in the development of U.S. healthcare.)

The 1950s: The Emergence of "Modern" Medicine

As American society entered a new period of growth and prosperity following the end of World War II, the modern U.S. healthcare system began to take shape. The economic growth of the period resulted in the demand for a wide range of goods and services, including healthcare. "Health"

Table 5–1.   The Stages of U.S. Healthcare

Pre-WWII	Premodern medicine
1950s	The emergence of modern medicine
1960s	The golden age of medicine
1970s	Questioning the system
1980s	The great transformation
1990s	The emerging healthcare paradigm
2000s	New millennium healthcare

was coming to be recognized as a value in its own right and considerable resources were expended on a fledging healthcare system that had lain dormant during the war.

The 1950s witnessed the first significant involvement of the federal government in healthcare, as the Hill-Burton Act resulted in the construction of hundreds of hospitals to meet the pent up demand resulting from the lack of domestic development during the war. Health insurance was becoming common and, spurred by the influence of trade unions, healthcare benefits became a major issue at the bargaining table.

World War II had also served as a giant "laboratory" for pioneering a wide range of medical and surgical procedures. Trauma surgery was essentially unknown prior to the war and trauma and burn treatment capabilities were now available to apply in a civilian context. New drug therapies were being introduced and formal health services were coming to be seen as a solution for an increasing number of problems.

The 1960s: The Golden Age of American Medicine

During the 1960s the healthcare institution in the U.S. experienced unprecedented expansion in personnel and facilities. The hospital emerged as the center of the system, and the physician—much maligned in earlier decades—came to occupy the pivotal role in the treatment of disease. Physician salaries and the prestige associated with their positions grew astronomically.

Private insurance became widespread, offered primarily through employer-sponsored plans. The Medicare and Medicaid programs were introduced, and these initiatives expanded access to healthcare (at government expense) to the elderly and poor, respectively.

New therapeutic techniques were being developed, accompanied by growth in the variety of technologies and support personnel required. New conditions (e.g., alcoholism, hyperactivity) were identified as appropriate for medical treatment, resulting in an increasing proportion of the population coming under "medical management". Complete consumer trust existed in the healthcare system in general and in hospitals and physicians in particular.

The only dissension was heard on the part of those few who had discovered that certain segments of the population were not sharing in this "golden age". Even here, though, there was virtually no criticism of the disease theory system that underlay the delivery system. It was felt that the infrastructure was sound and that only some improvement in execution by the system was required to address the deficiencies. (See Box 5-2 for a review of the assumptions that underlay the Golden Age of American medicine.)

Box 5-2

Assumptions from the Golden Age of Healthcare

The 1960's and 70s are considered by many as the "golden age" of American healthcare. The healthcare institution benefited from unprecedented prosperity and was rapidly expanding its influence within U.S. society. Hospitals had emerged as centers for care and physicians as the gatekeepers for the system. Both hospitals and physicians were accorded considerable prestige and high public trust. American healthcare was considered the best in the world and few objected to the expansion of the healthcare system to manage new conditions as fast they could be identified.

In retrospect, this golden age was founded on a number of assumptions, some of which would be considered suspect today. The following assumptions provided the basis for the disease theory system and the delivery system that characterized the U.S. during this period.

- "Health" is a state to strive after and can be reached by eliminating symptoms.
- Sickness can be cured (and life prolonged) through appropriate medical intervention.
- Allopathic medicine is the only appropriate approach to addressing sickness.
- Medical care is the primary contributor to the improved health status of the U.S. population.
- Treatment is a more appropriate use of resources than prevention.
- More care is better; when it comes to medical resources, overkill is better than "under kill."
- The healthcare system, not the individual, is responsible for the health of that individual.

The 1970s: Questioning the System

Entering the 1970s the healthcare system appeared to be continuing along a track of expansion and growth. New techniques continued to be introduced, and there appeared to be no limit to the application of technology. Even more new conditions were identified, and increasing numbers of Americans were brought under medical management financed through private insurance and government-subsidized insurance plans. The hospital was entrenched as the focal point of the system, and the physician continued to control more than 80% of the expenditures on health services.

During the 1970s a number of issues began to be raised concerning the healthcare system and its operation. Issues of access and equity that were first voiced in the 1960s reached a point where they could no longer be ignored. Large segments of the population appeared to be excluded from

- The individual, not the community, is the focal point of the healthcare system.
- One human life is worth whatever amount of money and effort it takes to save it.

Some of these assumptions may still be ascribed to today, although all have come under criticism as the U.S. system of care has evolved. The new paradigm that emerged in the late 20th century would take issue with many of these. The chief arguments would relate to the inordinate credit given to formal medical care in the improvement of health status. Proponents of the new paradigm would argue that: medical intervention alone is often not sufficient for the management of health problems; formal medical care only partly contributes to the improvement of health status; and there is more than one approach to the management of disease. They would also argue that: most contemporary health problems can be prevented and, in the long run, investments in prevention will yield better results than investments in treatment and that the marginal benefit derived from incremental services is limited. Proponents of the new paradigm would also contend that: the healthcare system cannot function efficiently without contributions from the patient; only by "treating" the community can overall health status be elevated; and, in a world of finite resources, the costs involved in the meaningless prolongation of life need to be weighed against the benefits of alternative uses of these scarce resources.

While certain of these assumptions from the golden age of American medicine may retain their validity, for the most part, the new healthcare environment demands new assumptions that are more in keeping with the emerging healthcare paradigm.

mainstream medicine. Further, the effectiveness of the system in dealing with the overall health status of the population was brought into question. Health status indicators were demonstrating that the U.S. population was lagging behind other comparable countries in improving health status.

The most critical issue that developed in the 1970s related to the cost of care. Clearly, the U.S. had the world's most expensive healthcare system. The costs were high and they were increasing much faster than those in other sectors of the economy. While it was once assumed that resources for the provision of healthcare were infinite, it was now realized that there was a limit on what could be spent to provide health services. Coupled with questions about access and effectiveness, the escalating cost of care was a basis for widespread alarm.

During this period the underlying foundation of the healthcare system was questioned for the first time. Earlier criticism had been directed at the operation of the system, and it was assumed that the disease theory system was appropriate. Hence, a "band-aid" approach had been advocated rather than major surgery. As the 1970s ended, more and more voices were being raised concerning the underlying assumptions of the system.

The 1980s: The Great Transformation

The 1980s will no doubt be seen by historians as a watershed for U.S. healthcare. The numerous issues that had been emerging over the previous two decades came to a head as the 1980s began. By the end of the decade, American healthcare had become almost unrecognizable to veteran health professionals. Virtually every aspect of the system had undergone transformation and a new paradigm began to emerge as the basis for the disease theory system.

The escalating—and seemingly uncontrollable—costs associated with healthcare care prompted the Medicare administration to introduce the prospective payment system. Other insurers soon followed suit with a variety of cost containment methods. Employers, who were footing much of the bill for increasing healthcare costs, began to take a more active role in the management of their plans.

The decade also witnessed the introduction of new financial arrangements and organizational structures. Experiments abounded in an attempt to find ways to more effectively and efficiently provide health services. The major consequence of these activities was the introduction of managed care as an approach to controlling the utilization of services and, ultimately, the cost borne by insurers. The managed care concept called for incentives on the part of all parties for more appropriate use of the system.

This transformation resulted in considerable shifts in both power and risk within the system. The power that resided in hospital administrators and physicians was blamed for much of the cost and inefficiency in the system. Third-party payors, employers and consumers began to attempt to share in this power. Large groups of purchasers emerged that began to negotiate for lower costs in exchange for their "wholesale" business. Insurers, who had historically borne most of the financial risk involved in the financing of health services, began shifting some of this risk to providers and consumers.

Developments outside of healthcare were also having significant influence. Chief among these was the changing nature of the American population. The acute conditions that had dominated the healthcare scene since the inception of modern medicine were being supplanted by the chronic conditions characteristic of an older population. The respiratory conditions, parasitic diseases and playground injuries of earlier decades were being replaced in the physician's waiting room by arthritis, hypertension and diabetes. The mismatch between the capabilities of the healthcare system and the needs of the patients it was designed to serve became so severe that a new disease theory system began to emerge.

The 1990s: The Shifting Paradigm

Although change occurs unevenly throughout a system as complex as American healthcare, many are arguing that by the late 1990s a true paradigm shift was occurring. Simply put, this involved a shift from an emphasis on "medical care" to one on "healthcare". *Medical care* is narrowly defined in terms of the formal services provided by the healthcare system and refers primarily to those functions of the healthcare system that are under the influence of medical doctors. This concept focuses on the clinical or treatment aspects of care, and excludes the non-medical aspects of healthcare. *Healthcare* refers to any function that might be directly or indirectly related to preserving, maintaining, and/or enhancing health status. This concept includes not only formal activities (such as visiting a health professional) but also such informal activities as preventive care (e.g., brushing teeth), exercise, proper diet, and other health maintenance activities.

Since the 1970s there has been a steady movement of activities and emphasis away from medical care toward healthcare, and the importance of the non-medical aspects of care has become increasingly appreciated. The growing awareness of the connection between health status and lifestyle and the realization that medical science is limited in its ability to control the disorders of modern society have prompted a move away from a strictly medical model of health and illness to one that incorporates more of a social and psychological perspective (Engel 1977).

Demographic factors have played no small role in this process. Unquestionably, the influence of the large baby boom cohort has been felt with regard to these issues. This population more than any other has led the movement toward a value reorientation as it relates to healthcare. It has been this cohort that has emphasized convenience, value, responsiveness, patient participation, accountability, and other attributes not traditionally found in the U.S. system of healthcare delivery. It has also been the cohort that has been instrumental in the emergence of urgent care centers, freestanding surgery facilities, and health maintenance organizations as standard features of the system.

Despite this changing orientation, an imbalance remained in the system of the 1990s with regard to the allocation of resources to its various components. Treatment still commanded the lion's share of the healthcare dollar, and most research was still focused on developing cures rather than preventive measures. The hospital remained the focal point of the system, and the physician continued to be its primary gatekeeper. Nevertheless, each of these underpinnings of medical care had been substantially weakened during the 1980s, with a definitive shift toward a healthcare-oriented paradigm evident during the 1990s.

At the close of the twentieth century, the healthcare institution continued to be beset by many problems. It could be argued that the system was too expensive, particularly in view of its inability to effectively address contemporary health problems and raise the overall health status of the population, and that large segments of the population were excluded from mainstream medicine. The fact that "administrative costs" accounted for 23 percent of the U.S. healthcare dollar (compared to less than 10 percent in socialized systems) suggested that there were considerable inefficiencies in the system.

2000–2010: New Millennium Healthcare

As the twenty-first century dawns, U.S. healthcare appears to be entering yet another phase, one that reflects both late twentieth century developments and newly emerging trends. The further entrenchment of the "healthcare" paradigm appears to be occurring, as the medical model continues to lose its salience. This trend is driven in part by the resurgence of consumerism that is being witnessed and the reemergence of a consumer-choice market. At the same time, financial exigencies and consumer demand are encouraging more holistic, less intensive approaches to care.

The new millennium is witnessing continued disparities in healthcare, exacerbated by the growing number of uninsured individuals and a depressed economy that turns healthcare into a "luxury" for many Americans. Disparities exist in health status among various racial and ethnic groups and among those of differing socioeconomic status. Disparities exist in the use of health services and even in the types of treatment that are provided individuals in different social categories.

The first decade of the twenty-first century is also witnessing a further reaction to managed care. Capitated reimbursement arrangements are becoming less common, the gatekeeper concept is being abandoned, and consumer choice is being reintroduced into the market. Baby boomers are increasingly driving the market, shaping patterns of utilization, and creating demand for new services. At the same time, the growing population of elderly Americans is creating a demand for senior services far greater than anything ever experienced in the past.

Information technology is an increasingly important driving force. The new healthcare calls for effective information management and data analysis. The demands of the Health Insurance Portability and Privacy Act (HIPAA) are bringing information technology issues to the forefront. This is being accompanied by the rise of e-health, perhaps the most significant development in healthcare in several years. The use of the Internet in the distribution of health information, the servicing of patients and plan enrollees, and the distribution of healthcare products promises to significantly change relationships within the healthcare arena.

THE ORGANIZATION OF U.S. HEALTHCARE

Healthcare is one of the more complex components of U.S. society. Its complexity is such that it is hard to define and even more difficult to describe in meaningful terms. Is healthcare an industry? A system? An institution? In actuality, it is all of these and more. As shall be seen, much of what healthcare *is* depends on one's perspective. The sections that follow view healthcare within an institutional context.

An encyclopedia would be required to fully describe the multiple dimensions of American healthcare, and that is certainly not appropriate here. The material that follows is restricted to the information necessary to appreciate the healthcare system relative to the field of medical sociology. While some will no doubt be critical of what has been included and excluded, the author has made his best efforts to restrict this material to that relevant within the context of the remainder of this book.

A useful starting point for attempting to examine the organization of U.S. healthcare would be an inventory of its component parts. The U.S. healthcare system has an incredible number of functioning units, including approximately 6,400 hospitals, over 15,000 nursing homes, and an estimated 300,000 clinics providing physician care. These figures do not include non-physician providers such as dentists, chiropractors, and mental health counselors.

The "providers" of care typically are autonomous parties operating under a variety of guises and means of control. Healthcare providers— whether facilities or practitioners—can be organized as private for-profit organizations, private not-for-profit organizations, public organizations, and quasi-public organizations, among others. Similarly, they may be owned by private investors, publicly held, local-government owned and operated, or run by a religious denomination, foundation, or some other nonprofit entity.

The complexity of the U.S. healthcare system is reflected in the proliferation of occupational roles, the levels and stages of care that are provided (along both vertical and horizontal continua), and the almost unlimited points at which a patient might enter the system. The end result, many observers contend, is a "non-system" that is poorly integrated, lacks centralized control and regulation, and is characterized by fragmentation, discontinuity, and duplication.

The Structure of Healthcare

A useful approach to understanding the healthcare system is to conceptualize it in terms of *levels* of care. (The framework is illustrated graphically in Table 5–2.) These levels are generally referred to as primary care, secondary care, and tertiary care. Additionally, some observers have identified a fourth category—quaternary care—to be applied to superspecialized services such as organ transplantation and trauma care. These levels can be viewed as the vertical dimension of the healthcare delivery system.

Primary care refers to the provision of the most basic services. These generally involve the care of minor, routine problems, along with the provision of general examinations and preventive services. For the patient, primary care usually involves some self-care, perhaps followed by the seeking of care from a non-physician health professional such as a pharmacist. For certain ethnic groups, this may involve the use of a "folk" healer.

Table 5–2.   The Levels of U.S. Healthcare

	Procedure	Site	Physician
	Quartenary Care		
	Organ transplant Complex trauma	Multi-institution medical centers	Teams of super- specialists
	Tertiary Care		
	Specialized surgery Complex medical cases	Large-scale comprehensive hospitals with extensive technological support	Subspecialists
	Secondary Care		
	Moderately complex medical and surgical cases	Moderate-scale hospitals Some freestanding surgery and diagnostic centers	Specialists
	Primary Care		
Complexity Severity Specialization	Routine care Standard diagnostic tests Simple surgery Preventive care	General hospitals Clinics Physician offices Urgent care centers	Primary care physicians Physician "extenders"

Primary care services are generally provided by physicians with training in general or family practice, general internal medicine, obstetrics/gynecology, and pediatrics. These practitioners are typically community based (rather than hospital based), rely on direct first contact with patients rather than receiving referrals from other physicians, and provide continuous rather than episodic care. Physician extenders like nurse practitioners and physician assistants are taking on a growing responsibility for primary care. In the mental health system, psychologists and other types of counselors constitute the primary level of care. Medical specialists also provide a certain amount of primary care.

Primary care is generally delivered at the physician's office or at some type of clinic. Hospital outpatient departments, urgent care centers, freestanding surgery centers, and other ambulatory care facilities also provide primary care services. For certain segments of the population, the hospital emergency room serves as a source of primary care. The home has increasingly become a site of choice for the provision of primary care. This trend toward home healthcare has been driven by a number of factors, including financial pressures on inpatient care, changing consumer preferences, and improved home care technology.

In terms of hospital services, primary care refers to those services that can be provided at a "general" hospital. These typically involve routine medical and surgical procedures, diagnostic tests, and obstetrical services. Primary care also includes emergency care (although not major trauma) and many outpatient services. Primary hospital care tends to be unspecialized and requires a relatively low level of technological sophistication. In actuality, there are few hospitals remaining today that could truly be considered to provide "primary care". Even the smallest hospital today is likely to have equipment that may not have been available in major hospitals only a few years ago.

Increasing attention is being paid to the role of self-care in the provision of basic medical services. Self-medication has long been an activity carried out by the American population. Now the availability of home diagnostic tests has further encouraged a "do-it-yourself approach" to healthcare. Research has now verified that much of what occurs under the umbrella of "primary care" actually takes place outside the formal medical arena. Self-care and other informal alternatives appear to be firmly entrenched in the American healthcare ethos.

Secondary care reflects a higher degree of specialization and technological sophistication than primary care. Physician care is provided by more highly trained practitioners such as specialized surgeons (e.g., urologists and ophthalmologists) and specialized internists (e.g., cardiologists and oncologists). Problems requiring more specialized skills and more sophisticated biomedical equipment fall into this category. Although much of the care is still provided in the physician office or clinic, these specialists tend to spend a larger share of their time in the hospital setting. Secondary hospitals are capable of providing more complex technological backup, physician specialist support, and ancillary services than primary care hospitals. These facilities are capable of handling moderately complex surgical and medical cases and serve as referral centers for primary care facilities.

Tertiary care addresses the more complex of surgical and medical conditions. The practitioners tend to be subspecialists, and the facilities highly complex and technologically advanced. Complex procedures such as open-heart surgery and reconstructive surgery are performed at these facilities, which provide extensive support services in terms of both personnel and technology. Tertiary care cases are usually handled by a team of medical and/or surgical specialists who are supported by the hospital's radiology, pathology, and anesthesiology physician staff. Tertiary care is generally provided at a few centers that serve large geographical areas. Frequently, a single hospital is not sufficient for the provision of tertiary care; a "medical center" may be required. These centers typically support functions not directly related to patient care, such as teaching and research.

The ability to extend this level of technology to the community is limited by the number of subspecialists and the availability of state-of-the-art technology. However, secondary facilities are increasingly performing what were previously considered tertiary procedures. The "routinization" of previously uncommon procedures reflects to a great extent improvements in technology and the increased numbers of specialists with advanced surgical training.

Some procedures often performed at tertiary facilities may be considered as *quaternary care*. Organ transplantation—especially involving vital organs like heart, lungs and pancreas—and complicated trauma cases are examples. This level of care is restricted to major medical centers often in medical school settings. These procedures require the most sophisticated equipment and are often performed in association with research activities.

This review of the levels of care ignores some other important structural aspects of the system that are not as directly related to patient care. In addition to physicians' offices, clinics, and acute care hospitals, mention should also be made of specialty hospitals and nursing homes. Specialty hospitals include facilities for the treatment of specific categories of conditions such as mental illness, substance abuse, or tuberculosis. They also are established for the treatment of certain categories of patients such as women, children, or geriatric patients. Federally-operated facilities such as those run by the Veterans Administration should also be considered as a special category of facilities. The various specialty facilities are operated under different guises, ranging from poorly funded state-operated facilities to upscale, privately owned for-profit facilities. The nation's 15,000 nursing homes provide extensive custodial care to nearly two million residents each year. Add to these the growing number of newly-defined care settings (e.g., assisted living facilities, extended care facilities), and the variety of care settings continues to grow.

The Healthcare Process

The discussion so far has focused on the vertical organization of the healthcare system. The system can also be viewed as having a horizontal dimension in that healthcare episodes can be viewed as linear phenomena that proceed through a variety stages. If the assumption is made that individuals are naturally in a state of "health," a scenario can be developed whereby prevention, screening, and routine self-care represent the initial stage. With the onset of symptoms, the individual makes a transition to the point of diagnosis and treatment at an outpatient facility. This may result in assignment to the patient category (sickness), whereby the stages of the vertical axis (primary, secondary, tertiary, and quaternary) come into play. Assuming the patient survives the illness episode, he or she may move out of the patient care model back into the community as a "well" person. Alternatively, the patient may require follow-up care or chronic disease management (e.g., by a home care agency), temporary institutionalized care (e.g., a subacute facility), long-term nursing care (e.g., a nursing home), or rehabilitative services of some type (e.g., physical or occupational therapy). These post-patient services extend the model horizontally.

This patient "career" could actually be thought of as involving three stages: pre-patient, patient, and post-patient. Significant aspects of the pre-patient and post-patient stages fall outside the vertical dimension of the model. Some of the structural components that are involved in these stages are noted above; others would include public health agencies (for prevention and screening) and hospices (for care of the terminally ill).

Because of the emphasis historically placed on treatment and cure by the healthcare system, the components in the horizontal integration model not involving direct patient care have not been emphasized until recently. However, research has now demonstrated that much of the care received by Americans takes place outside the mainstream of formal care.

Most of the encounters in which patients participate take place at the practitioner's office or the clinic. These practitioners include physicians (which account for the bulk of the encounters), dentists, optometrists, chiropractors, and various other practitioners. Encounters also take place in the offices or clinics of mental health providers, such as psychologists, psychological social workers, or other therapists. Thus, both public and private organizations may establish clinics to serve a particular population and these exist independent of any specific practitioners.

Additional encounters take place at other freestanding facilities such as urgent care centers, freestanding diagnostic and imaging centers, ambulatory surgery centers and other facilities. These facilities may be sponsored by a variety of different organizations.

The site most associated with the provision of healthcare is the hospital. The hospital clearly symbolizes healthcare in the United States and accounts for a major share of healthcare expenditures. However, in terms of patient encounters (rather than dollars) hospitalization is a rare event. Some Americans go their entire lives without a hospitalization, while they may visit physicians scores of times. In fact, the hospital declined as a setting for care during the waning years of the twentieth century. Everything that could be handled on an outpatient basis was moved out of the hospital, and hospitalization became an even rarer event for U.S. healthcare consumers.

Other institutional settings for the provision of care are nursing homes, residential treatment centers, and assisted living centers. Aggressive medical care is not typically provided in any of these settings, with custodial functions often being more important than curative activities. While assisted living facilities have become more common in recent years, few new nursing homes have been established. None of these settings for care accounts for a significant number of patients relative to other settings. Home health services, along with hospice care, continue to account for a growing portion of the care provided, although the growth in this sector has been slowed by limitations in reimbursement.

Health services of various types may also be provided at employment sites and schools. The "factory nurse" has long been a fixture in U.S. industry and the recent emphasis on environmental safety has prompted more involvement of clinical personnel in the corporate world. Medical personnel have long been found in school systems, with school nurses and mental health counselors being common fixtures in the school house.

REFERENCES

Ackerknecht, Erwin H. (1982 [1955]). *A Short History of Medicine*. Baltimore: Johns Hopkins Press.

Kuhn, Thomas S. (1970). *The Structure of Scientific Revolutions*. Chicago: University of Chicago Press.

ADDITIONAL RESOURCES

Rosen, George (1993). *History of Public Health*. Baltimore: John Hopkins University Press.
Rosen, George (1973). *From Medical Police to Social Medicine: Essays on the History of Health Care*. Canton, MA: Watson Publishing.
Starr, Paul (1982). *The Social Transformation of American Medicine*. New York: Basic Books.

Chapter 6

Social Groups in Society and Healthcare

THE NATURE OF SOCIAL GROUPS

For medical sociologists an understanding of group dynamics is critical to the analysis of the healthcare setting. Human beings are group animals and virtually all social development occurs within the group context. We learn to become human beings from the groups in which we participate, and the group represents the cradle of culture for us. The experience of group membership provides a sense of belonging for individuals.

A social group is defined as two or more people who identify with others in the group and interact with one another. Human beings interact as couples, families, circles of friends, neighborhood residents, church members, and members of clubs and other organizations. Regardless of the type of group, groups contain people with shared experiences, loyalties, and interests. Members of social groups come to identify with the group and think of group members as "we."

Social groups represent organized behavior (as opposed to unorganized behavior) within a society. An appropriate view of society would, in fact, see it not as a collection of individuals but as a collection of groups to which these individuals belong. In a complex society such as the United States, it could be argued that there are more groups than individuals, since virtually every individual belongs to more than one group.

In every society, individual members (except those who are totally alienated or perhaps mentally disordered) relate to society through the groups in which they participate. These groups are the context for human behavior. Society members seldom act alone but in relation to a group. Even when acting as individuals in isolation, group affiliation is likely to influence these individual actions. We are "group animals", often deferring to group consensus even if we are convinced we are right and the group is wrong.

Social groups, especially small, primary groups, are particularly important for the individual. The group is, after all, the individual's link to the larger society. Within the small group uniqueness counts and everyone is accepted for what they are. It is within the small group that one's self-concept develops, safe from the threats of the larger society. The small group serves as a protective buffer for the individual and helps to interpret the norms of society for its members. Finally, the small group provides the social and psychological support required by the individual.

Not every collection of individuals forms a group, and sociologists distinguish between social groups and other groupings of society members. Some of these groupings may be thought of as social "categories" such as children, senior citizens, and immigrants. While members of these categories may have some things in common, they do not have the attributes associated with true groups and are typically strangers to one another. Similarly, sociologists may speak of social "aggregates" or crowds of people gathered together for a particular purpose. The audience at a theatre or a college class may be thought of as an aggregate but not a group. The concept of group, thus, does not apply to groupings of individuals who simply have one or more common characteristics, groupings of individuals who are in the same place at the same time, or groupings of individuals who may interact regularly but have limited involvement with each other.

A social group, then, involves a plurality (two or more) of persons who interact to the point of developing social relationships. Further, group members take one another into account and have something significant in common. Groups are also characterized by informal or formal boundaries that set them apart from other groups and the rest of society. Thus, the insignia worn by gang members clearly designates who is in the group and who is not, and the lab coat and stethoscope indicate that their bearer belongs to the medical "fraternity".

GROUP SIZE

Groups can range in size from two people to any number as long as they maintain the characteristics of groups. Social scientists think in terms of small groups and large groups. Small groups can range from two persons up to perhaps as many as twenty or more. However, at some point the grouping will become too large to maintain the characteristics of the group and come to be defined as some other grouping. After a certain point it becomes impossible to know all members of the group well or to interact with everyone. As groups grow in size, there is a tendency for subgroups to arise that are more appropriate for maintaining the characteristics of a true group.

As group size increases, the potential number of relationships increases. Two people form a single relationship; adding a third person results in three relationships; a forth person yields six. Thus, by the time seven people join one conversation, twenty-one "channels" connect them. As groups grow beyond three people, they become more stable and able to survive despite the loss of members or turnover in membership. On the other hand, as groups increase in size, the opportunities for personal interaction are reduced. With so many possible channels of communication, the group usually divides at this point.

Small groups tend to be more closely knit, more intimate and involve more intense feelings of association and loyalty than larger groups. Interaction is more intense and more frequent in small groups. Individuals feel more allegiance to small groups than to large groups. Small groups tend to be ones we are born into (e.g., the family) or that we choose to participate in (e.g., play groups, school cliques). For these reasons, we tend to have much more invested in the small group than in the large group.

While large groups share basic characteristics with small groups, there is a qualitative difference between the two. Large groups tend to be more formal with more structure and organization. Thus, the large committee forms subcommittees. The roles in the large group become more specialized and "officers" must be elected, while in the small group everyone is the same and no special offices are required. Further, more formal means of communication must be developed as the group grows in size.

TYPES OF SOCIAL GROUPS

Various types of social groups have been identified by sociologists. Two of these are primary and secondary groups. A primary group is a small group whose members share personal and enduring relationships.

Interconnected by means of personal relationships, members of primary groups spend a great deal of time together, engage in a wide range of activities, and tend to know one another very well. Primary group members demonstrate a concern for each other's welfare.

Sociologists consider these personal and tightly integrated groups "primary" because they are among the first groups we experience in life. Thus, in every society, the family is the most important primary group. In addition, family and friends have primary importance in the socialization process, shaping attitudes, behavior and social identity.

Primary groups have characteristics that make them qualitatively different from secondary groups. Primary groups are small in terms of numbers and tend to be personal and informal. They involve long-term interaction of an on-going nature, and the members know each other well. This knowledge is likely to be multidimensional in that they know a lot about various aspects of other group members' lives. The goals of the primary group tend to be more generalized and may simply involve the emotional satisfaction of the participants (as in a friendship group). Primary groups are also characterized by honest displays of emotion. Membership in primary groups is typically based on kinship, proximity and shared interests.

Members of primary groups help one another in many ways, but they generally think of their group as an end in itself rather than a means to other ends. Thus, these individuals want to be together for the sake of being together rather than for some other purpose. Moreover, members of a primary group tend to view each other as unique and irreplaceable. Especially in the family, we are bound to others by emotion and loyalty.

Secondary groups, on the other hand, are larger in size and tend to be more impersonal and formal. Participation in the group may be temporary and sporadic. The large group is likely to have a more specialized goal-oriented function supported by formal by-laws. Interaction is typically indirect and may take the form of formal communication (e.g., the corporate "memo"). Members of large groups are not likely to know other members well (except for those who form small groups within the larger group), and their interest in other members is not likely to extend beyond the immediate business of the group. Large groups tend to be based on professional affiliation, although they may also be based on shared interests (as with a civic organization). Often individuals may be assigned to a large group as in a department within a corporation and may have no interest in other group members beyond their role in the department.

In most respects, secondary groups have precisely the opposite characteristics of primary groups. Secondary relationships involve weak emotional ties and little personal knowledge of one another. Many secondary groups are short term, beginning and ending with no particular significance. Students in a college course, for example, who may or may not see each other after the semester ends, exemplify the secondary group. Students enrolled in professional schools are often an exception to this and may constitute a primary group over time. Medical students, dental students and students in other health professions often enter the program as a cohort and spend much of their time together over a period of years. Unlike most students who do their class time and then get on with the rest of their lives, students in professional programs leave class, go to the laboratory, go to the library, and then to study groups, all with the same people. By sharing educational experiences on almost a seven-day-a-week basis, these classes often turn into true groups.

Secondary groups include many more people than primary groups. Hundreds of people may work together in the same office as members of a secondary group, but few of them are likely to know each other well. Sometimes time transforms a group from secondary to primary, as with co-workers who share an office for many years. Members of a secondary group usually do not think of themselves as "we," although competition between universities or corporations may create a team spirit that pits "us" against "them".

As the U.S. has become industrialized and urbanized, the basis for relationships has changed. Two or three generations ago, relationships were based on family, geographic proximity (i.e., community), and perhaps the work environment. In a world that is increasingly impersonal, relationships are likely to be based on interests and professional associations. Society members are often isolated from their families and do not have ties to the community. Even the experience of work may be isolating, and social ties are sought outside of work that reflect the individual's interests.

Primary relationships are motivated by individual needs (personal orientation), while secondary relationships are motivated by organizational needs (goal orientation). Interaction among family members or friends is likely to be highly personal. Interaction among students and business associates is likely to be impersonal even if cordial. Primary group members define their relationships in terms of kinship or personal qualities (i.e., who they are), while members of secondary groups define each other in terms of the functions they perform (i.e., what they are). The goal orientation of secondary groups means that their members usually remain formal and polite. It would be inappropriate, for example, to ask personal questions of individuals in secondary groups.

While sociologists have identified the traits that characterize "ideal types" of primary and secondary groups, in the real world most groups contain elements of both primary and secondary groups. Table 6–1 summarizes the characteristics of primary and secondary groups.

Table 6–1. Characteristics of Primary and Secondary Groups

	Primary group	Secondary group
Quality of relationships	Personal orientation	Goal orientation
Duration of relationships	Usually long-term	Variable, often short-term
Breadth of relationships	Broad, involving many activities	Narrow, involving few activities
Nature of relationships	As ends in themselves	As means to an end
Typical examples	Families, circles of friends	Co-workers, political organizations

SOURCE: John Macionis (2000). *Society: The Basics.* Upper Saddle River, NJ: Prentice Hall.

Another type of group is the reference group. A reference group is a social group that serves as a point of reference for individuals in making evaluations and decisions. Reference groups are groups that the individual "refers" to and accepts the values of. Typically, these are groups of which the individual is a member. Groups like the family, peer groups and work groups exert inordinate influence on the individual, and the individual looks to these groups for guidance in behavior and attitudes. Indeed, every parent worries about the influence of the peer group as a reference group for their children. (Note that "group" here is used in a loose sense, since we may talk about a social category in terms of a reference group.)

The reference group may not be a group that one is a member of but one to which the individual aspires. Historically, Americans have taken as a reference group the social stratum right above them on the social ladder. Thus, working class individuals have aspired to be middle class and have taken their cues for behavior from that reference group. Generations of immigrants have used native-born Americans as their reference group, often becoming more "American" than native-born citizens.

In healthcare, a great deal of research has focused on the training of physicians and the extent to which they adopt the behaviors, mannerisms, and attitudes of their main reference groups—medical school faculty and practicing physicians. Indeed, research has found that idealistic medical students typically go through a transformation during medical school training in which they adopt the more pragmatic attributes of those in their reference groups. (This topic is covered in more detail in the chapter on occupations and professions.)

There is also such a phenomenon as negative reference groups. These are groups that individuals shun and whose behavior serves as an example of how not to act, dress and think. Parents are good at pointing out negative reference groups and admonishing their children not to act like the reference group's members. Individuals moving up the social ladder may view their previous social group as a negative reference group and be careful to avoid the behaviors associated with that previous group. Indeed, some second-generation immigrants may even see their parents (first-generation immigrants) as a negative reference group.

Like other groups, reference groups may be primary or secondary in nature. They may be primary groups to which we belong or secondary groups which we revere or disdain. Members of desirable groups influence aspirants to those groups by providing an example of behavior to emulate. Thus, would-be group members imitate this behavior as a strategy to win acceptance by the group. Medical students' success, for example, depends on winning the acceptance of their medical school mentors and, as physicians, that of their colleagues.

Sociologists also make a distinction between in-groups and out-groups. An in-group is a social group commanding a member's esteem and loyalty. An out-group, by contrast, is a social group toward which one feels competition or opposition. In-groups and out-groups are based on the idea that the traits associated with the in-group are positive and desirable and those associated with the out-group are negative and undesirable. For example, orthopedic surgeons may show disdain for chiropractors and refuse to practice in the same setting with them. People in virtually every social setting develop such positive and negative evaluations.

CHANGING GROUP STRUCTURE

One of the major trends in U.S. society over the past century or so has been the shift from an emphasis on primary groups to an emphasis on secondary groups. Generations ago in small town and rural America, everyone tended to know everyone else (and everyone else's business). Virtually all interactions were of a primary nature, with people that one knew well or at least a lot about. The grocery store clerk was perhaps the son of a friend or a fellow church member, and social interaction involved more than a simple business transaction. Relationships were based on traditional associations, family ties, and neighborhood proximity. Except for the occasional traveling salesman, virtually all interactions were of a primary nature. Customs and mores were usually sufficient to maintain social order due to the powerful influence in the social group on the individual.

The industrialization and urbanization of American society in the twentieth century contributed to the shift from primary to secondary relationships. An agrarian economy with its emphasis on extended families, the family farm, and multi-generational ties to the community gave way to an industrial society that valued nuclear families and geographic mobility, thereby destroying the traditional ties to the community. The urbanization that accompanied industrialization drew individuals and families to urban areas and broke the hold of family and community. Individuals were typically placed into situations where they had few primary relationships, and most of the people with whom they came in contact were quite different from themselves.

These developments resulted in a preponderance of secondary interactions over primary interactions as the twentieth century progressed. In this new urban environment, one seldom knew the persons they interacted with very well, and interactions were of necessity impersonal. Urbanites didn't know much about the people they conducted transactions with and, frankly, they didn't want to know much about them. People did not speak to each other on the street and few knew their neighbors. Relationships became transitory and short-lived. The associations that existed were typically not based on family or geographic proximity, but on common work experiences or personal interests (e.g., sports, music). Customs and mores were no longer sufficient to assure social control since the "agents" of social control—family members, neighbors, church members—were no longer around to assure compliance. Laws became increasingly important for maintaining order in a society based on secondary relationships.

Likewise, U.S. healthcare has experienced a shift from a primary orientation to a secondary orientation during the last half of the twentieth century. What could be more intimate than the doctor-patient relationship—especially when the doctor may know more about the patient than his or her spouse. Even as recently as the post-World War II years, doctors typically knew their patients well and, indeed, often visited their homes. They were aware of their family situations, their social circumstances, and the environments in which they lived.

As the U.S. healthcare system has evolved, the relationships between the various participants have become increasingly secondary. The family physician has been replaced by the corporate employee/physician, and even then there is no guarantee that the patient will get to see this physician. Most patients complain that they have been reduced to a number and that intake personnel are more concerned about their insurance information than their symptoms. The hospital patient has become "the gall bladder in room 316" rather than "John Smith". The mediator for health problems has become the faceless insurance clerk that determines what treatments can be covered.

This trend toward impersonality in healthcare has been prompted by the urbanization of U.S. society, the increasing formalization of all institutions including healthcare, and medical training that emphasizes the importance of impersonality on the part of the physician. These trends illustrate the influence that large social structures have on individual behavior. Today a physician who wanted to take the time to know his patients well would potentially be censured by his managed care plan, face a salary reduction, and/or be derided by his colleagues.

This type of impersonal treatment is, of course, nothing new to the millions of Americans who have had to depend on "charity" for their healthcare. Those forced to use hospital emergency rooms for their care, for example, are used to being treated as non-persons and being known by numbers rather than names. The assembly-line manner in which they are typically processed mitigates against any semblance of personal care. The need to process a large number of patients typically overrides any possibilities for personal attention. This is not to diminish the dedicated work of generations of emergency room personnel who no doubt did everything they could to be empathetic with their patients. Unfortunately, the "system" has mandated an approach that requires an emphasis on secondary relations. Medical education emphasizes the maintenance of objectivity (i.e., impersonality) on the part of physicians, and the greater the social distance between clinicians and patients, the greater the impersonality.

By the end of the twentieth century, a significant backlash with regard to the impersonality of medicine had surfaced. Healthcare "consumers" (that is, patients with the attitudes of customers) were spawned by the Baby Boom generation, and they were used to higher level of service than that available through the healthcare system. They began demanding more attention from practitioners and more of a partnership in the therapeutic process. They spearheaded an attack on the perceived impersonality of managed care plans.

In response to this backlash some physicians have re-instituted house calls, and others have established "concierge" practices wherein patients pay extra for personal care. Medical schools have attempted to make their curricula more patient centered. Much of the reaction on the part of the medical community reflects the higher rate of malpractice claims resulting from the impersonal behavior of physicians vis-à-vis their patients.

SOCIAL SUPPORT AND HEALTH

The importance of the social group for health status and health behavior cannot be overemphasized. To this end, sociologists have expended considerable research effort on the study of social support. According to Pilisuk and Parks (1966), "'social support' is a general term for the many different resources that aid persons in times of crisis and help them cope with life. It is a general term used to describe different aspects of social relationships, including those mechanisms that may protect the individual from the negative effects of stress.

Social support has been found to be an important variable in the development of feelings of well-being and the relieving of symptoms and tension. The social support rendered by families and friendship networks helps reduce the potentially harmful effects of stress on the body and mind. Social support tends to function as a buffer or intervening variable between an individual and his or her sense of stress. Persons with the strongest levels of social support typically report fewer health problems than those with little or no support (Cockerham and Richey, 1997).

Pearlin (1983) emphasizes that social support reduces strain by preventing the loss of self-esteem and aiding a sense of mastery that stressors can erode. Social support can also serve an instrumental purpose, such as financial aid and other assistance. Social support can encourage recovery from an illness, for example by encouraging a family member to do therapeutic exercises. Those enjoying strong social ties appear to be at low risk of psychosocial and physical impairment, whereas a lack of social support has been found to be associated with depression, neurosis and even mortality. Social networks can promote such health habits as regular exercise, good eating habits, and adequate sleep (Freund and McGuire, 1999). In general, social support seems to be an important moderating factor in the stress process.

Various studies have found that the more people were involved socially with family, friends, and groups, the lower the death rate. This was true for both sexes across ages 30 to 69. Having meaningful social contacts through friends, family, and the community was found to help people control stress, solve problems, and cope with setbacks.

A recent study found social butterflies get fewer colds than loners. When 276 health volunteers had their noses sprayed with common cold viruses, people who had six or more types of social relationships, such as being a friend, a parent or a neighbor, were almost half as likely to come down with a cold as people with only three or fewer such relationships. The researchers found this social factor was more important even than good health practices in helping people resist colds, perhaps because being needed by others improves the immune response. Close-knit communities also have the resilience to bounce back in the face of adversity such as a flood, loss of an industry, or a rail line closure.

SOCIAL NETWORKS

A network is described by sociologists as a web of weak social ties or as a "fuzzy" group containing people who come into occasional contact but lack a sense of boundaries and belonging. A network might be considered a "social web" expanding outward, often reaching great distances and including large numbers of people. Some networks come close to being groups, as is the case of college friends who stay in touch years after graduation. More commonly, however, a network includes people who know each other but interact seldom if at all.

Networks may involve weak ties, but they can be a powerful resource for their members. Unlike many social groups, networks are not tied to geography and typically are far flung. New information technology has now generated a global network of unprecedented size in the form of the Internet.

Networks may be based on individuals' affiliations with colleges, clubs, neighborhoods, political parties, and so forth. The networks in which people participate determine to a certain extent the social resources to which they have access. Some people have denser networks than others in that they are connected to more people. Typically, the most extensive social networks are maintained by people who are young, well educated, and living in large cities.

Although the networks of men and women have been found to be generally the same size, women include more relatives (and other women) in their networks, while men include more co-workers (and other men). In this regard, women's ties historically have not carried the same clout as the "old-boy" networks. As gender inequality lessens in the United States, it appears that the networks of men and women are becoming more alike.

An insightful early study examined the influence of different types of social networks on the utilization of various services for mental symptoms (Suchman, 1965). In his study of various ethnic groups in New York, Suchman sought to relate individual medical orientation and behaviors to specific types of social relationships and their corresponding group structures. Based on his analysis of sickness behavior and network affiliation, Suchman categorized people as belonging to either "parochial" or "cosmopolitan" networks. Persons involved in a parochial network were found to have close and exclusive relationships with family, friends and members of their ethnic group. These networks were quite limited in their scope. Network members displayed limited knowledge of disease, skepticism of the benefits of medical care, and high dependency during illness. They were more likely than the cosmopolitan group to delay the seeking of medical care and more likely to rely upon a lay referral system in coping with their symptoms of illness. This lay referral system consisted of family members, friends and/or neighbors who assist individuals in interpreting their symptoms and in recommending a course of action. Parochial networks were most common in lower-class neighborhoods characterized by a strong ethnic identification and extended family relationships (Cockerham, 2001).

By contrast, those involved in cosmopolitan social networks demonstrated low levels of ethnic identification, less limited friendship systems, and fewer authoritarian family relationships. Their networks tended to be far-flung, unrestricted by geography and extending beyond the immediate area to become nationwide and even international. (This analysis was carried out, of course, well before the advent of the Internet.) The relationships within the cosmopolitan network were likely to be looser than those in the parochial network and based not on family relations and geographic proximity but on business associations, school ties, and common interests. While the parochial network was essentially a "closed" network, restricted to a few well-known individuals, the cosmopolitan network was open-ended in the sense that each contact represented a link to additional potential relationships. Those in cosmopolitan networks were more likely than the parochial network members to know something about disease, to trust health professionals, to be familiar with the healthcare system, and to be less dependent on others while sick (Cockerham, 2001).

Network membership, Sutherland found, has significant implications for the help-seeking process for those with psychiatric symptoms. Those in parochial networks turned to members of their close-knit network for feedback on and interpretation of their symptoms. They called on members of the network for access to resources. Sources of help first consisted of family and friends who had some knowledge of or experience with such conditions, followed by referral to clergyman or other lay counselors who may provide some insights. Turning to the formal healthcare system—particularly for psychiatric care—was virtually never a consideration for members of this network.

Members of cosmopolitan networks, on the other hand, looked beyond family and friends to their more far-flung network when seeking help for their symptoms. Access to a cosmopolitan network provided exposure to a wide range of alternatives and ample feedback on possible options for care. Members of this group were likely to be channeled into the formal healthcare system and referred to psychologists, psychotherapists, psychiatrists or other clinically oriented personnel. Clearly, they were encouraged to pursue an institutional response, in contrast to the informal solution pursued by members of the parochial social network.

GROUP INFLUENCES ON HEALTH BEHAVIOR

Group affiliation plays an important part in many types of health behavior. The type of response one makes in the face of symptoms, the choice of provider, and even the decision to do nothing typically reflects the influence of the group on the individual. While Americans like to think that they are in control of their destiny, many of their health-related decisions are made or at least greatly influenced by family, friends and associates.

Healthy behavior is greatly influenced by the social group. In fact, many individuals attempting to lose weight, become more fit, and generally live healthier lifestyles depend on members of their social groups for support and assistance. Peer pressure is often an important influence on the individual's pursuit of healthy or unhealthy behaviors.

The influence of the group is clearly seen in the help-seeking process in the face of the onset of symptoms. The help-seeking process essentially involves a series of decisions in response to the condition. The first decision involves an initial recognition of symptoms on the part of the individual. Then, a decision as to the seriousness of the symptoms is likely to follow. Beyond this, there are decisions as to whether to take action or to wait and see what develops, what type of informal response to make, what type of formal response to make, which provider to choose, whether to submit to surgery, and so forth. A decision may even be made on whether to follow doctor's orders or not.

These decisions are not made in a vacuum but are heavily influenced by the social group. The influence may be direct in that family members or friends counsel the individual on his situation. Indeed, family members may actually make the decision on behalf of the individual. Every step of the way, there is the option for input from significant others.

The influence of the social group may be indirect as well, in that the individual is likely to be influenced by group affiliations even if acting in a solitary manner. An individual's decision to seek care, to select a particular provider, or to follow doctor's orders will reflect the demographic, socioeconomic and psychographic characteristics of the individual (whether he realizes it or not). The fact that one is a member of a particular ethnic group, a particular subculture, or a particular religion will influence the decisions that are made during the help-seeking process.

FORMAL ORGANIZATIONS

Formal organizations are established in all societies and are particularly a feature of modern societies. They represent an extension of large social groups as they take on a more formal structure. A century ago, most people lived in small groups of family, friends, and neighbors, but in contemporary America, our lives revolve more and more around formal organizations, or large secondary groups.

Large, complex societies rely upon formal organizations to perform the necessary functions of the society. These organizations develop an existence of their own so that, as members come and go, their operation can continue unaffected. Formal organizations, such as corporations and government agencies, differ from small primary groups in their impersonality and controlled environment. The evolution of healthcare as a set of formal organizations reflects the institutionalization of the healthcare function during the twentieth century.

Although formal organizations date back thousands of years, their history in the U.S. is limited. The industrialization and urbanization that occurred in the United States during the twentieth century involved a transformation from a traditional, agrarian society to a complex, modern society in which change, not tradition, is the central theme. This transformation clearly influenced the direction of development for the healthcare system, as the traditional managers of sickness and death—the family and church—gave way to more complex responses to health problems.

The formal organization is based on rationality and the deliberate calculation of the most efficient means to accomplish a particular task. A rational worldview eschews the past and is open to change in whatever way seems likely to get the job done better and more quickly (until, as will be seen below, they take on some of the negative attributes of bureaucracies). This tendency toward formalization led to the rise of the "organizational society". In modern society sentimental ties give way to a rational focus on science, complex technology, and a bureaucratic organizational structure. (Box 6-1 describes the extent to which hospitals, as they become more formalized, become "total institutions.")

TYPES OF FORMAL ORGANIZATIONS

Social institutions (except for the family) rely on formal organizations to achieve their goals in modern societies. The religious institution relies on large, bureaucratic denominational offices for managing the operation of the particular religion. The political institution relies on complicated court systems at many levels of government for the accomplishment of its goals. Healthcare relies on hospitals as formal organizations for performing much of its work, assisted by other large-scale organizations such as the American Medical Association, medical schools, and multinational pharmaceutical companies.

Sociologists identify three types of formal organizations, distinguished by the reasons that people participate in them (Etzioni 1975). "Normative" organizations pursue goals their members consider morally worthwhile, personally satisfying, perhaps socially prestigious, but not monetarily rewarding. Sometimes called voluntary associations, they include community service groups (such as the League of Women Voters and the Red Cross), political parties, and religious organizations. Americans tend to be much more involved in voluntary associations than members of others societies.

"Coercive" organizations force members to join as a form of punishment (e.g., prisons) or treatment (e.g., mental hospitals). With their locked doors and barred windows, these settings segregate people as "inmates" or "patients" for a period of time and sometimes radically alter their attitudes and behavior.

"Utilitarian organizations" (e.g., business enterprises) grant more individual freedom than coercive organizations, but less than normative organizations. Most people have little choice but to spend half of their waking hours at work, where they have limited control over their jobs.

A formal organization may fall into one or all of these categories. A mental hospital, for example, is a normative organization to a hospital volunteer, a coercive organization to a patient, and a utilitarian organization to a security guard.

The epitome of the formal organization is the "bureaucracy". The bureaucracy is an organizational model rationally designed to perform tasks efficiently. Bureaucratic officials regularly enact and revise policy to increase efficiency. Sociologists identify six key elements of the bureaucratic organization. The relevance of bureaucratic structures for the modern hospital can be clearly seen in the core traits of the bureaucracy:

1. *Specialization.* Individuals in a bureaucracy are assigned specialized roles. Medical specialties among physicians tend to be the most visible form of specialization within a hospital, but the entire hospital workforce is highly specialized with distinct roles characterizing the various occupations.
2. *A hierarchy of offices.* Bureaucracies arrange personnel in a vertical ranking of offices and the administrative structure of the hospital reflects this. Each individual in hospital management is supervised by "higher-ups" in the organization while, in turn, supervising others in lower positions.
3. *Rules and regulations.* Rationally enacted rules and regulations guide a bureaucracy's operation and the hospital is run on strict protocols. Not only are there rules and regulations that guide the behavior of clinical staff, but rules are put into place the specify what patients and their families can do. These rules serve to allow physicians and administrators to retain control of the situation and assure at least some level of predictability within the organization.
4. *Technical competence.* Perhaps no other bureaucracy emphasizes technical competence to the extent a hospital does. There are few "routine" tasks in a hospital for which anyone can be hired off the street. Virtually all positions require at least some level of technical competence. The emphasis in hospital hiring, thus, focuses inordinately on credentials.
5. *Impersonality.* Bureaucracy puts rules ahead of personal whim so that clients as well as workers are all treated uniformly. Despite the caring mission of the hospital, the need to "process" large numbers of patients and even larger numbers of transactions mandates a certain level of impersonality. Indeed, a major complaint of patients is their being reduced to a number by hospital staff.
6. *Formal, written communications.* Rather than casual, face-to-face talk, a bureaucracy relies on formal written memos and reports,

---

Box 6-1

The Hospital as a "Total Institution"

Sociologists have identified a type of social entity that they refer to as a "total institution." A total institution is a setting in which individuals are isolated from the rest of society and put under the complete control of the institution's staff. ("Institution" is used here to refer to an organizational type rather than a component of social structure.) Prisons, the military and mental hospitals are all examples of total institutions. Prisons and mental hospitals, for example, physically isolate inmates behind fences, barred windows, and locked doors, and control their access to the telephone, mail and visitors. Cut off in this way, the institution is the inmate's entire world, making it easier for the staff to produce lasting change—or at least immediate compliance—in the inmate. As will be seen, the general hospital can also be considered to have many characteristics of a total institution.

As a total institution, the hospital has the mission of restoring the individual to a functioning role in society, and this involves a two-part process. First, the staff erodes the new residents identity through various processes designed to subordinate the patient to the operation of the institution. When patients present themselves for treatment in a hospital, they bring with them a particular social identity representing their attitudes, beliefs, values, concept of self, and social status, all of which form the basis for their manner of presenting themselves to the world. Through a process of "stripping", the hospital systematically divests the person of these past representations of self. The patient's clothes are taken away and replaced with a hospital gown. The gown serves as a uniform that identifies that person as sick and restricts his movement to those areas of the hospital in which patient dress is authorized. Personal belongings of value are taken away and locked up for safekeeping by the staff. Once inside the hospital, individuals also give up their privacy as staff routinely monitor patient rooms.

One result of this process is the depersonalization of the patient. Patients tend to be devalued by hospital personnel because they are sick and dependent, and they are offered thought of as "non-persons" by staff. Patients are given a number and subsequently referred to by staff in terms like "the gall bladder in 305."

Personnel in hospitals do not have the express goal of making their patients feel depersonalized, but the organization of the hospital's work favors rules and regulations that reduce patient autonomy and encourage patient receptivity of the hospital routine. The process of depersonalization is further enhanced by the need of the physician or nurse to have access to the patient's body.

A second aspect of total institutionalization is loss of control. The staff takes control over the patient's body and his environment. First, staff members supervise all spheres of daily life, including how residents eat, sleep, and participate in the organization's activities. Second, the environment is highly standardized, with institutional food, uniforms, and one set of rules for everyone. Third, rules and schedules dictate when, where, and how inmates perform their daily routines.

This control by staff extends to the control of physical items like bed-clothes and toilet paper, as well as the control of information about the patient's medical condition. Visitation regulations control not only when patients are allowed to have visitors, but also who is allowed to visit (with children under a certain age typically excluded). In addition, the staff super-vises the patient's diet, decides when the patient should be asleep or awake, and in essence controls the general conduct of the patient's social life in the hospital. The hospital routine for one patient is very similar to the routine of others having the same or similar health problems.

The third aspect of depersonalization is the restriction of the patient's mobility. In most hospitals patients are not allowed to leave their nursing units without permission. When patients do leave the unit to travel to another area of the hospital, they are generally accompanied by hospital staff. When patients are admitted to or discharged from the hospital, they are taken in a wheelchair between the unit and the hospital entrance regardless of their ability to walk because the hospital is "responsible" for them whenever they are inside its walls. The result is that even the ability of patients to move about is supervised and controlled.

Once the patient has been depersonalized, the staff tries to restore the patient to some level of functioning through a series of treatments. As in the prison environment, the patient turns himself over to the institution "heart, body and soul." The staff subjects the patient to numerous "mortifications," including physical examinations, diagnostic tests and often-invasive treat-ments, all without the input of the patient.

While hospital services are oriented toward a supportive notion of pa-tient welfare, hospital rules and regulations are generally designed for the benefit of hospital personnel so that the work of treating large numbers of pa-tients can be more efficient and easier to perform. Consequently, the sick and the injured are organized into various patient categories (obstetrics, neurol-ogy, orthopedics, urology, pediatrics, psychiatry, etc.) that reflect the medical staff's definition of their disorder and after which they are subject to stan-dardized, staff-approved medical treatment and administrative procedures.

Despite the purported beneficence of the hospital, the typical hospital has many of the attributes of a total institution. Ultimately, the hospital op-erates for the convenience of its staff while subjecting the patient to what the staff determines is appropriate treatment. While the general hospital may not be as "total" as a prison or a mental hospital, it is clear that the patient in a general hospital is subjected to many of the same conditions as prisoners and mental patients.

Sources: William C. Cockerham (2001). *Medical Sociology* (8th edition). Upper Saddle River, NJ: Prentice Hall; John Macionis (2000). *Society: The Basics*. Upper Saddle River, NJ: Prentice Hall; M. Rodney Coe (1978). *Sociology of Medicine* (2nd edition). New York: McGraw-Hill.

which accumulate in vast files. In fact, the importance of written records is carried to extremes within the context of the hospital. Everything must be documented, not only to assure reasonably efficient operation of a complex institution but in response to ethical and legal requirements.

Despite the tendency—indeed, the necessity—for the creation of bureaucratic organizations for the operation of large, complex institutions, there are always anti-bureaucratic tendencies in society. Individuals cannot deal effectively with large, impersonal structures and, just as large groups tend to break down into small groups, individuals devise various ways of coping with bureaucratic structures. Although the ideal bureaucracy deliberately regulates every activity, in actual organizations human beings are creative (and stubborn) enough to resist bureaucratic blueprints. Despite the rigid protocols involved in patient care, even physicians find ways to cut corners or otherwise infuse the flexibility that every bureaucratic organization requires.

One source of informality is the personalities of organizational leaders. Studies of U.S. corporations document that the qualities and quirks of individuals—including personal charisma and interpersonal skills—have a great impact on organizational performance. Authoritarian, democratic, or laissez-faire types of leadership reflect individual personality as much as any organizational plan. Clear differences in the personal operating styles of hospitals have been noted, particularly since hospitals have historically been "local" operations, unaffected by the dictates of national systems. Indeed, hospitals have often been studied as examples of variations in corporate cultures.

Bureaucracies can dehumanize and manipulate their members, Bureaucracies like hospitals are often characterized by worker alienation, ritualism and "red tape", inertia, and a certain level of waste and incompetence. They also display a tendency toward oligarchy, with a handful of individuals, say, on the medical staff exhibiting an inordinate amount of control over the institution.

With regard to incompetence, hospitals like other bureaucracies suffer from the Peter Principle (Peter and Hull, 1969). According to Peter and Hull, bureaucrats are promoted to their level of incompetence. Employees competent at one level of the organizational hierarchy will be promoted to a higher position where they are in over their heads, perform badly, and become ineligible for further advancement. This is particularly true in the hospital, where individuals with technical skills (e.g., clinicians and technologists) are elevated to managerial positions for which they have little or no training. (Box 6-2 addresses the issue of dual authority in the hospital.)

Reaching their level of incompetence dooms officials to a future of inefficiency. Adding to the problem is the fact that, after years in the organization, they almost certainly have learned how to "work the system" and make themselves appear irreplaceable. Until the hospital shakeouts of the 1980s and 1990s, it was not unusual for administrators to rise up in the ranks of the hospital until they were ineffective.

THE CORPORATIZATION OF HEALTHCARE

The last two decades of the twentieth century witnessed a rapidly growing trend in the United States toward the corporatization of healthcare facilities. "Corporatization" is the process by which a relatively small number of investor-owned corporations control a greater concentration of proprietary interests. Regional and national chains of hospitals, nursing homes, psychiatric facilities, and outpatient surgery centers were established. At the same time, a significant proportion of healthcare institutions were being converted from not-for-profit organizations to for-profit operations.

Between 1977 and 1982, while the total number of U.S. hospitals declined by 2 percent, the number of investor-owned chain hospitals increased by 40 percent (Gray, 1983). Furthermore, the ownership was highly concentrated, with only four firms controlling approximately 70 percent of the more than 700 investor-owned hospitals (Berliner and Burlage, 1987). Even though the number of non-profit hospitals acquired by for-profit companies grew from 15 in 1992 to 347 in 1995, 85% of U.S. hospitals remain non-profit. The proportion of investor-owned specialty hospitals, such as short-term psychiatric hospitals and nursing homes, has continued to grow, however.

Perhaps the most detailed account of the early stages of the corporatization of American medicine was provided by Paul Starr (1982). Star describes how America was on its way to a major change in its system of healthcare delivery through the emergence of increasingly large corporations. The 1980s and 1990s subsequently witnessed a wave of mergers, acquisitions and diversification by healthcare corporations in which not only hospitals and nursing homes were acquired but also urgent care centers, hospital supply companies, medical office buildings, health spas, psychiatric hospitals, home health agencies, and hospital management systems.

For the first time in the United States, healthcare became regarded as a major business arena. For-profit corporations expanded either into markets that were underserved or into areas where their services could successfully compete with existing not-for-profit organizations. In corporations, physicians are likely to have a less prominent role in decision making, resulting

---

Box 6-2

The Dual Authority Structure of the Hospital

The operation of most hospitals is complicated by the existence of a dual authority structure. The overall supervision of the general hospital comes under the auspices of its governing body. In most nonfederal hospitals, that governing body is a board of trustees. Whereas the medical director and the hospital administrator are linked to the governing body by a direct line of responsibility, they are only indirectly responsible to each other. Thus, the authority structure of the general hospital operates as a two-headed creature. This arrangement is the primary contributor to the organizational conflict in the hospital between bureaucracy and professionalism.

The essence of the conflict between the bureaucrat and the professional consists of the professional's insistence on exercising autonomous individual judgment within the limits prescribed by the profession itself. The work norms of the professional (in this case, the physician) emphasize self-determination for each practitioner and minimizes control by those outside the profession. The bureaucrat (here, the hospital administrator), in contrast, seeks to follow a rationalistic management approach that favors the efficient coordination of the hospital's activities through formal rules and impersonal regulations applicable to all persons in all situations. This is complicated by the fact that, except for the medical director and a relative handful of other physicians, the physicians that practice at the hospital are independent practitioners who use the hospital without being formal employees. They are driven much more by the need to practice what they consider appropriate medicine (and by their own self-interest) than by any concern for the success of the hospital.

In the late 1800s and early 1900s the voluntary general hospital was dominated by its board of trustees, because this was an era when securing capital funds and gaining community recognition were critical hospital goals. Since community involvement was the pivotal factor, individual

---

in less personal autonomy for physicians practicing in a corporate facility. In the context of corporate healthcare, the physician is often an employee rather than an independent practitioner. The doctor is bound to the rules and regulations of the corporation that, in all probability, is managed by people trained in business not medicine.

Since Star's work in the early 1980s, the corporatization trend in health care has accelerated. Not only has the system experienced numerous mergers and acquisitions of healthcare organizations, even physician practices were consolidated during a period of aggressive empire building by physician practice management organizations. This short-lived movement

members of boards of trustees were usually laypersons selected at large from the community. Legally they were responsible for protecting the community's interests, but they also sought to incorporate hospital services into the general pattern of community life. By the 1930s trustee domination had been supplanted by medical domination. A number of factors contributed to this shift but the most important was the increasing body of knowledge characterizing the medical profession.

During the 1940s and 1950s the role of the hospital administrator gained in importance. Through a constitutional system, the administration was able to define the medical staff's official power, standardize the hospital's administrative procedures, and establish a level of quality for the hospital's medical services. These early administrators were often physicians who could be expected to further the interests of the medical staff but, in doing so, began to curtail their power. As authority became centralized in the administrator's office, communication between the medical staff and the board of trustees was inhibited. This period was characterized by a complex power struggle that eventually led in the 1950s to the dual authority system common among general hospitals today.

This system of dual authority, one administrative and the other medical, is predictable in a situation such as a hospital. The organization has multiple goals and various parties have different interests. Since the physician's professional norms can set specific limits on the hospital administrator's authority and vice versa, the result has been to reconcile the physician-professional with the administrator-bureaucrat by establishing a system of dual authority.

The board of trustees still remains the nominal center of authority in the general hospital. It usually meets on a periodic basis to review the hospital's operations and act upon matters that are brought to its attention. But despite their position as the hospital's ultimate source of authority, the trustees have only limited de facto authority over the medical staff, who usually make all clinically oriented decisions. The board of trustees typically concerns itself with administrative matters and public relations while working closely with

(continued)

illustrated the difficulties in corporatizing physician practices. Nevertheless, growing numbers of physicians work in corporate settings, in large group practices, or as employees of managed care organizations.

The purchasers of healthcare have also become corporatized, with the emergence of large groups of consumers who negotiate for the provision of care. This may take the form of self-insured employers who bargain with providers on behalf of their employees or groups of businesses who join together to gain greater negotiating leverage with providers in an attempt to control their healthcare costs. Although in the late 1990s there was a backlash against the high level of corporatization in healthcare, it is still the hospital administrator, who acts as their agent in exercising authority and supervising the day-to-day routine of the hospital.

The occupational groups in the hospital most affected by its system of dual authority are the nurses and other clinical hospital staff who perform tasks on the hospital's nursing units. Nurses are responsible to the physician for carrying out the physician's orders, but they are also responsible to the nursing supervision and the upper echelons of the hospital's administration. Even though the communication and allegiance of ward personnel tend to be channeled along occupational lines within and toward the "administrative channel of command", medical authority can and does cut across these lines.

Some researchers have found that the social order of the hospital is not fixed or automatically maintained, but is the result of continual negotiation between the administration, the medical staff, other hospital employees, and patients. The individuals involved have varying degrees of prestige and power, are at different stages in their careers, and have their own particular goals, reference groups, and occupational ideologies. In addition, hospital rules governing physicians' conduct are not clearly stated, extensive or binding. The hospital administration tend to take a tolerant position

appropriate to argue that most of the interaction on the business side of healthcare takes places between large corporate bodies rather than between individuals like doctors and patients.

The corporatization of healthcare has involved both horizontal and vertical integration. "Horizontal integration" is the process by which a corporation acquires large numbers of productive facilities, such as hospitals or nursing homes, across widespread markets. These chains are transforming healthcare into a large-scale high-stakes industry, described by some as the "medical-industrial complex" (Relman, 1980).

"Vertical integration" describes the conglomerate control over several levels of production, such as hospitals, nursing homes, hospital supply companies, pharmaceutical companies, prosthetic supply companies, medical office complexes, and home health agencies (Salmon, 1985). Vertically integrated industries have increased capacity to control diverse aspects of the market and to shift resources when one part of the business becomes less profitable. One particular form of vertical integration portends great structural change in the healthcare industry. When hospitals or clinics are owned by the same corporation as insurers or payment managers, considerable market control is concentrated. Such concentration greatly reduces the autonomy of professionals working in the system, reducing their ability to serve as advocates for patients. Patients too

toward institutional rules in the belief that good patient care requires a minimum of regulation and a maximum of discretion. Hospital administration and medical staff share a common goal of restoring patients to a better condition than when they entered the hospital.

To make this social organization function effectively, it has been necessary to construct a decentralized system of authority organized around a generally acceptable objective of service to the patient. While the administrator directs and supervises hospital policy, the medical staff retains control over medical decisions.

In the light of recent malpractice developments and liability cases, hospital administrators are likely to exercise greater control over the clinical aspects of hospital operation, imposing more of rules and regulations on the physicians, verifying the credentials of medical staff, and generally reducing the amount of professional discretion and autonomy physicians have traditionally been allowed to exercise.

Source: William C. Cockerham (2001). *Medical Sociology.* Upper Saddle River, NJ: Prentice Hall.

are severely limited in the affordable options open to them (Freund and McGuire, 1999).

REFERENCES

Cockerham, William C., and Ferris J. Richey (1997). *The Dictionary of Medical Sociology.* Westport, CT: Greenwood.

Etzioni, Amitai (1975). *A Comparative Analysis of Complex Organizations: On Power, Involvement and Their Correlates.* New York: Free Press.

Freund, Peter E.S., and Meredith B. McGuire (1999). *Health, Illness and the Social Body*, 3rd ed. Englewood Cliffs, NJ: Prentice Hall.

Pearlin, Leonard I. (1983). "Role Strains and Personal Stress," pp. 3–32 in H.B. Kaplan, ed., *Psychosocial Stress: Trends in Theory and Research.* New York: Academic Press.

Pearlin, Leonard I. (1989). "The sociological study of stress," *Journal of Health and Social Behavior*, 30:241–256.

Peter, Laurence J., and Raymond Hull (1969). *The Peter Principle: Why Things Always Go Wrong.* New York: William Morrow.

Pilisuk, Marc, and Susan H. Parks (1966). *The Healing Web: Social Networks and Human Survival.* Hanover, NH: University Press of New England.

Relman, Arnold S. (1980). "The new medical-industrial complex," *New England Journal of Medicine* 303:963–970.

Salmon, J. Warren (1985). "Profit and health care: Trends in corporatization and proprietarization," *International Journal of Health Services* 15:395–418.

Starr, Paul (1982). *The Social Transformation of American Medicine.* New York: Basic Books.

Suchman, Edward A. (1965). "Social patterns of illness and medical care," *Journal of Health and Social Behavior* 6:2–16.

ADDITIONAL READINGS

American Hospital Association (1998). *Hospital Statistics.* Chicago: Healthcare InfoSource.

Stevens, Rosemary (1989). *In Sickness and Wealth: American Hospitals in the Twentieth Century.* New York: Basic Books.

INTERNET RESOURCES

American Hospital Association (AHA) homepage: www.aha.org.

American Medical Association (AMA) homepage: www.ama-assoc.org

Occupations and Professions in Healthcare

THE SOCIOLOGY OF OCCUPATIONS AND PROFESSIONS

The types of work people do and the occupations they pursue have profound effects upon all aspects of their lives. Their livelihood, their life chances (including their mental and physical health), their social and political views, their social standing (status), their family life and numerous other aspects of their lives are strongly influenced by their occupations. This is not surprising when we consider that for the average person work occupies the majority of his or her waking hours through most of their lives. Further, in contemporary U.S. society, our personal identities are tied inextricably to our work, and the perceptions others develop of us are shaped by the occupations we pursue. For that reason the first question we typically ask someone to whom we are introduced relates to where they work. The influence of our occupations on ours lives is made even more significant because of the central role of the economic institution in American society.

The character of the American labor force and the major changes taking place within it are of particular interest to sociologists. The factors affecting the healthcare occupational structure are topics of study for medical sociologists and there are many aspects of occupations that are of interest. People must obtain training, formal or informal, and acquire specific occupational skills for their jobs. They are socialized into specific occupations and many become members of occupational communities and learn to function within occupational cultures. They also must adapt to the organizations in which they are employed—learning the "corporate culture" and the expectations of the work groups within them. They also have to learn how to mediate between occupational demands and the demands of the other statuses they occupy.

The professions represent a special category in the study of occupations. There are certain unique characteristics associated with professions that distinguish them from ordinary occupations. Health professions represent a special case in that they involve a component of helping and caring not associated with other occupations. Professional occupations like healthcare often exert major control over other occupations.

The importance of occupational standing in the U.S. is reflected in the relative status accorded various professions. Society accords high prestige to occupations,—such as physicians, lawyers, and engineers— that require extensive training and generate high incomes. By contrast, less prestigious occupations—a waitress or janitor or hospital orderly, for example—not only pay less, but require fewer skills and less education. Occupational prestige ratings—as displayed in Table 7–1—are much the same in all industrial societies.

In any society, high-prestige occupations are accorded to privileged categories of people, and the highest-ranking occupations are typically dominated by men. Only after passing a dozen jobs on the prestige scale do we find "registered nurse", an occupation where most workers are women. Similarly, most low-prestige jobs are commonly performed by minority group members.

THE OCCUPATIONAL STRUCTURE OF HEALTHCARE

Relative to other occupations, the occupational history of healthcare is short. Until World War II, a handful of statuses accounted for virtually everyone who labored in the provision of health services. The doctor and nurse were the foundation of the occupational structure, supported on occasion by some other type of worker, perhaps a nursing assistant or laboratory technician. Generally, the doctor labored in isolation allowing for direct contact with the patient. There was little enough for

Table 7–1. Occupational Prestige Ranking for
the Highest Prestige Occupations in the U.S.

Occupation	Prestige score
Physician	86
Lawyer	75
College/university professor	74
Architect	73
Chemist	73
Physicist/astronomer	73
Aerospace engineer	72
Dentist	72
Clergyman	69
Psychologist	69
Pharmacist	68
Optometrist	67
Registered nurse	66
Secondary-school teacher	66
Accountant	65
Athlete	65
Electrical engineer	64
Elementary-school teacher	64
Economist	63
Veterinarian	62
Airplane pilot	61
Computer programmer	61
Sociologist	61
Editor/reporter	60
Police officer	60
Actor	58
Radio/TV announcer	55
Librarian	54
Aircraft mechanic	53
Firefighter	53
Dental hygienist	52
Painter/sculptor	52
Social worker	52
Electrician	51
Computer operator	50

SOURCE: National Opinion Research Center.

the doctor to do prior to World War II, much less for an assistant of any type.

The transformation of the occupational structure of healthcare into its modern configuration required a number of developments both inside and outside of healthcare. Outside of healthcare, the social environment had to change to create a context in which medicine in its modern form could flourish. Society members had to be willing to turn over the management of their health to a formal organization and develop a level of trust in its agents that had never existed in the past. On the cultural side, health as a value had to emerge to provide the motivation necessary to drive people to the doctor for care. Inside of healthcare, the institution had to demonstrate some level of success in dealing with sickness and that use of its practitioners was better than doing nothing at all. This required not only the development of modern therapeutic modalities but the reorganization of medical education in the United States.

None of these prerequisites were in place at the time of World War II, but many of the necessary supporting conditions rapidly appeared in the aftermath of the war. Formal institutions of all types were gaining ascendancy, and healthcare followed in their wake. Numerous breakthroughs in surgery and medicine, to a great extent initiated by wartime medicine, gave a new confidence to medical practitioners. Medical schools were upgraded, and student physicians actually had something of substance to learn. The nation went on a hospital building binge to make up for the lack of construction during the war. These new hospitals became "cathedrals" for the physician-priest caste that was evolving. The notion of "health" as a value in its own right, one that was worth aggressively pursuing, caused citizens to turn to the healthcare system as never before. And for the first time in U.S. history, most people had the discretionary income to spend on healthcare. These resources were soon supplemented by the widespread availability of health insurance.

These developments provided the foundation for the emergence of the modern healthcare occupational structure. The expansion and newfound acceptance of medical practitioners, coupled with expanding knowledge and biomedical technology, had a dramatic effect on the occupational component of the institution. Suddenly there was tremendous demand for the traditional health professionals as medical and nursing schools struggled to keep up with society's needs. Perhaps more important was the proliferation of new statuses in healthcare beginning in the 1960s. New therapeutic modalities and new technology, coupled with the increasing specialization characterizing healthcare, resulted in the creation of dozens of new occupations within the institution. Doctors and nurses were joined by therapists of all types and by the growing plethora of technicians to handle the rapidly expanding technology component of the healthcare system. The core occupations were joined by an army of paraprofessionals and allied health personnel to handle the ever-expanding responsibilities associated with the healthcare system.

The "medical imperialism" of the 1960s and 1970s led to the identification of more and more problems as "health problems" requiring the development of new occupations to address these conditions. The explosion in the mental health field during this period resulted in a whole new group of professionals devoted to the management of mental disorders.

Clinical personnel were needed to staff factories and schools as health professionals made incursions outside the walls of the hospital.

Two new categories of health workers emerged during the 1970s that further added complexity to the occupational structure. A class of health care administrators emerged to manage the increasingly bureaucratic operation of the system. The hospital came to be recognized for its "administrators" who were taking over responsibilities for management from clinicians, as the physician/administrator gave way to the professional administrator trained by formal hospital administration programs. As medical practices grew in size, they required managers and, as is the case with any institution undergoing formalization, a distinct administrator class evolved.

The other category of health worker that emerged during this period involved the "supportive" occupations. As hospitals became larger and more complex, they required a growing army of non-clinical personnel for their operation. The expanding facilities required physical plant managers, materials managers, medical records departments, and information technology support. They added restaurants, parking garages, and gift shops and these required staffing. The growing financial complexity of healthcare required the establishment of extensive financial management departments that could not only oversee finances but handle the increasingly complicated billing and collections activities associated with hospital care. The shift toward more of a business orientation also contributed to the need for more financial managers, accountants and lawyers.

By 2000, according to the Healthcare Resources and Services Administration (HRSA), there were over 200 different healthcare occupations and professions. Increasing from one million employees in 1970, the health sector now accounts for over 11 million U.S. workers and nine percent of the workforce. If health professionals working outside of healthcare settings are counted, healthcare accounts for 10.5% of the workforce. While the number of clinical and technical occupations in healthcare continued to grow during the last quarter of the twentieth century, the major growth occurred in non-clinical areas. Eventually, the numbers of health workers involved in patient care in the hospital were matched by the non-clinical staff. Thus, at the height of hospital utilization in the 1980s, hospitals that reported six employees per bed were likely to have three involved in-patient care and another three involved in non-patient-care activities.

HEALTH PROFESSIONS

An examination of the structure of the healthcare system requires a discussion of the personnel involved in the provision of care. The U.S. healthcare system is highly labor-intensive and involves millions of workers.

The healthcare sector, in fact, accounts for more employees than almost any other sector of the economy. The typical hospital has three or more employees per hospital bed, and there are enough physicians in practice to staff several hundred thousand clinics nationwide.

The complexity of the U.S. healthcare system is reflected in the proliferation of occupational roles, the levels and stages of care that are provided (along both vertical and horizontal continua), and the almost unlimited points at which a patient might enter the system. In terms of those who provide patient care, the key player is the physician. There were over 750,000 licensed physicians (including approximately 20,000 osteopaths) in active practice in the United States in 2000, most of whom are in direct patient care (National Center for Health Statistics, 2002, table 103). Most of this number were in office-based practices, with about one-fifth in hospital-based positions. About 16% are residents in training, and small segments of the physician pool are involved in research, teaching or administration.

Although not the largest occupational category in numerical terms, physicians constitute the key occupation in healthcare. For this reason, their characteristics are of great importance in determining the nature of the healthcare delivery system. The physician is considered the key player within the system because of the control he or she maintains over the utilization of health services. Only physicians are allowed to diagnose illness, perform most procedures, hospitalize patients, and prescribe drugs. It is the physician who determines what type and length of treatment is appropriate, when the patient should enter and leave the hospital, and what other types of specialists or services the patient needs.

Most office-based physicians are self-employed, even when part of a group practice. Some physicians are hospital based, and these are often employed by the hospital rather than practicing independently. Hospital-based physicians include specialists like radiologists, anesthesiologists, and pathologists, who generally do not have their own patients but provide related services such as x-ray interpretation or laboratory analysis. Many hospital-based physicians (e.g., radiologists, pathologists) practice under a contract with the hospital. Increasing numbers of patient care physicians are becoming employees of large physician groups, health maintenance organizations, and other corporate entities. In fact, the increasing "corporatization" of the providers of care is one of the major features of U.S. healthcare today. (See Box 7-1 for a discussion of the changing characteristics of physicians.)

Physicians are considered independent practitioners because they are licensed to practice without supervision or oversight. Other practitioners who, although less important in the system, are considered independent practitioners are chiropractors, optometrists, podiatrists, dentists, and some "marginal" practitioners such as mental health counselors. All other health workers are dependent upon physicians or these other providers in that they cannot act independently but only under the supervision of one of these. In fact, the dependent workers often cannot be paid for their services unless a physician "signs off" on them. The degree of independence of a practitioner is typically a reflection of the licensing practices of the particular state.

As of the 2000, approximately one-third of the physicians providing patient care were involved in primary care; this includes general and family practice, general internal medicine, obstetrics/gynecology, and pediatrics. These practitioners are considered primary because they usually serve as family doctors, are the initial point of entry into the system, and generally treat routine, less complex conditions. The remainder of the nation's physician pool is divided among 13 major specialties. Despite greater interest in "family medicine" in the 1980s and 1990s, and the trend toward increased specialization is only starting to abate. Changes in reimbursement, more than any other factor, have contributed to the beginning of a shift in training priorities away from the specialties and toward primary care.

By far the largest group of healthcare employees is registered nurses (RNs). In 1999 there were nearly 2.3 million employed RNs in the U.S. healthcare system. If the nearly 700,000 licensed practical nurses (LPNs) are included, the significance of this employment category becomes even greater. These are joined by nursing assistants and nurse's aides. Nurse practitioners—registered nurses with graduate training—have become more common and often perform some of the functions usually reserved for physicians.

Most nurses and related personnel are employed by hospitals, and some of these positions are found only within hospital settings. However, as the focal point for care has shifted to the outpatient arena, a growing proportion of nurses and other personnel have moved outside the hospital. In fact, the fastest growing health professions tend to be concentrated in outpatient settings.

The healthcare industry has periodically faced nurse shortages and the current situation appears to be the worst in history. The conditions surrounding the nursing profession have been widely studied by medical sociologists, and this situation represents a case study in the factors that constitute acceptable working conditions for professionals. The industry clearly has not historically addressed the needs of nurses, and there appears to be no obvious solution to the current nurse deficit. (See Box 7-2 on the nature of the nursing shortage.)

Physician assistants and other physician extenders (including nurse practitioners) have been introduced into the healthcare system over the past two decades. The intent has been to "extend" the capabilities of the physician through lesser trained mid-range medical professionals. For a variety of reasons, this level of care has never been well accepted by the medical community. It is likely, however, that the continued pressure from

--- Box 7-1 ---

The Changing Characteristics of American Physicians

The characteristics of the physician personnel pool in the United States changed significantly during the last two decades of the 20th century. Not only has the number of physicians and their distribution among specialties changed, but the demographic composition of this category of professionals has been radically modified. In 1960, there were fewer physicians in the United States per 100,000 population than there were in 1900. However, between 1960 and 2000, the number of physicians per 100,000 population increased from 150 to around 260. This represents a rate of growth much greater than that for the population as a whole. This increase in the physician pool was attributable partly to the establishment of new medical schools and growth in the size of medical school classes during the 1960s and 1970s. It was also attributable to a relaxing of immigration and eligibility policies that resulted in the influx of tens of thousands of foreign-trained physicians.

The change in the demographics of the physician pool have been equally dramatic. Once the almost exclusive province of upper middle-class white Anglo-Saxon males with close relatives who were physicians, the medical community has clearly taken on a different flavor. Between 1980 and 2000, the number of licensed physicians who were women increased by 360 percent, compared to 61 percent for males. In 2000, the proportion of licensed physicians that were female stood at over 24 percent, over twice the proportion recorded in 1980 (11%). Females accounted for 39% of the medical residents in 2000. African Americans who—at one time almost totally excluded from all except the few African American medical schools—still only accounted for around 5 percent by the late 1990s. Starting in the 1980s, medical students

managed care interests for the provision of care by lower level professionals along with other developments in healthcare, will further boost the interest in physician extenders.

Among the healthcare occupations tracked by the federal government, pharmacists account for the next largest group, accounting for 208,000 workers in 2000. They are followed by dentists, with 168,000 clinicians in the dental area practicing in 2000. Other occupations accounting for a significant number of health workers include physical therapists (144,000 in 2000), nutritionists/dieticians (97,000 in 2000) and speech therapists (97,000 in 2000) (National Center for Health Statistics, 2002, table 103).

An analysis of the distribution of healthcare *employees* (which excludes most physicians, dentists and other independent practitioners) finds that hospitals account for nearly half of health services employment. Thus,

were less likely to be drawn exclusively from science majors or to have come from affluent backgrounds that included physician relatives.

Because of the manner in which the physician pool increased, today's active practitioners are younger and more likely to be foreign born and/or educated. The grandfatherly family doctor is an endangered species, since the largest single age cohort of physicians is those 35–45 years of age (26%). Those under 35 accounted for 17 percent of the total in 2000, meaning that nearly half of practicing physicians were under 45.

Until the 1960s, the physician manpower pool included few non-Americans. Foreign physicians who did enter practice in this country came from the traditional bastions of medical education in England, Scotland, and Germany. The 1970s and 1980s witnessed the influx of tens of thousands of additional foreign physicians, a trend that only moderated slightly in the 1990s. Today, international medical graduates (IMGs) are more likely to originate from India, the Philippines, and different European countries; to them are added the new immigrant physicians from Iran, Southeast Asia, and Latin America. By 2000, international medical graduates in the U.S. totaled 197,000 out of a licensed physician pool of 813,000. IMGs accounted for 24 percent of active physicians in America in 2000

What are the implications of this new physician manpower pool—one that is more female, is younger, is more ethnic, and comes from different socioeconomic backgrounds? These new doctors have different priorities than the "good old boys" of the past. They are more likely to emphasize primary care and have helped resurrect the concept of the family doctor. They are less interested in big incomes and want security, stable working conditions, and time for their families. They are much more likely to become employed as physicians in clinics, health maintenance organizations, or other corporate settings. Finally, they bring a diversity—demographically and otherwise—to medical science that it has never experienced.

while the number of hospital encounters is much lower than office encounters, the intensity of hospital care calls for a higher ratio of staff to patients. (Thus, we find that hospitals average from three to six employees per bed.) The next largest group (more than 15 %) is found in nursing and personal care facilities. Again, while admission to these facilities is rare, they do require around-the-clock care with all that implies for staffing. Nearly as many personnel (13%) are employed in the offices and clinics of medical practitioners and, when dentists and certain other independent practitioners are included, this proportion increases to around 20 percent. The diversity of healthcare settings is indicated, however, by the fact that another 20 percent of health workers is spread over other sites.

The annual projections of growth in occupations published by the Bureau of Labor Statistics within the U.S. Department of Labor typically

———— *Box 7-2* ————

The Nursing Shortage: A Social Problem?

The U.S. healthcare system has periodically experienced shortages of qualified nursing personnel. Since the evolution of the modern health care system following World War II, the U.S. has undergone cycles of shortages and surpluses of nurses. As the demand for care would increase, nurse production would lag behind. Eventually, the system would react and step up production of nurses. Typically, by the time supply caught up with demand, the crisis had passed and a surplus would result.

Unlike most professions, the number of nurses trained far exceeds the number of nurses employed in healthcare. This fact reflects the historical vulnerability of an essentially all-female workforce to the demands of family life. More recently, the availability of opportunities in other fields has also contributed to the decline in the attractiveness of nursing as a profession.

At the beginning of the 21st century, the nursing shortage had reached unprecedented proportions, with hundreds of thousands of nursing positions in the U.S. going unfilled. And unlike previous periods of shortage, the system does not appear capable of remedying the problem. Nursing schools have been unable to make up for the gap through stepped up production, and, in any case, nursing school applications have leveled off. The traditional source of nursing personnel (i.e., educated, ambitious young women) is now seeking to take advantage of opportunities in other industries and other professions in healthcare. As a result, in 2002 the average age of active nurses was 47 years. Shortages are such that healthcare organizations—especially hospitals—must compete for a declining pool of qualified nurses. This has resulted in high personnel turnover, higher personnel costs, and severe understaffing at most hospitals.

In many ways, this situation represents more than a technical training issue. The existence of a severe (and now persistent) nursing shortage reflects social factors on at least two different levels. At the macro level, broad social trends have had an impact on the perceived desirability of nursing as an occupation for young women entering the labor force. The last quarter of the 20th century witnessed the opening up of numerous unprecedented job opportunities for women. More prestigious occupations offering more opportunity for advancement channeled qualified students away from what was increasingly considered a "technical"occupation relative to other job opportunities. At the same time, nursing salaries failed to keep pace with the overall salary structure.

At the micro level, other developments have affected the attractiveness of nursing as an occupation. The primary employers of nurses, hospitals, have probably contributed, however unwittingly, to the growing nursing shortage through their own actions. The conditions of employment of nurses have been criticized for decades by those inside and outside of nursing.

Hospitals, for the most part, have been unresponsive to concerns for better conditions of employment, and efforts by organized nursing to improve these conditions have met with limited success.

From the hospital's perspective, nurses are hourly laborers who can be assigned to units and shifts at the convenience of the hospital. They are not expected to contribute to the planning or administration of the facility, despite the fact that they provide the bulk of the care provided and increasingly are trained at the master's level.

The structural subordination of nurses relative to both physicians and hospital bureaucracies has worked severely against the economic interests of nurses. Employers of nurses try to keep wages low and to maximize the labor they can extract for those wages. Relative to other professions with comparable years of training, hospital nurses experience several important occupational disadvantages: unfavorable hours and shift work, high stress, and little opportunity for advancement in status or pay. In fact, the maximum average salary for nurses is only around 36 percent higher than the average starting salary, whereas other professionals can expect to double or triple their salaries before reaching the upper limit.

Most idealistic nurses find they have been given significant responsibility with little authority. At the same time, they feel like they are not allowed the latitude to practice care in the manner in which they were trained. Now, with chronic shortages of nurses, the historically high stress level for nurses has further increased.

The abuse of nurses by physicians is legendary. Nurses are treated for the most part like hired hands by physicians (despite the fact that nurses are employees of the hospital and not the physicians). The role of nurses in patient care is belittled by physicians and their input, even if sometimes grudgingly accepted, is seldom recognized. Adequate or even excellent levels of performance are seldom noted but mistakes—real or imagined—are always reported. The chronic tension between nurses and physicians only adds to the stressful relationship that exists between nurses and administrative staff.

While financial incentives are important to nurses, study after study has found that money is not adequate incentive for improving performance and loyalty. Today's nurses want responsibility and authority commensurate with their training. They want more autonomy in the management of patients and input into the operation of their unit. They want to be treated with respect and with the degree of professionalism their training demands.

Ultimately, the changes required to restore nursing to an attractive position as an occupation have less to due with financial and technical aspects than they do with social factors. While improvements in the structural aspects of employment (e.g., wages, hours, benefits) are important, social factors such as the attachment of value to the role of nurse, respect from physicians and administrators, participation in planning and administration, and the freedom to provide care as they see appropriate are even more important.

Table 7–2. Projected Fastest Growing Occupations in the U.S. 1998–2008

Occupation	Projected growth rate
Computer engineers	108
Computer support specialists	102
Systems analysts	94
Database administrators	77
Desktop publishing specialists	73
Paralegals and legal assistants	62
Personal care and home health aides	58
Medical assistants	58
Social and human service assistants	53
Physician assistants	48
Data processing equipment repairers	47
Residential counselors	46
Electronic semiconducter processors	45
Medical records/health information technicians	44
Physical therapy assistants	44
Science/computer managers	43
Respiratory therapists	43
Dental assistants	42
Surgical technologists	42
Securities, commodities and financial services sales agents	41
Dental hygienists	41
Occupational therapy assistants and aides	40
Cardiovascular technologists and technicians	39
Correctional officers	39
Speech-language pathologists and audiologists	38
Social workers	37
Bill and account collectors	35
Ambulance drivers and attendants	35
Biological scientists	35
Occupational therapists	34

SOURCE: U.S. Department of Labor.

include numerous healthcare occupations among the fastest growing occupations and/or the occupations expected to require the most new re-
cruits. (Table 7–2 presents the most recent projections of the fastest growing
occupations.) The numbers and types of health professionals grew steadily
through the end of the twentieth century but during the 1980s and 1990s a
couple of new trends emerged.

Because of the financial retrenchment commencing in the early 1980s,
ways to save on the most expensive component of healthcare, personnel,
were sought. One solution was to substitute lower-level and less expensive personnel for higher-level staff. One ill-fated approach involved sub-
stituting LPNs for nurses in the care of patients. While this ploy was

unsuccessful, the numbers of highly trained personnel were reduced and their responsibilities spread among lower-level personnel.

The demands of managed care reinforced this trend as newly enacted policies called for patients to receive care from the lowest possible level of practitioner as long as adequate quality was maintained. Thus, optometrists were favored over ophthalmologists, psychologists over psychiatrists, nursing assistants over home health nurses, and primary care physicians over specialists. The trend toward expansion at the lower levels of the occupational structure were so marked by the 1990s that virtually all of the patient care occupations that were projected to grow rapidly were at the lower end of the spectrum. (See Table 7–2.) While moderate growth in demand was expected for physicians and nurses, dramatic growth was expected for nursing assistants, personal care assistants, physical therapy assistants, and social workers.

The other trend initiated in the 1980s was the shift in the setting of care from institutional to non-institutional settings. The wholesale discharge of mental patients from psychiatric hospitals and from the care of psychiatrists to community-based facilities and the care of psychologists and social workers in the 1970s was a preview of what was to occur in medical care during the 1980s. During that decade, there was a dramatic shift away from inpatient care to outpatient care. Hospital censuses declined and new ambulatory facilities could not be built fast enough to meet the demand. The number of hospital workers was reduced dramatically (from about six employees per bed to around three) and these displaced workers mostly took up residence in ambulatory care settings. Many functions of the hospital were replicated in outpatient settings, as urgent care centers served minor emergency needs, freestanding diagnostic centers took over hospital diagnostic functions, and ambulatory surgery centers captured a large share of the outpatient surgery business. Most of the growth in the healthcare labor pool was absorbed by the outpatient setting and very little by hospitals.

The shift from institutional care to non-institutional care did not stop with movement out of the hospitals. There was a shift in emphasis from specialty clinics to community-based facilities, from psychiatrists' offices to community mental health centers. There was a further shift from any type of facility to the home, as home healthcare and hospice services became increasingly common.

SOCIAL STRATIFICATION WITHIN HEALTHCARE

The occupational structure of healthcare in the U.S. is often depicted as a microcosm of the larger social system, particularly in terms of social stratification. In this sense, the healthcare occupational structure replicates the patterns of interaction between various groups in society. The racism, sexism and class discrimination that exists in society are reflected in the occupational structure of healthcare.

Historically, women and non-whites have held the lowest status positions in healthcare and white males have held the highest. The medical staff and hospital administration were dominated by white males with little opportunity for women or minority group members to break in. The medical community has been the epitome of the "old boy" network. The educational system historically reinforced the stratification within healthcare by encouraging girls to become nurses and boys to become doctors. The educational pathways made available routed minority group members away from healthcare and into other "technical" trades.

At the beginning of the twenty-first century, white males still predominate among physicians, white females among nurses, and minority group members among the lowest level healthcare jobs. However, this situation has been undergoing a dramatic shift. Females are beginning to become a numerical majority in medical school and their numbers among practicing physicians have increased dramatically over the past two decades. The number of women also has increased significantly among the rolls of healthcare administrators. African-Americans, Hispanics and Asian-Americans have achieved more than "token" status among both medical staffs and hospital administrators. International medical graduates—physicians who received their M.D. degrees outside the United States—have gained grudging acceptance by the medical community (after long being accepted by patients). (See Box 7-3 for a discussion of the role of international medical graduates.)

Despite these changes, much of the traditional power structure remains in place, with women and minority group members continuing to face limitations on their ability to advance. This situation has been perpetuated through the recruitment processes of the various occupations and professions in healthcare. While medical students are no longer drawn almost exclusively from the upper strata of society, they still reflect an upper-middle class ancestry. Nurses continue to be drawn from working class or middle class segments of society, and lower-level personnel are drawn from the working class and lowest income groups. Low SES individuals may escape the community to become a hospital orderly but few make it as hospital administrators. Few people from upper-middle-class backgrounds are recruited for the low level positions in health care.

All of these factors have combined to create a rigid occupational structure in healthcare. An occasional hospital administrator may work himself up from the mailroom, but that is rare given the professionalization of hospital administration. On the clinical side, there is virtually no opportunity for crossing stratum boundaries and, even within a stratum such as nursing, there are likely to be rigid lines between, say registered nurses and nursing assistants.

THE SOCIOLOGY OF THE PHYSICIAN

Although doctors constitute less than 10 percent of the total healthcare workforce in the United States, they maintain disproportionate influence over the operation of the system. Physicians generally control the conditions of their own work and the work of most of the other members of the health professions as well. Consequently, the status and prestige accorded to the physician by the general public is recognition of the physician's expertise concerning one of society's most essential functions. Further, by maintaining control over diagnosis, the ordering of tests, hospital admission and discharge, and drug prescribing, physicians extend their influence far beyond their direct participation in care. The social importance of the medical function and the limited number of people with the training as physicians go a long way toward explaining their professional dominance.

A particularly important factor in physician domination is the organization of the medical profession itself. William Goode (1956, 1960) noted that two basic characteristics are sociologically relevant in explaining professionalism: prolonged training in a body of specialized, abstract knowledge and a commitment to service. Once a professional group becomes established, it begins to enhance its power by formalizing social relationships that govern the interaction of the professionals with their clients, their colleagues, and official agencies outside the profession. Recognition on the part of clients, outside agencies, and the wider society of the profession's claim to competence, as well as the profession's ability to control its own membership, is necessary to prevent outside authorities from reviewing professional decisions.

Professions have the following characteristics:

- A profession determines its own standards of education and training.
- A student professional goes through a more stringent socialization experience than students in other occupations.
- Professional practice is often legally recognized by some form of license.
- Licensing and admission boards are staffed by members of the profession.
- Most legislation concerned with a profession is shaped by the profession.

Box 7-3

The Role of International Medical Graduates in the U.S. Healthcare System

A major controversy in American medicine relates to the participation of foreign-trained doctors in the U.S. healthcare system. Referred to as international medical graduates (IMGs), these doctors account for over 20% of the physicians practicing medicine in the United States today. This situation and the controversy that surrounds it has been scantily covered by the popular press, so that except for an occasional newspaper article, the average American knows little about this aspect of U.S. medical care. However, if one requires the services of an anesthesiologist, a psychiatrist, or certain other specialists, there is a good chance that the care will be provided by someone who went to medical school in another country.

In medical circles the continued influx of IMGs and the implications of their presence in American healthcare remain highly controversial issues. Organized medicine has always voiced concern over the quality of training that foreign physicians receive, contending that it does not meet American medical school standards. In the 1980s, with physicians facing increased competition for patients and revenue, the threat of additional competition from foreign-trained doctors led to attempts to limit immigration, introduce more difficult qualifying examinations, and preclude foreigners from specialty training and licensure.

Since World War II, IMGs have become an increasingly significant component of the U.S. physician pool. At present, over 120,000 IMGs are in practice in this country. Another 17,000 IMGs are annually enrolled in residency training programs at various hospitals and other health care facilities. An undetermined number of IMGs (possibly in the tens of thousands) are in this country attempting to obtain residency positions or licenses to practice. Most of these are "alien IMGs," who are typically citizens of foreign countries who have received their basic training (i.e., the M.D. degree) in their homelands and subsequently immigrated to the United States for specialty training and, for most, the establishment of practices. Some are "U.S. IMGs," American citizens who have received medical school training overseas and subsequently returned to the U.S. for residency training. Some of these have been educated at long-established medical schools in Europe; most, however, have attended newly created medical schools in the Caribbean or Mexico. The numbers of U.S. IMGs, however, remain small compared to alien IMGs.

In the United States and in most other countries, individuals enter medical school with an undergraduate degree. The medical school curriculum includes approximately two years of basic science training, followed by two years of clerkship. These third and fourth years are spent essentially as apprentices, with students rotating through various clinical departments in addition to attending classes. At the end of this program, ranging from three and one-half to five years, medical students are awarded an M.D. degree.

In the United States, at least two years of postgraduate or residency training are required for licensure. While in residency training, physicians provide much of the charity care that is offered and staff hospital emergency rooms. Thus, in today's medicine the actual training in patient care takes place primarily during the residency program.

Although there has been some influx of IMGs into the United States throughout this century, the size of the current pool is primarily the result of national policies formulated during the 1960s. At that time, it was widely held that a severe physician shortage existed. Measures were taken to facilitate the immigration of IMGs to fill the gap until an adequate supply of American-trained physicians could be established. These policies resulted in an influx of large numbers of IMGs, with several thousand entering practice annually from the early 1970s to the present. By the mid-1970s, however, concerns over a shortage were replaced by fears of a physician surplus. The number of domestically trained physicians had increased dramatically, and large numbers of alien physicians had been added to the physician pool. In response to these developments, immigration policies were made more restrictive, and more difficult qualifying examinations were introduced for IMGs. Both formal and informal measures were introduced to discourage entry of IMGs into training and practice, and legislation was proposed to limit the entry of U.S. IMGs into the market.

During the 1970s and 1980s, the circumstances under which immigration occurred changed significantly. Previously, immigrant physicians entered under temporary visas, and most returned to their homelands. By the 1970s, however, the majority of IMGs were seeking permanent immigration status with the intention of practicing medicine in this country. The earlier immigrants typically entered by means of a formal exchange program, while the later ones were more likely to obtain entry though a nonmedical status, such as tourist, student, family reunification, or even refugee. Even those who entered on a temporary exchange basis often subsequently petitioned for a change of status once here. During the late 1970s, this flow was augmented by thousands of U.S. IMGs.

The changing basis for admission was accompanied by a change in the national origin of the IMGs. This, perhaps, contributed to the controversy as much as issues of quality and competition. In the years immediately following World War II, the typical physician-immigrant was from Europe. However, by the late 1960s, the influx was dominated by Asian immigrants, particularly those from India and the Philippines. While both of these groups continue to be important, they have been joined by large numbers of physicians from Southeast Asia and the Middle East. By the 1980s, increasing numbers of immigrant-physicians were arriving from Latin America. Many of these newer immigrants entered as refugees, often without complete documentation of their medical background.

There are numerous subissues involved here that relate to testing, training requirements, licensure requirements, and even the issue of

(*continued*)

discrimination, which is currently being explored by the legal system. What is important to focus on for this brief discussion is the significance of physician-immigrants for the U.S. healthcare system. Opponents of IMGs argue that foreign-trained physicians are less qualified to provide care than American-trained physicians. They are increasingly arguing that they are contributing to a physician oversupply and causing unnecessary competition. These opponents are primarily representatives of organized medicine—presenting the view of medical schools, specialty associations, and practicing physicians—that have a vested interest in limiting physician supply.

On the other hand, IMGs and their supporters contend that foreign-trained physicians have historically made important contributions to U.S. medical teaching, research, and practice. There is evidence that IMGs enter

- As a profession gains income, power, and prestige, it can demand high-caliber students.
- The practitioner is relatively free of lay evaluation and control.
- Members are strongly identified by their profession.

The professionalization of medicine would not have been possible without control over the standards for medical education (Stevens 1971). By the mid-1920s, the medical profession had consolidated its professional position to the point that it clearly had become the model for professionalism. The medical profession had not only met the basic criteria of being a service occupation supported by prolonged training in specialized knowledge, it had established its own standards for education and training, successfully demanded high-caliber students, staffed its own licensing and admission boards, shaped legislation in its own interests, developed stringent professional standards, and insulated itself from formal lay evaluation and control (Cockerham, 2001).

PROFESSIONAL SOCIALIZATION

One of the most important aspects of socialization of interest to medical sociologists involves the professional socialization of physicians and other health personnel. The training offered would-be physicians, nurses and other health personnel involves both an objective and a subjective component. Extensive classroom training and clinical exposure provide the "content" component of the socialization process. Observation and imitation of mentors and established practitioners provide the "attitude" component of the process. (See Box 7-4 for an overview of the socialization process.)

specialty areas that are considered undesirable by domestic medical school graduates. Further, they are found to practice in areas (such as inner cities and rural communities) in which American-trained physicians are reluctant to practice. Many residency programs contend that IMGs are essential for the provision of care to their indigent patients, particularly in inner-city hospitals that are not attractive to U.S. medical school graduates.

Regardless of the merits of the above arguments, one fact is clear. IMGs will continue to be a major factor in U.S. medical care for the foreseeable future. Each year thousands of IMGs enter practice, despite increasing restrictions. The estimated tens of thousands who are in "limbo" seeking training and practice opportunities must be dealt with. Regardless of one's perspective on international medical graduates, a significant portion of the care received by American patients will be provided by IMGs.

Medical school didactic training involves the acquisition of knowledge in the basic sciences and in the techniques employed in the practice of medicine. Basic medical science studies consist of courses in anatomy, biochemistry, physiology, pathology, pharmacology, microbiology, physical diagnosis, clinical laboratory procedures, and often behavioral science. The clinical programs focus on the application of basic medical science in solving clinical problems by working with patients under the supervision of the faculty. The students also rotate through clerkships in various medical services, such as medicine, surgery, pediatrics, obstetrics-gynecology, psychiatry and other specialties. Included in this process is the internalization of ethical and moral principles that are essential if the physician is to be trusted by patients, colleagues, and the community and is to maintain his or her professional status (Cockerham, 2001).

Sociologists frequently speak of "anticipatory" socialization, or training in advance of expected future roles. An example of this anticipatory socialization can be seen in the play of children, as American children play "house" or children in traditional societies play at "hunting". While the family and other informal agents of socialization provide some anticipatory training, this job falls primarily to more formal agents of socialization— the schools and work groups. The task of preparing future workers for the economic system begins in elementary school by instilling values of hard work, punctuality, and obedience to authority. Higher education, while often touted as a value in its own right, is designed to prepare students for future employment if not teach job skills outright.

Professional schools such as medical schools are established with the intention of teaching the skills required for a future vocation. Their curricula are geared toward instilling the knowledge, skills and values that will prepare physicians, dentists and other health professionals for their future occupations. In medical school, this involves classroom instruction

---

Box 7-4

The Role of the Socialization Process in Society

Sociologists contend that humans come into the world as a "blank slate", unformed as human beings and susceptible to imprinting by society. Unlike other species whose behavior is biologically set, humans need "training" in order to learn about their culture and acquire the necessary tools for survival. The training that human infants undergo in order to become participating members of society is referred to as "socialization".

The socialization process begins at birth and usually continues throughout one's lifetime. Initially, the infant is taught the basics of social interaction through this process. Later the family and other agents of socialization teach the child how to relate to the outside world. Formal agents of socialization such as schools provide more advanced training, and work groups introduce the worker to the skills necessary to not only do the job but to survive in the particular work environment. Outside of these formal contexts, family, friends, and associates continue the socialization process throughout life.

This process serves to create a "group animal" out of this as-yet-undeveloped creature, introducing the process of social interaction and teaching the basic skills for participating in group life. This not only involves learning how to act appropriately in social settings but the importance of taking others into consideration. Newborn babies are of necessity self-centered, and this natural disposition must be tempered through socialization to allow for the feelings and interests of others to emerge. The socialization process also serves to instill a degree of conformity of behavior within the new society member. The efficient functioning of society requires a high level of conformity to the rules of that society, and other society members expect the new member to act in a predictable manner.

The socialization process, within the family and in other settings as well, utilizes two means of training. One might be thought of as direct admonition, or the direct teaching of cultural patterns. During informal training this would include the admonishments of parents to do this but don't do that—the "shalts" and "shalt nots" of behavior. Sometimes these admonitions are codified into specific rules, but most of the time members of the

---

and "on the job" training through clinical rotations and subsequent resident training. In addition to information transfer, medical students are also inculcated with the values appropriate for medical practitioners. These come not through classroom lecture but through observation and imitation of professional referents in the form of medical school faculty and practicing physicians.

Professionalism in American medicine has resulted in at least three undesirable consequences (Rasmussen 1975). First, it has fostered the

socializing group admonish the new society member as the situation arises. Rules might be useful in situations where the circumstances are foreseeable; for example, "Wash your hands before every meal". In other cases, the circumstances might be unpredictable and the parent might have to suddenly warn: "Don't touch that stove!" In either case, much of what we learn comes through direction admonition on the part of the agents of socialization.

The second means of demonstrating appropriate behavior is by example. In fact, it is argued that much more is learned though imitation than through direct admonition. By imitating the behavior of those around them, fledgling society members begin to take on the behavior patterns of the social group. Imitation does not end with childhood socialization, however, and much of the "attitude" that is developed by physicians in training, for example, results not from direct admonition but from observation and imitation. Indeed, attitudes are seldom taught but result from observing the attitudes and behavior of others. The socialization that takes place within the family is not all deliberate. Children learn from the kind of environment that adults create. How children learn to see themselves and whether they see the world as trustworthy or dangerous, largely depends on their surroundings.

Adult socialization continues the process began with the child. Adult socialization generally serves to reinforce and refine the training provided to children. At the same time, the teachings from childhood socialization may be modified or even contradicted for adults. The university and the employer become the new formal agents of socialization. Informal socialization is carried out by work groups and friendship groups. Earlier agents of socialization such as the family and the church group may continue to hold some influence but, many Americans physically move away from these childhood influences early in life.

Individuals in U.S. society are faced with a variety of often competing agents of socialization, perhaps more so than any other society. Other spheres of life beyond family, school, peer group, and the media also play a part in socialization. For most people in the United States, these include religious organizations, the workplace, the military, and various social clubs. As a result of these varying influences, socialization may offer inconsistent or conflicting viewpoints as the society members are bombarded with different information from different sources.

development of a view of disease that is largely confined to specific organs and physiological systems but that fails to consider a more holistic view of patients as people. This conflicts directly with a wide spectrum of disorders related to problems of living rather than to specific biochemical and physical abnormalities of the body. Second, professionalism has led to the development of a highly rigid stratification system in medical practice that has promoted an increasingly large gap between physicians and non-physician medical personnel. And for certain functions the non-physician health worker may have a more important service to provide the patient than the physician (Cockerham, 2001).

Third, professionalism has resulted in the separation of professional training so that a common educational base is lacking between physicians and paraprofessionals that might allow a healthcare team to work more effectively as a cohesive group. Further, while the healthcare needs of American society are those of the early twenty-first century, organized medicine continues to pursue a pattern of professional behavior based upon the image of medical practice in the early twentieth century when the physician worked on a solo basis as an independent, fee-for-service practitioner (Cockerham, 2001).

Increased consumerism on the part of patients and greater government and corporate control over medical practice indicate that the professional authority of physicians is in a state of decline. Doctors are moving from being the absolute authority in medical matters toward a state of lessened authority and the requirement to share authority with other parties. With many patients insisting on greater equality in the doctor-patient relationship and health organizations that employ doctors seeking to control costs, maximize profits, and provide efficient services that are responsive to market demand, physicians continue to face a loss of power (Cockerham, 2001).

Ritzer and Walczak (1988) indicate that medical doctors toward the end of the last century began experiencing a process of "deprofessionalism" as a result of these developments in healthcare. They define the process as "a decline in power which results in a decline in the degree to which the professions possess, or are perceived to possess, the constellation of characteristics denoting a profession" (1988:6). Deprofessionalization essentially means a decline in a profession's autonomy and control over clients. In the case of physicians, they still retain the inordinate authority in medical affairs but that authority is no longer absolute, and medical work is subject to greater scrutiny by patients, healthcare organizations, and government agencies. The result is that greater external control over physicians by the government and corporations now exists, there by lessening the professional power and authority of doctors. The pressure on physicians from below (consumers) and above (government and corporate medicine) forecasts a decline in their professional dominance. Doctors are still powerful in health matters but not to the extent they were for most of the second half of the twentieth century.

One other dimension of socialization that should be mentioned is the "resocialization" process. For various reasons, society members may require resocialization. This may be voluntary as in a career change or imposed by an agent of society such as a mental hospital. Resocialization involves the retraining of individuals through modification of earlier socialization or replacement of existing patterns with new, more appropriate (in someone's mind) behavior patterns, values and attitudes. The resocialization process may be relatively mild and only affect certain aspects of the individual's persona. This might occur, say, when a nurse leaves a job at a physician's clinic to work as a floor nurse in a hospital, or when a hospital executive leaves a not-for-profit health facility to work for a for-profit hospital chain. These changes are likely to require some resocialization but even here it is likely to be limited to the work environment.

Resocialization is utilized in healthcare for a variety of purposes. On a basic level, individuals undergoing rehabilitation after amputation, paralysis or some other traumatic experience must be retrained to operate with their new limitations. More extensive resocialization is involved in drug and alcohol rehabilitation programs and in the operation of psychiatric facilities. In the case of drug and alcohol abuse treatment, resocialization is fairly extensive in that it attempts to not only discourage the abuse of substances but a modification of lifestyle in order to eliminate the factors that contributed to the situation in the first place. This may involve cutting ties with friends (and perhaps families in some cases), adopting new behavior patterns, and even moving to a different community. Thus, the resocialization process serves to reduce the opportunities for relapse to the extent possible.

Participants in the healthcare system—whether patients, physicians, or hospital administrators—are socialized by their society and this process is reflected in the their attitudes and behavior. The socialization of health professionals—especially physicians—represents an area of particular interest. Health professionals are expected to have certain attributes beyond their clinical skills, and even individuals in lower-level healthcare occupations are presumed to have some of these traits of service and caring. These skills and traits are inculcated during the socialization process.

The socialization of the physician has been studied a great deal over the years. To understand how the physician is socialized into the profession, it is important also to consider the manner in which physicians are selected and trained as medical professionals. The process actually begins prior to acceptance into medical school, since most medical students in the past came from families that featured one or more physician members offering early opportunities for anticipatory socialization. The courses taken in the undergraduate pre-medical curriculum and the counseling received as an undergraduate initiate the process. Thus, formal medical this training was not the first exposure to medical practice for these students. Even the process of being accepted to medical school contributes subtly by indicating to the student that he or she has what it takes to become a doctor.

A study of the medical education process shows that both the structure of medical training and professional ideology work against the development of humanistic doctor-patient relationships. New physicians are taught to avoid interaction with patients, to restrict time spent with them, and to limit the patient input they listen to in medical interviews (Mizrahi, 1986: 118–119). This study concluded that the very structure of internship and residency experiences teaches doctors to avoid non-interesting patients. Interns and residents, for example, were informally rewarded for quickly and efficiently taking patient histories, and they learned not to bother with inquiring about social aspects of the cases because there were no incentives for doing so.

Medical students learn, formally and informally from their professors and supervisors to narrow their clinical findings to biophysical data relevant to possible pathology. These attitudes reflect the medical model's separation of the disease from the socio-emotional aspects of the patient's illness; doctors are socialized to view the non-biophysical aspects as "fuzzy", "soft" facts that are ultimately irrelevant to their essential task (Freund and McGuire, 1999).

Although traditionally beyond the influence of the non-medical world, a number of factors inside and outside of healthcare are having an impact on the physician socialization process. The socialization process for doctors is slowly changing as medical education adjusts to the new realities of medical practice. These include the shift in orientation from an emphasis on medical care to one on healthcare, with all that implies in regard to doctor/patient relationships. The importance of "bedside manner" is being revisited, and research has demonstrated the therapeutic benefits of treating the patient like a person and involving the family in the treatment process.

The push to take a more "business-like" approach to the practice of medicine and the influence of managed care organizations and other corporations that employ physicians are also factors. The changing characteristics of physicians themselves are playing a role, as less and less medical students are drawn from the traditional pool. From a more practical perspective, experience with malpractice suits has found that quality relationships with patients is a protection against malpractice claims. These transformations in the medical education environment have been hard won in the face of the traditional conservatism of medicine.

THE EMERGENCE OF ALTERNATIVE THERAPISTS

By the 1990s, it was clear that Americans were increasingly turning to "alternative therapists" for a large portion of their healthcare. Alternative therapies have been "officially" labeled "complementary and alternative medicine" (CAM) by the National Institutes of Health (NIH). According to NIH, complementary and alternative medicine is a broad domain of healing resources that encompasses all health systems, modalities, and practices and their accompanying theories and beliefs, other than those intrinsic in the politically dominant health system of a particular society or culture in a given historic period.

The categorization of these therapies as "alternative" is problematic in that the term implies non-standard or marginal care. However, what allopathic physicians might consider "alternative" is often the mainstream form of care in some other society. Some of these therapies are alternative in the sense that they might be utilized in place of conventional Western medicine. They could be considered "complementary" as well, in that many are utilized as adjuncts to standard medical treatment.

The array of complementary therapies is vast, unsystematized, and largely unregulated. Nonetheless, these treatments carry a widening appeal and, especially in the face of chronic illness, merit investigation by both consumers and medical professionals. Traditional approaches can address quality of life and prevention of opportunistic infections, as well as relieve end-of-life suffering. Perhaps most importantly, they usually involve a quality of interaction between caregiver and client that is emotionally satisfying to both, and which engages people in their own care. Patients who are actively involved in their healing often enjoy better outcomes.

Whereas conventional physicians reduce the body to separate components attended to by specialists (reductionist philosophy), traditional therapists typically address the entirety of a person's being (holistic philosophy). A complementary therapist is a specialist in taking care of a whole person with a particular technique (such as reflexology or homeopathy) or system of techniques (such as Traditional Chinese Medicine and Ayurveda). Strictly speaking, holistic therapies do not address side effects or specific symptoms separate from the whole person. Two people may have identical symptoms for different reasons. Each person is evaluated and treated as an individual.

Holistic therapy extends into the person's environment and relationships, including that between practitioner/teacher and client/student. In evaluating a client's nutrition, for example, a nutrition specialist would limit his attention to what the client is eating. By contrast, a truly holistic practitioner would also discuss how, when and with whom—the entire emotional/social/spiritual climate of nurturance. Holistic practitioners of any modality value the quality of the practitioner/client relationship as a powerful ally in healing. Such a relationship expects the practitioner and client to work together toward a common goal, empowering the patient as co-healer. Being a holistic practitioner is as much about manner as modalities.

In modern Western societies, people may use alternative healing systems simultaneously with biomedicine. A study of middle-class Americans who used certain alternative healing approaches (e.g., Christian faith healing, psychic healing, and Eastern or occult healing) found that virtually all adherents used both biomedical and alternative systems (McGuire, 1988). Furthermore, their beliefs shaped how they combined these various approaches. Adherents of the various alternative healing approaches felt that medical doctors were not necessarily the best source of help for such problems as chronic pain and illness, because they treat the symptoms, not the cause. These adherents believed that the "real" causes of such illnesses were spiritual (or the socioemotional by-products of spiritual problems). Thus, by definition, modern medicine alone was not a sufficient source of help (McGuire, 1988).

Probably the best-known alternatives in the United States are chiropractic and osteopathy, therapeutic systems based on the idea that misalignments of the musculoskeletal system also produce problems in the neuro-endocrine system. Osteopathy has become largely subordinated within regular (allopathic) medical practice and licensing. Until the 1980s, chiropractic was actively suppressed by the AMA through licensing legislation. Chiropractic treatment has gained greater legitimacy and recognition is now covered by much health insurance. It is still viewed by many medical practitioners as an unacceptable alternative to treatment by a medical doctor.

Homeopathy, a holistic form of pharmacological therapeutics developed in the early nineteenth century, is now more common in Europe and Latin America than in the United States. In England, for example, homeopathic physicians are licensed to practice and are reimbursed under the National Health Service. The homeopathic movement also encourages laypersons to self-treat certain illnesses and to learn to use some of the homeopathic medicines.

Some traditional Asian medical practices have recently been introduced into Western societies. The paradigms of illness and healing of such therapies as acupressure, acupuncture, and Asian herbal medicine are very different from those of Western biomedicine. Acupressure, or shiatsu, is generally administered like a massage, so it is not in direct competition with licensed medicine, but neither is it typically covered by medical insurance. Acupuncture, which involves the insertion of needles, is under tighter legal control. In most of the United States non-physician acupuncturists are required to work under the supervision of licensed doctors, although some states have made allowances for licensing non-physician acupuncturists (who, ironically, are often better trained as acupuncturists than physicians who took relatively brief training in the method).

Because these alternative medical systems are in direct competition with allopathic medicine, political and legal maneuvers regarding their practice have concrete economic effects. Like allopathic medicine, these alternative are organized as professional practices, with their own body of knowledge, training and certification standards, code of ethics, and organizations. Like biomedicine, they rely largely upon learned diagnostic and therapeutic techniques, which do not require the patient to understand or agree with the underlying paradigm in order to be effectively treated (Freund and McGuire, 1999).

There is another category of alternative therapists that should be mentioned, although they are not widely utilized by the general population. This is the category of folk or indigenous healers that are utilized by various ethnic groups. Immigrants from Latin American, African, and Asian countries often import traditional therapies when they enter the United States. Perhaps the most widely practiced system of this type involves the curanderos utilized by Mexican-Americans in the United States. These and other folk healers are frequently utilized for minor or routine conditions that affect these ethnic populations. Modern Western medicine might be utilized for more serious conditions. The healers in these systems typically do not take on the characteristics of a separate occupation.

Faith healers are also found among certain "native" subcultures in the United States such as in Appalachia and other rural communities. These healers pursue a therapeutic regimen rooted in religion and often rely upon the healing powers to the supernatural rather than more secular therapies. They vary in the extent to which these cult-like healing systems coexist with conventional medicine. More so than the folk healers, a separate formal status for healers is rare in these systems.

OCCUPATION, HEALTH STATUS, AND HEALTH BEHAVIOR

Medical sociologists have documented a strong relationship between occupation and health status. Occupation can be examined in terms of occupational status (e.g., blue-collar, white-collar, professional) or in terms of specific occupations. In the first case, there is a relatively direct and positive relationship between the relative importance of the occupation one holds and health status. In general, the higher the occupational prestige, the better the health status. Those at lower occupational levels tend to be characterized by higher rates of morbidity and disability. Like the poor and the uneducated, they tend to be characterized both by more health problems and by more serious conditions. Levels of disability (as measured by restricted-activity days and lost days from work and school) are higher for lower occupational levels as well (Marmot et al. 1991).

At the same time, mortality rates and longevity vary directly with occupational status. Past research has consistently found a clear link between mortality and occupational status, with age-standardized death rates for the lowest occupational group (unskilled laborers) being considerably higher than those of the highest (professionals). Recent research (Rogers et al. 2000) has reaffirmed this finding, showing mortality rates for those with the lowest occupational status to be considerably higher than those for the highest. The causes of death for those lower in terms of occupational status are similar to those for the poor and uneducated noted above.

A second approach to examining the relationship between the conditions of employment and health status involves an analysis of health status in terms of specific industries and occupations. Although this is a highly complex process, it is found that certain industries tend to be characterized by inordinately high levels of both morbidity and mortality. Among the standard industry categories utilized by the Department of Labor, the industry with the highest rate of injuries involving work loss is the transportation/communications/utilities industry. In 2000, the mining industry reported the highest rates or occupational injuries, followed closely by the manufacturing and construction industries. This contrasts vividly with the "safest" industry (finance, insurance and real estate) that reported an occupational injury rate of less than one per 100,000 workers (National Center for Health Statistics, 2002, table 50).

A similar pattern was found for occupation-related deaths. In 2000 the highest rate of occupational injury deaths was recorded for mining, with 30 deaths per 100,000 workers. This was followed by agriculture, forestry and fishing was a rate of 21 per 100,000. This compares to the finance, insurance and real estate industry which recorded an occupational injury death rate of less than one per 100,000.

High-morbidity occupations often include those whose workers are exposed to environmental risks. Similar patterns have been identified for mortality, although the occupations most affected may be different. The single most dangerous occupation is fisherman, followed by lumberjacks and airplane pilots.

Researchers on this issue have been successful at establishing that both prevalence and types of disorders may be to a certain extent occupation specific. Based on data from treatment records, self-reports, and even suicide records, it has been determined that certain occupations carry varying risks of mental disorder.

One other consideration when examining occupational categories is the issue of employment status. This issue may, in fact, be more significant than occupational differentials. When the employed are compared to the unemployed, clear-cut differences surface in terms of physical and mental illness. The unemployed appear to be sicker in terms of most health status indicators; they have higher levels of morbidity and higher levels of disability than the employed. While it could be argued that poor health leads to unemployment, it has been found that otherwise healthy individuals who have undergone loss of employment often develop symptoms of health problems (Catalano, 1991). In fact, even perceived threats to job security have been found to be associated with an increase in morbidity (Ferrie, 1998). It has also been suggested that, among those who cannot find employment, developing an illness serves as something of a rationale for a failure to find work.

Apart from evidence linking unemployment to high suicide rates, little research has been conducted on the relationship between the lack of employment and mortality. However, the recent work by Rogers et al. (2000) has demonstrated that the employed tend to have a lower risk of mortality than the unemployed. Interestingly, the analysis also found that individuals who were not in the labor force (i.e., neither employed nor looking for employment) were at the greatest risk of mortality of all employment statuses.

The same pattern holds for employment status and mental illness. The unemployed tend to be characterized by higher levels of mental illness symptoms than the employed. In fact, for both physical and mental disorders, it has been suggested that the lack of social integration resulting from unemployment serves as a "trigger" for various health problems.

Occupational status is related not only to levels of service utilization but to the types of services utilized and the circumstances under which they are received. This is true whether the indicator is for inpatient care, outpatient care, tests and procedures performed, or virtually any other measure of utilization.

To a limited extent, the use of health services by members of the various occupational status categories corresponds with the differentials in health status identified. In general, those in higher occupational categories require fewer health services because they are healthier. Yet, they utilize more of certain types of services because they are more aware of the need for preventive care and tend to have better insurance coverage. The higher occupational groups have somewhat higher hospital admission rates.

The lower-status occupational categories make up for any differences in admissions by recording more patient days. Some differences are found in the use of other types of facilities on the basis of occupational status. Income and educational levels no doubt play a role here, and the type of insurance coverage available (which is primarily a function of employment status) is important in the type of service utilized.

Some differences related to occupational status exist in the utilization of physician services. Despite the higher incidence of health problems among the lower occupational statuses, these individuals tend to use physicians, dentists and other health professionals less often than higher occupational groups.

Some selectivity does occur with regard to certain health professionals. While those in lower-status occupations utilize less outpatient mental health services than those at higher statuses, despite greater identified need, the counselor of choice is seldom a psychiatrist. Less formal sources, such as social workers or clergymen, are likely to be utilized. Here, as above, income, education, and insurance coverage play an important role in the use of physician services.

Differences in sickness behavior based on employment status are probably greater than those among the various occupational categories. When the employed and unemployed are compared, the employed have significantly higher admission rates, despite the greater level of morbidity identified for the unemployed. The unemployed, in fact, use less of all types of health services. The only exception might be higher use of hospital emergency rooms and public health facilities. The primary explanation for this differential, of course, is the lack of insurance on the part of the unemployed.

There are several reasons for the close association between occupation and sickness behavior in its various forms. Different levels of morbidity are associated with each occupational status category, resulting in demands for differing levels and types of services. An important factor related to occupational status is its implications for lifestyle. Because of the importance of the economic system in U.S. society, occupation becomes a key factor in the shaping of the individual's worldview. The attitudes and perceptions components of lifestyles, as well as values, vary with occupational status.

REFERENCES

Albrecht, Gary L, and Judith A. Levy (1982). "The professionalization of osteopathy: Adaptation in the medical marketplace," *Research in the Sociology of Health Care* 2:161–202.

Catalano, Ralph (1991). "The Health Effects of Economic Insecurity," *American Journal of Public Health* 81(9): 1148–1152.

Cockerham, William C. (2001). *Medical Sociology* (8th edition). Upper Saddle River, NJ: Prentice Hall.

Ferrie, J.E., Shipley, M.J., Marmot, M.G., Stansfeld, S.A., and J.D. Smith (1998). "An uncertain future: The health effects of threats of employment security in white-collar men and women," *American Journal of Public Health* 88(7):1030–1036.

Freund, Peter E.S., and Meredith B. McGuire (1999). *Health, Illness and the Social Body*, 3rd ed. Englewood Cliffs, NJ: Prentice Hall.

Goode, William J. (1960). "Encroachment, Charlatanism, and the Emerging Professions," *American Sociological Review*, 24:38–47.

Marmot, M.G., Davey Smith, G., Stansfeld, S., Patel, C., North, F., Head, J., et al. (1991). "Health inequities among British civil servants: The Whitehall II study," *Lancet* 337:1387–1393.

McGuire, Meredith B. (1988). *Ritual Healing in Suburban America* (with the assistance of Debra Kantor). New Brunswick, NJ: Rutgers University Press.

Mizrahi, Terry (1986). *Getting Rid of Patients: Contradictions in the Socialization of Patients.* New Brunswick, NJ: Rutgers University Press.

National Center for Health Statistics (1997). *Health, United States, 1997.* Hyattsville, Maryland.

National Center for Health Statistics (2002). *Health, United States, 2002.* Hyattsville, Maryland.

Rasmussen, Howard (1975). "Medical education—Revolution or reaction," *Pharos*, 38:53–59.

Ritzer, George, and David Walchak (1988). "Rationalization and the deprofessionalization of physicians," *Social Forces*, 67:1–22.

Rogers, Richard G., Robert A. Hummer, and Charles B. Nam (2000). *Living and Dying in the USA: Behavioral, Health, and Social Differentials in Mortality.* New York: Academic Press.

Stevens, Rosemary (1971). *American Medicine and the Public Interest.* New Haven, CT: Yale University Press.

ADDITIONAL RESOURCES

Aguirre, B.E., F.D. Wolinsky, J. Niederauer, V. Keith, and I.J. Fann (1989). "Occupational prestige in the health care delivery system," *Journal of Health and Social Behavior* 30:315–329.

Allen, Davina (1997). "The nursing-medical boundary: A negotiated order?" *Sociology of Health and Illness.* 19:398–498.

Katz, Pearl (1999). *The Scalpel's Edge: The Culture of Surgeons.* Boston: Allyn and Bacon.

Rothstein, William (1996). *American Medical Schools and the Practice of Medicine: A History.* London: Oxford University Press.

U.S. Department of Labor (1998). *Occupational Injuries and Illnesses: Counts, Rates, and Characteristics.* Washington, DC: U.S. Department of Labor.

Waitzkin, Howard (1991). *The Politics of Medical Encounters.* New Haven, CT: Yale University Press.

INTERNET RESOURCES

American Medical Association (AMA) homepage: www.ama-assn.org.

Health Resources and Services Administration (HRSA) homepage: www.hrsa.gov.

National Center for Complementary and Alternative Medicine (NCCAM), National Institutes of Health, homepage: http://nccam.nih.gov.

Chapter **8**

Social Epidemiology

THE FIELD OF SOCIAL EPIDEMIOLOGY

Social epidemiology is the branch of epidemiology that deals with the social distribution of disease and the social determinants of health and illness. The field incorporates the concepts and methods of sociology, psychology, political science, economics, demography, geography and biology. Social epidemiologists examine the origin and spread of various health conditions and examine the ways in which health is tied to different social factors.

Social epidemiology has its roots in medical epidemiology. As the term implies, the medical specialty "epidemiology" was originally devoted to the study of communicable diseases with epidemic potential. The "social" dimension was added in the twentieth century and social epidemiology now, more appropriately, applies to virtually any health problem that affects a population. The expanded perspective offered by social epidemiology owes its existence in no small part to the work of medical sociologists during the last half of the twentieth century.

Contemporary social epidemiologists take particular interest in the relationship between populations and their environments; the spatial distribution of health-related phenomena; and the social correlates of health conditions. Functions that social epidemiologists perform include: understanding the causation of disease, disorders, and conditions; defining the mode of disease transmission; defining and measuring contributing factors in disease; and identifying and explaining geographic patterns of disease.

Social epidemiology differs from epidemiology and other clinical sciences in that it focuses on the community or group rather than the individual. In keeping with the medical sociology perspective, the community is thought to be more complex than the sum of the individuals that comprise it. This approach represents a conceptual shift in epidemiologic research and theory and has directed researchers to features of the sociocultural context neglected by traditional epidemiology. Physicians have long known that the way people live affects their health. Indeed, the Hippocratic treatise enjoined those who pursue the "science" of medicine to consider the mode of life of their patients. Two thousand years later, medical sociologists and other researchers have documented the relationships about which the Greeks could only speculate.

A number of developments during the twentieth century encouraged the incorporation of a social dimension into traditional epidemiology. A major factor in this regard was the growing (or, in a sense, the resurrected) appreciation of the role of non-biological factors in the onset and progression of health conditions. Lifestyles, for example, were found by researchers to have much more influence on health status than heredity. At the same time, a broadened definition of health conditions was emerging. Prompted both by the expansionist tendency of twentieth-century medicine and the growing expectations of the American healthcare consumer, an increasing number of conditions was brought under the aegis of medical care during the twentieth century. Longstanding "conditions" like alcoholism, homosexuality and menopause were redefined as health problems, while newly identified conditions such as hyperactivity in children and eating disorders were identified.

The importance of the social dimension of epidemiology was further promoted through the epidemiological transition that affected the United States during the second half of the twentieth century. This involved a shift in the predominance of health problems from acute conditions to chronic conditions. This shift fostered not only a change with regard to treatment modality, but a total rethinking of the nature of disease, its causation, and its management. Much more so than acute conditions like bronchitis, colds, and digestive tract problems, chronic conditions like diabetes, hypertension, and emphysema represented the cumulative

Table 8–1. Characteristics of Acute and Chronic Conditions

	Acute condition	Chronic condition
Etiology	Simple/biological	Complex/multiple
Rate of onset	Rapid	Slow/insidious
Distinctiveness of onset	Clear-cut	Difficult to diagnose
Duration of illness	Short-lived	Perpetual
Treatment	Counter pathogens	Manage symptoms
Course of disease	Recovery or death	Slow progression
Goal of care	Cure	Management
Duration of care	Short-term	Lifelong
Contribution to mortality	Direct	Indirect

affect of various sociocultural factors and behavior patterns on the part of affected individuals. In effect, the growing preponderance of chronic conditions could be attributed primarily to social rather than biological factors. (See Table 8–1 for a comparison of acute and chronic conditions.)

Another consideration in the incorporation of a social dimension into epidemiology relates to the growing appreciation of the importance of spatial relationships in healthcare. The documentation of variations in the distribution of conditions based on geography and community-to-community differences in physician practices have raised important questions about the link between health status and geography. It has become apparent that the spatial distribution of various social, demographic and economic attributes played an important role in the distribution of health problems. While geography could not be said to "cause" health problems, spatial analysis provides a useful tool in the study of "social epidemics".

The major contribution of research by medical sociologists, social epidemiologists, health demographers, and others during the last quarter of the twentieth century was the linking of various social, demographic and economic attributes of individuals and groups with health conditions. It was found that the overall physical and mental well-being of members of U.S. society was a reflection of the social attributes of these members. A correlation between health status, regardless of how it is measured, and a range of non-biological attributes revolutionized thinking with regard to the nature of disease. The link between health conditions and age, sex, race and ethnicity were clearly established, along with correlations with marital status, income level, educational level, occupational category, and even type of community. Even when a biological dimension can be considered— as in the case of age, sex, or race—we find that the correlations do not reflect the fact that males are biologically different from females or whites from

---
Box 8-1

What Happened to the Epidemics: Medical Science
or Social Change?

During the twentieth century the United States, along with the rest of the world's developed nations, experienced a dramatic decline in mortality. From 1900 to 1973, the mortality rate (adjusted for age and sex) in the United States dropped from nearly 17.5 per 1,000 population to barely 5 per 1,000. Over this period, a 69.2% decrease in overall mortality was recorded, with most (92.3%) of this occurring during the first 50 years of the twentieth century. It is likely that the decline in mortality, for some causes of death at least, actually commenced during the 1800s. Due to a lack of data, however, the "documented" decline in mortality is usually reported to have occurred during the first half of the twentieth century.

The most direct explanation for the decline in mortality is well documented. This period of history witnessed the virtual eradication of several of the contagious diseases that had been the leading causes of death since the Middle Ages. In the United States in 1900, 40% of the deaths were attributable to 11 major infectious conditions. These included measles, tuberculosis, pneumonia, diphtheria, scarlet fever, typhoid, influenza, whooping cough, poliomyelitis, smallpox, and diseases of the digestive system. By 1973, these conditions combined accounted for only 6% of the nation's deaths. While death rates due to these conditions were dropping precipitously, little decline was seen in the rates for other, non-contagious conditions. In fact, chronic conditions were dramatically increasing their share of the mortality rate.

---

blacks, but that these subgroups are *socially* different. While these correlations do not fully *explain* the etiology of contemporary health conditions, they point us in the right direction for further explanatory research.

A growing appreciation of the role that social behavior plays in the etiology and progression of disease was also a major contributor. As we have come to better understand chronic conditions. It became obvious that the clue to disease causation was not under the microscope but in our behavior. Whether it involves risky behaviors that result in HIV infection, tobacco-induced lung cancer, or alcohol induced cirrhosis, or simply "sins of omission"—the failure to practice prevention, get exercise, or make healthy dietary choices—the implications of social behavior for health status are clear. Even acute conditions, we are now realizing, are likely to be triggered by or otherwise affected by social factors. (See Box 8-1 for a discussion of the role of medical science and social conditions in the eradication of disease.)

What, then, was responsible for the virtual elimination of these killer diseases during the first half of the twentieth century? This question is conventionally answered by pointing to breakthroughs on the part of medical science that led to the eradication of these diseases. Many cite this period as conclusive proof for the efficacy of medical science in dealing with these nearly universal health threats. Medical science has perpetuated the notion that its efforts in the development of cures for these killers were the primary factors in reducing their threat to the population. The general public has accepted this argument and become a willing supporter for this explanation of the elimination of epidemic diseases.

An increasing number of researchers in both Europe and the Untied States, however, have argued that medical science had a limited impact on these killer diseases and, therefore, made little contribution to the reduced mortality experienced since 1900. While conceding that some major breakthroughs occurred during the late 1800s and early 1900s in terms of our understanding of the causes and cures of these epidemic diseases, it is argued that factors other than medical care were responsible for the dramatic drop in mortality.

McKinlay and McKinlay (1977) contend, after examining the relationship between mortality trends and developments in medical science, that the timing of the development of "cures" for these conditions virtually eliminates them as an explanation for the recorded reduction in mortality. The McKinlays argue that, for the 10 infectious conditions for which there is adequate information available, the therapeutic agents developed to counteract them were introduced long after declines in mortality had begun

(continued)

MAJOR TOPICS IN SOCIAL EPIDEMIOLOGY

Social epidemiologists, medical sociologists, health demographers, and others spend considerable time studying the demographic processes that are critical to an appreciation of the social aspects of health conditions. Fertility, morbidity, and mortality are important areas of concern for such analysts. The study of these processes has broadened our understanding of the correlates of the incidence and prevalence of health conditions. Although fertility per se does not constitute a morbid state, many aspects of reproduction have implications for the distribution of health conditions. Thus, a discussion of fertility is included in this chapter.

Fertility

Fertility refers to the reproductive experience of a population, and its study subsumes all factors related to sexual behavior, pregnancy, and birth occurring. For example, by the time a vaccine had been developed in 1943 to combat influenza, this condition had virtually ceased to be a significant cause of death. In fact, 75% of the decline in mortality from influenza between 1900 and 1973 had occurred by the time the cure was introduced in 1943.

Similar scenarios can be constructed for most of the other major infectious diseases. It is further noted that most of the reduction in mortality in the United States overall occurred prior to 1950—that is, before expenditures for health services reached an appreciable level. The McKinlays contend that "3.5 percent probably represents a reasonable upper-limit estimate of the total contribution of medical measures to the decline of mortality in the United States since 1900" (McKinlay and McKinlay 1977, p. 425).

If medical science cannot be credited with the elimination of these epidemic diseases, what can? There is now widespread support for the notion that changes in the sociocultural characteristics of the population, rather than medical care, accounted for the bulk of the mortality decline documented. Changes in the political, economic, and social environment in the United States had brought about changes in the demographic structure of the population. This was accompanied by general improvement in socioeconomic conditions and educational levels, as well as improvements in nutrition. A similar pattern of social change characterized industrialized European countries as well.

McKeown et al. (1972) concluded that the decline in mortality in several European countries during the second half of the nineteenth century was

outcomes. The emphasis here is on the health-related aspects of pregnancy, childbirth, and infant care. The fact that fertility is ultimately a "social" process cannot be overemphasized. Fertility behavior is viewed broadly and includes prenatal care, health-related activities during pregnancy (e.g., cigarette smoking), pregnancy outcome (e.g., birth, miscarriage, induced abortion), as well as postnatal care. The reproductive process involves the biological interaction of two persons in an economic, social, and/or political context. This perspective involves understanding how factors such as culture, technology, and economic conditions relate to fertility behavior.

Fertility patterns and related behavior have numerous implications for health and healthcare. The obvious linkage involves the healthcare needs of mothers and children prior to, during, and after birth. Historically, factors such as the quality of care given during the prenatal, birthing, and postnatal periods, have been shown to be related to birth outcomes (Harvey and Satre 1997), although some recent evidence indicates that prenatal care has a limited effect on factors such as birth weight (e.g., Huntington and Connell 1997, Rogers et al. 1996). A number of studies indicate that lesser amounts and lower quality of care in the postnatal period substantially increase the likelihood that a young child will be less healthy and require more postnatal

attributable to rising standards of living (especially improvements in diet), improvements in hygiene, and a healthier environment. Therapy, it was argued, made virtually no contribution to this improvement. Dubos (1959) argued convincingly for nonmedical—primarily demographic—explanations for the decline in mortality and Fuchs (1974) clearly implicates rising incomes, not medical technology, in the reduction in mortality, beginning in the middle of the nineteenth century.

While conventional beliefs concerning the elimination of the epidemic diseases are still maintained by many within both medical circles and the general public, by the 1970s the research emphasis had substantially shifted away from its focus on the medical factors involved in the reduction of morbidity and mortality. The importance of demographic and sociocultural characteristics as factors associated with the nation's mortality levels has now become widely recognized.

References: Renè Dubos (1965). *Man Adapting.* New Haven: Yale University Press; Victor R. Fuchs (1974). *Who Shall Live?* New York: Basic Books; T. McKeown, R. G. Brown, and R. G. Record (1972). "An Interpretation of the Modern Rise of Population in Europe." *Population Studies* 9: 119–141; John B. McKinlay, and Sonja J. McKinlay (1977). "The Questionable Contribution of Medical Measures to the Decline of Mortality in the United States in the Twentieth Century." *Milbank Memorial Fund Quarterly/Health and Society* (Summer), 405–428.

services (Clark et al. 1993). Ultimately, the likelihood of receiving prenatal (and postnatal) care is linked to a variety of sociocultural factors.

The fertility level is measured in its simplest form through a simple count of births for a particular geography. In the U.S., this information is typically extracted from birth certificates which, by law, must be filed for every birth that occurs. These counts of births tend to be highly accurate due to the complete reporting that occurs. The birth certificate contains a considerable amount of information on the characteristics of the mother and, to a lesser extent, of the father.

Counts of births by themselves often do not provide the information required by researchers, so a variety of fertility rates have been developed. The *crude birth rate* (CBR) is the most basic measure of fertility. The calculation of rates facilitates the comparison of fertility across areas that differ in size and/or other characteristics. This measure of fertility divides the total number of births for a given year (or the average over three years) by the midyear total population for that year (the midyear in the range if a three-year average of births is taken). This quotient is then expressed as the number of births per 1,000 population. The crude birth rate for the U.S. was 23.7 births per 1,000 persons in 1960 and fell to 14.8 by 1995.

While the CBR is adequate for making very general comparisons and has the advantage of requiring only two pieces of information, it has two major shortcomings. First, the denominator includes people who are not *at-risk* of having a birth. Males, very young females and females beyond menopause are not at-risk of giving birth, yet they appear in the denominator of the rate. Second, the CBR masks differences between the age composition of populations. Fertility rates are greatly affected by age composition, particularly for women, and the CBR cannot account for this. As a result of these shortcomings, more refined measures of fertility have been developed.

The *general fertility rate* (GFR), sometimes referred to simply as the fertility rate, represents a refinement of the CBR. It adjusts the denominator of the rate by focusing on the *population at risk*. It is expressed in terms of births per 1,000 females aged 15 to 44 (or 15 to 49).

Additional information can be provided by calculating *age-specific birth rates*. Age-specific birth rates are essential in that changes in fertility levels specific to certain ages provide the analyst with much needed information regarding trends in service demand. For example, the recent increases in birth rates for young ladies under age 15 and women over age 30 point to the rising need for specialized services. Demographers typically calculate age-specific fertility rates using five-year age intervals.

The *total fertility rate* (TFR) is sometimes utilized as a summary measure for age specific fertility rates. The TFR reflects hypothetical completed fertility for a population. Technically, the only way to accurately determine how many children a cohort of young women (e.g., those currently under age 15) will have over their lifetimes is to wait 30 or more years until they have completed their childbearing. Therefore, hypothetical measures that allow an analyst to project the completed fertility of a specified cohort without the long wait have been developed. The calculation of the TFR assumes that a group of 15-year-old females will experience the some age-specific fertility rates throughout their lifetimes. While this hypothetical rate may be somewhat at variance with the actual fertility experience, the TFR represents a good estimation of completed cohort fertility as long as ASFRs remain fairly stable.

At the same time, social epidemiologists have found that the formal care associated with the pregnancy process is not as important a predictor of birth outcome as are various sociocultural characteristics. The demographic characteristics of women who bear children, such as age, race, marital status, income and education, are useful predictors of both fertility levels and birth outcomes. The same factors affect fertility levels and the health status of mothers and their children. These factors also include the nutritional level, age at conception, and the lifestyles characterizing the mother. Indeed, the likelihood of compliance with prenatal and postnatal medical regimens is dependent upon sociocultural traits.

The mother-related social factors important in explaining fertility outcomes in the United States today are age at first birth, race/ethnicity, educational attainment, and marital status among others. At least two of these factors, age at first birth and race/ethnicity, are closely associated with economic factors such as employment and income. In fact, it can be said that each time one social factor is discussed in regard to patterns of fertility, interaction with many others is implied.

The marital status of mothers is of concern for researchers, given the implications of out-of-wedlock childbearing for both mothers and babies. Babies born out of wedlock tend to suffer from a higher prevalence of both physical and mental disorders and are at greater risk of death during infancy. Considering that the proportion of births accounted for by unmarried women has been increasing, this situation presages continued high costs for society and the healthcare system (National Center for Health Statistics, 2002, table 9).

Large racial differences in the marital status of mothers exist as well. In 2000, nearly 70% of all African American births were to unmarried women, but only 27.1% of white births were (National Center for Health Statistics, 2002, table 9). The racial difference in premarital birth rates is explained largely by differences in socioeconomic status, although there has been a rise in this percentage for both racial groups over the last decade. African American women with low socioeconomic status are two and one-half times more likely to have a premarital birth than African American women with high socioeconomic status (Bumpass and McLanahan 1989). When the age of the mother is accounted for the differential narrows. At age 16, for example, 83% and 98% of all white and African American births, respectively, in 1999 were to mothers who are unmarried (Ventura et al. 2000, table 4).

As noted earlier, numerous social factors are associated with the conditions of birth. While 6.6% of white newborns were classified as low birth weight in 2000, 13.1% and 6.4%, respectively, of African-American and Hispanic newborns are classified the same way (National Center for Health Statistics, 2002, table 12). The percent of babies who are of low birth weight is about twice as high for unmarried women (10.4% versus 5.7%). Moreover, the percentage of all births classified as low birth weight declines from 9.8% for those women with 9 to 11 years of education to 6.2% for those with a college education or more (National Center for Health Statistics, 2001, table 1–27).

A statistical correlation can be demonstrated between fertility levels and health status that resembles a J-shaped curve. It appears that the healthiest segments of the population (the most fecund) are not the most prolific (the most fertile). In fact, subpopulations that demonstrate moderate levels of health status tend to have the highest birth rates. However, once health status drops below a certain level, biological factors come into play to reduce the level of fecundity or the physical ability to reproduce.

This mechanism operates with regard to the individual's ability to conceive, the ability to carry the fetus to term, the potential for a positive pregnancy outcome, and the potential for producing a healthy child. This relationship, more than anything else, reflects the non-biological aspects of reproduction.

Those who are in the best health are also likely to be those who are best educated, most affluent, most knowledgeable about contraception, and most responsive to social expectations with regard to reproduction. Those with less favorable characteristics—the poorly educated, the working poor, the least knowledgeable about contraception-are characterized by high fertility levels.

Certain racial and ethnic minorities have the highest fertility rates in U.S. society today. Members of these groups generally suffer disadvantages that have either a direct or indirect impact on the health of mother and child. Since the mothers are likely to be in relatively poor health themselves, this has implications for the children during gestation. In general, these high-fertility populations suffer from high rates of infant mortality, maternal mortality, birth complications, low birth-weight babies, birth defects, and mental retardation. Further, these children are likely to be born into environments that are relatively unsafe and/or unsanitary, to be exposed to poor nutritional levels, and generally to suffer from a lack of the resources necessary to maintain a healthy lifestyle. These conditions essentially assures that many individuals end up as multi-problem persons. This results in the creation of large numbers of individuals whose health is impaired from before birth and many who are never given the opportunity to improve.

Given racial/ethnic differences in fertility and the younger age structures of the African-American and Hispanic populations, the proportion of all births that are African American or Hispanic are projected to increase sharply in the next decade. Moreover, given that the rates for early prenatal care are lower African Americans and the incidence of low birth weight is higher in this population, the proportion of low-birth-weight babies can be expected to rise.

MORBIDITY

Morbidity, or the level of sickness and disability within a population, historically has been an area of study for both clinicians and population-oriented scientists such as epidemiologists. In recent years, however, increased activity on the part of social scientists has been observed, as researchers apply various methodologies and perspectives to the study of sickness and disability.

The study of morbidity is perhaps the most important dimension of social epidemiology, particularly in modern industrialized societies. Death is a relatively rare event in such societies, so the health of the population must be measured based on the incidence and prevalence of various health conditions. Indeed, the health profile of U.S. society today compared to a century ago is a function of shifts in the major contributors to morbidity.

In looking at morbidity from a health services perspective, the morbidity profile of a population can be translated into healthcare needs. Healthcare needs can be defined in terms of the level and types of conditions existing within a population that require some type of health service response. These are the health conditions that an objective evaluation—e.g., a physical examination—would uncover within a population. A population with certain characteristics can be expected to experience a specified level of various health conditions based on these characteristics. These might be thought of as the *absolute* needs that exist in "nature" without the influence of any other factors.

All things being equal, the absolute level of need should not vary much from population to population. Researchers working independently should draw the same conclusions with regard to the level and types of healthcare needs characterizing a specific population. The concept of healthcare needs is more closely related to the concept of "illness" described previously rather than what we have defined as "sickness." Despite the research that has now been conducted on the health status of the population, we are still a long way from determining the "true" prevalence of health problems within U.S. society. We do not, in fact, have an epidemiologically based model for examining a population and determining the absolute level (and types) of extant health problems. While a lack of such a model has been a nuisance in the past, the inability to measure health status effectively based on morbidity indicators is an increasingly serious problem for researchers.

The study of morbidity is made more complicated and important as a result of the sometimes-subjective nature of health problems. Earlier chapters dealing with the nature of health and illness and the distinction between illness and sickness illustrate the complexity of the study of morbidity. Ultimately, to understand the health status of a population, one must analyze the clinically identifiable conditions affecting that population, as well as the conditions that society members themselves identify.

Several measures have been developed for use in morbidity analysis. The first involves the simple counting of officially recognizable conditions for the nation or sub-national units of geography. Although little success has been achieved in establishing a summary measure of morbidity for individuals or populations, indicators for specific conditions are frequently used. Some of the indicators that are used include incidence and prevalence statistics for specific conditions, symptom checklists, and various measures of disability. Assuming that high-quality morbidity data are available, several other measures can be utilized.

Two of the most useful measures are incidence and prevalence rates. An *incidence rate* refers to the number of new cases of a disease or condition occurring over a certain time period expressed as a number per 1,000, 10,000, or 100,000 population at risk. A *prevalence rate* divides the total number of persons with the disease or condition in question by the population at risk with respect to a specific point in time. Again, the population at risk is the number of persons who have some nonzero probability of contracting the condition in question.

The prevalence rate includes, for example, the total number of persons with AIDS divided by the population at risk. In this instance the population at risk is the total population, since this is a prevalence rate and the entire population is theoretically at risk. In 2001, the AIDS prevalence rate was 14.3 cases per 100,000 population (National Center for Health Statistics, 2002, table 54). The prevalence rate always exceeds the incidence rate, since the former involves but a fraction of the latter. The only time the two rates are nearly comparable is when the condition is acute and of very short duration. For example, the incidence rate would almost equal the prevalence rate at the height of a 24-hour virus epidemic since victims recover almost as quickly as they are affected.

Incidence and prevalence rates are both used in the study of the distribution of disease. If the analyst knows, for example, that the incidence rate for a certain medical procedure is 17 per 1,000 population aged 65 years and over and has reason to believe that the incidence rate for that procedure will remain nearly constant for the next five years (data must support this assumption), then the demand for that procedure five years in the future can be determined by multiplying the incidence rate by the projected population of persons age 65 and above. The prevalence rate can be used in much the same way when the condition is a chronic one.

The incidence rate is also a valuable measure in epidemiological investigations. If a new or mysterious condition afflicts a population, epidemiologists can trace the spread of the condition through the population by backtracking using incidence data. The cause or population of origin of a new disease can often only be determined by identifying the characteristics of the victims and the conditions under which the disease was contracted. The exact date of occurrence becomes crucial if the epidemiological detective is to link the onset to a particular set of circumstances. Quite often the key is the sociocultural characteristics of the victims. AIDS is a case in point wherein the means of transmission is identified based on the non-biological characteristics of the victims.

The National Notifiable Diseases Surveillance System (NNDSS) is the mechanism by which notifiable disease data, such as those for gonorrhea,

Table 8–2.   Selected Notifiable Diseases for the United States, 1970–1996

Disease	1970	1985	1996
AIDS	N.A.	8,249	65,475
Hepatitis A	56,300	23,200	29,024
Hepatitis B	8,300	26,600	9.994
Animal rabies	3,224	5,565	6,676
Malaria	3,051	1,049	1,542
Syphillis	91,000	68,000	11,110
Gonorrhea	600,000	911,000	308,737
Tuberculosis	37,000	22,200	19,096
Measles	47,400	2,800	295
Mumps	105,000	3,000	658
Pertusis	4,200	3,600	6,467

SOURCE: Centers for Disease Control and Prevention.

hepatitis, Lyme disease, and pertussis (whooping cough) are gathered. It should be recalled that these particular diseases have been singled out primarily because of their communicable nature. A *notifiable disease* is one for which regular, frequent, and timely information on individual cases is considered necessary for the prevention and control of that disease. Public health officials are particularly interested in these conditions since they have the potential to spread to epidemic proportions. Note that they are virtually all acute conditions, at a time when the major health problems are chronic conditions. For this reason, reportable morbid conditions have become increasingly less useful as indicators of health status. (See Table 8–2 for a listing of major notifiable diseases and their occurrence.)

There are some other conditions that are monitored through reports from health facilities, sample surveys, and ongoing panel studies. Federal health agencies conduct periodic surveys of hospital inpatients and ambulatory patients utilizing clinics and other outpatient services. In addition, databases have been established for the systematic compilation of information on inpatient and, to a lesser extent, outpatient utilization. These data collection efforts allow for the identification of cases for a wide variety of conditions and the monitoring of the level of these conditions over time. While this information is invaluable, coverage is far from complete at this point. It also should be remembered that these compilations include only reported cases. If individuals afflicted by various disorders are not diagnosed and treated, they will not show up in these studies.

There have been considerable fluctuations in the number of cases of various communicable diseases over the 26-year period covered by the table. While there were approximately 47,000 reported cases of measles in 1970, for example, there were less than 100 in 2000. This same downward trend can be seen over the same time period in the data for mumps

(105,000 to 338 cases); hepatitis A (56,797 to 13,397 cases); and primary and secondary syphilis (21,982 to 5,979 cases). At the same time, increased incidence is seen for AIDS, animal rabies and pertussis (whooping cough) (National Center for Health Statistics, 2002, table 53).

Another approach to the development of morbidity indicators is the use of symptom checklists in sample surveys. A list of symptoms that has been statistically validated is utilized to collect data for the calculation of a morbidity index. These are utilized to derive health status measures for both physical and mental illness. Usually there are 15 or 20 symptoms, since it is hard to retain respondents' attention much longer. While the symptoms are sometimes examined individually, the main use is in the calculation of an index. Typically, the number of symptoms is simply summed and this becomes the index score for that individual. In some cases, the symptoms may be weighted on the grounds that some symptoms may be more important in the determination of morbidity levels than others.

A primary rationale for the utilization of symptom checklists is the fact that much of the population is free of clinically identifiable disorders but is likely to have some, albeit minor, manifestations of ill health. Virtually everyone has vaguely defined symptoms of some type at various times. It is further argued, with regard to both physical and mental conditions, that these "everyday" symptoms are more significant measures of health status than are comparatively rare clinical conditions. Symptom checklists are also attractive because of their objective nature and generally agreed-upon definitions. Virtually everyone is going to agree as to what constitutes an "occasional cough" or "occasional dizzy spells," but clinical diagnoses are often misunderstood by patients or obscured by the terminological complexity of the healthcare setting.

Symptom checklists usually are based on answers directly obtained from survey respondents. Respondents either complete a questionnaire that contains the checklist or provide responses to an interviewer who records them. In some rare cases, the checklist will include signs as well as symptoms, and clinical personnel will be involved in the data collection process to obtain test results. This approach is occasionally utilized, for example, in studies of psychiatric morbidity, in which case the clinician will typically administer various psychiatric tests. The index calculated in this manner generally reflects a combination of symptoms reported by the respondent and signs observed by the clinician.

Another group of health status measures might be generally referred to as disability measures. Even more so than other aspects of morbidity, disability is difficult to operationalize. While it would appear simple to enumerate the blind, deaf, or otherwise handicapped, the situation is actually quite complex. A wide variety of other conditions that are not so clear-cut cloud the picture. Does lower back pain that interferes with work constitute a disability? When does an arthritic condition become disabling? How is mental retardation classified, and at what point? Even those disabilities that appear obvious defy easy categorization due to the subjective dimension of disability. There are many hearing impaired individuals, for example, that would take exception to being classified as disabled.

This definitional problem is partly resolved by the utilization of more objective and easily measured indicators as proxies for disability. One category of indicators focuses on "activities of daily living" (ADLs). ADLs constitute a series of indicators related to the ability of individuals to care for themselves, solely or with assistance. Thus, the respondent is asked to what extent he can feed himself, dress himself, and go to the bathroom unassisted. Other indicators may address mobility, as in the ability to climb stairs, walk a certain distance without discomfort, and so forth. ADLs offer a fairly effective means of getting at the overall disability status of individuals by combining their responses into a score that indicates the individual's relative level of disability.

Another category of disability measurement might be referred to as "restriction" indicators, since they reflect the extent to which affected individuals are restricted in terms of work or school activities. Measures in this category include: work-loss days, school-loss days, and bed-restricted days. The number of days missed from work or school and the number of days individuals are restricted to bed can all be calculated and used as proxy measures of morbidity. While such measures are being used increasingly, it should be remembered that much of this information is available only from sample surveys. It is possible that many "cases" go undiscovered and uncounted. Nevertheless, significant variations have been identified in terms of the demographic correlates of disability as measured in this manner.

Chronic illness and disability are likely to have more significant consequences for interpersonal relationships, role performance, and sense of self than acute conditions. Thus, they involve a different sickness experience than acute illness. Although some people with chronic illnesses are impaired and disabled, chronic illness does not inevitably lead to disability. For example, diabetes may interfere only minimally with some people's functioning. Some people with impairments (for example, from an automobile accident) are not sick and may object to being defined as such. The sick role is meant to temporarily exempt affected individuals from normal activities, but the disabled find themselves prevented from participating in normal social activities and placed in a state of perpetual dependence. For this reason, the traditional conceptualization of the sick role is less applicable to chronic conditions and disability than to acute conditions.

Box 8-2

Accidents: Not So Accidental?

In the United States, accidents are a common occurrence and, led by motor vehicles fatalities, "unintentional injuries" are one of the ten leading causes of death. Accidental injuries are a major cause of lost workdays and schooldays and contribute significantly to the cost of healthcare in the U.S. Because accidents are not closely associated with old age—unlike heart disease and stroke, for example—they account for a disproportionate share of productive years of life lost due to premature death.

It would be natural to assume that accidents, by their very nature, are unpredictable and random in occurrence. It is reasonable to assume that motor vehicle accidents, firearms accidents, and sports injuries would be no respecter of age, sex, race or class. While most other health conditions might be expected to display patterns of distribution that reflect the demographic and sociocultural traits of the population, one would expect accidents to be randomly distributed throughout the population.

While the distribution of accidents may be more often attributed to chance than most other conditions, the distribution is far from random. Accidents are more common for males than females, for certain age groups, for certain racial and ethnic groups, and even for certain socioeconomic categories. Children, adolescents, young adults *and* the elderly suffer more accidents than other age groups, while nonwhites experience a higher rate of accidents than whites. The lower income groups appear more susceptible to accidents than the more affluent. In fact, injuries do not occur randomly to professional athletes, but can be linked to certain sociocultural characteristics.

One might argue that, if motor vehicle and firearm accidents account for a significant portion of accidents, it makes sense that certain segments of the population—who drive more and handle firearms more—are likely

---

Chapter 9 on the social dimensions of health status further examines the circumstances surrounding morbidity in the U.S. Box 8-2 examines one factor in morbidity that is, interestingly enough, influenced by sociocultural factors.

MORTALITY

Mortality refers to the death process characterizing a population. The study of mortality examines the relationship between death and the size, composition, and distribution of the population. Furthermore, mortality studies investigate the who, how, why, and when issues related to dying. Medical

to be at higher risk. Although there is some truth to this, the pattern of accident distribution cannot be attributed to fast driving or careless use of firearms: accidental falls.

Falls are the most common cause of accident-related deaths. Some 17,000 people die from falls in the U.S. each year. The leading cause of death for children is accidents and, for this age group, that usually involves a fall. In fact, the very young and the very old are the most affected by fall-related injuries. In addition, the distribution of falls within the population is associated with social class and other demographic and sociocultural factors. Further, the occurrence of falls varies by the month of the year, the day of the week and the time of day, reflecting an extremely non-random pattern.

It might be worthwhile to examine falls among children, since the rate is high and falls account for 42% of emergency room visits by children. Among children, males account for 53% of the fall-related injuries. In terms of age, the highest rate of falls is for those 65 and over, with a rate of 400 per 100,000 individuals each year. The second highest age cohort, those less than ten years of age, reported a rate of 175. The reported rate of fall-related injuries for the low-income population is 250 per 100,000, compared to 80 per 100,000 for the high-income population.

The greatest number of fall injuries for children are reported for May and June and the fewest number for November and December. A full 45% of falls occur on Saturday or Sunday. The highest fall rates are from 6 p.m. to midnight.

If a pattern can be discerned for the distribution of falls within the population, even clearer distinctions can be expected for conditions that are directly related to lifestyle and social characteristics. The fact that a decreasing number of conditions can be linked to biological factors means that the importance of demographic and sociocultural factors in the distribution of disease, disability and mortality within the population will be only continue to grow.

sociologists have contributed greatly to the understanding of the factors contributing to mortality and the distribution of mortality within the population.

The study of mortality is an important area of social epidemiology, particularly in societies that are less developed and are affected more by acute conditions than chronic conditions. The common causes of death in such societies typically reflect the common health problems, making the mortality profile a reasonable approximation of the morbidity profile.

Cause-of-death analyses are utilized in modern, industrialized societies in the examination of health status, partly because such data are readily available. However, mortality analyses are less useful for determining the illness profile in developed societies because of the preponderance of chronic conditions. Thus, the conditions that people die from (e.g., heart disease, cancer, and stroke) are not necessarily the conditions that characterize most of the population. Chronic diseases are typically not killers, so the link between disease prevalence and cause of death is not very direct.

Mortality like fertility is significantly influenced by sociocultural factors and even age-specific deaths are to a certain extent a function of nonbiological factors. These include such characteristics as: marital status and family structure, socioeconomic status, occupation, industry and employment status, lifestyle and even religion.

The primary source of mortality data in the United States is the governmental registry based on certificates filed at the time of death. Death certificates must be filed by law, typically with the county health department. These certificates are, in turn, aggregated at the local, state, and national levels. The information available generally includes primary cause of death, contributing causes, and individual social and economic characteristics such as sex, age, race/ethnicity, last occupation, place of residence, and place of death. Using these data, analysts can begin to study the relationship between the cause of death and a variety of sociocultural variables.

The most basic measure of mortality is simply a count of the deaths occurring within a particular area or population. Death counts compiled over a period of years indicate trends with regard to increases or decreases in mortality. Deaths are also cross-classified by the medical, social, and economic characteristics of the deceased.

Utilizing a simple count of deaths in the analysis of mortality has several shortcomings. As in the case of fertility analysis, the comparison of deaths for different geographic areas or over time is generally not very useful given the various population sizes generating these deaths. It may be of little value to compare the number of deaths in Community X (population 10,000) with the number of deaths in Community Y (population 100,000). Therefore, other measures of mortality have been developed that allow for both area-to-area and longitudinal comparisons.

The simplest measure used is the *crude death rate* (CDR). This rate expresses deaths as the number per 1,000 population. In the U.S., the CDR was 8.6 in 1990, 8.8 in 1980, 9.5 in 1970, 9.6 in 1950, and 10.8 in 1940. However, since not everyone in the population is at the same risk of death, lumping all deaths into one crude rate limits this measure's usefulness. Thus, *age-specific death rates* (ASDRs) are often generated. ASDRs are usually calculated for five-year age intervals, though for more detailed analyses three- or even one-year intervals may be used. Recent figures for the U.S. indicate that age-specific death rates are lowest at the ages 5 to 9 (0.2), stay relatively low through ages 45 to 49 (3.8) and rise again at the ages 65 to 69 (20.6).

Another measure, the *infant mortality rate* (IMR), is used to determine the death rate during the first year of life. It is always expressed as a one-year rate because of the greatly increased probability of dying during the first year of life as compared with subsequent ages. Persons under age one, for example, are 20 times more likely to die in a given year than someone in the 1- to 4-year-old category. The infant mortality rate is considered an important indicator because it does more than simply reflect the number of infant deaths. It serves as a proxy for a number of variables, reflecting the characteristics of the mother, the infant's environment, access to healthcare, and other factors.

The infant mortality rate declined steadily in the U.S. during the twentieth century, with the decline leveling off toward the end of the century. While occurrences of infant deaths have become rare enough that it is difficult to attribute various sociodemographic variables to variations in rates, infant mortality continues to be a consideration among low-income minority groups within the U.S. population. More importantly, it appears that medical science has done all it can to reduce the infant mortality rate in the U.S. Any further reduction must be derived from changes in lifestyles, improvements in socioeconomic status, and/or modification of other non-clinical factors.

While researchers rely heavily on the data collected by means of death certificates, there are several potential problems with these data. The first is one of correct specification of the primary cause of death. While identifying the cause of death may seem relatively easy to the layperson, in practice it is often difficult and the result is that sometimes incorrect data are recorded. Some deaths are complicated in that more than one condition is present (e.g., cancer and pneumonia) with several bodily systems affected (e.g., lungs and heart). The second problem is closely related to the first in that it is often difficult to distinguish between and among the primary and contributing causes.

Epidemiologists often calculate *cause-specific death rates* in order to decompose the overall death rate. The method is similar to that of the CDR, with the number of deaths from a specific cause comprising the numerator and the total population as the denominator of the rate. Cause-specific rates can be calculated for specific age intervals as well. These figures, which are derived by dividing the number of deaths from one cause by the total number of deaths, represent the proportion of the population dying of a specific cause.

The leading causes of death are used frequently to describe the health status of the nation. Over the past 100 years, the U.S. has seen a great deal

Table 8–3. Selected Causes of Death for the United States (Rate per 100,000
Population), 1900–1995

Year	Major cardiovascular diseases	Influenza and pneumonia	Tuberculosis	Gastritis, duodenitis, enteritis, colitis	Malignant Neoplasms
1995	340.8	31.6	<1.0	<1.0	204.9
1990	368.3	32.0	<1.0	<1.0	203.2
1980	436.4	24.1	<1.0	<1.0	183.9
1970	496.0	30.9	2.6	0.6	162.8
1940	485.7	70.3	45.9	10.3	120.3
1920	364.7	207.3	113.1	53.7	83.4
1900	345.2	202.2	194.4	142.7	64.0

SOURCE: Center for Disease Control and Prevention.

of change in the leading causes of death. At the beginning of the 1900s, infectious diseases ran rampant in the United States and worldwide and topped the leading causes of death. A century later, with the control of many infectious agents and the increasing age of the population, chronic diseases top the list.

A very different picture emerges when the leading causes of death are viewed for various population groups. Unintentional injuries, mainly motor vehicle crashes, are the fifth leading cause of death for the total population, but they are the leading cause of death for people aged 1 to 44 years. Similarly, HIV/AIDS is the 14th leading cause of death for the total population but the leading cause of death for African-American men aged 25 to 44 years.

Table 8–3 presents death rates for selected causes for various time intervals since 1900. These causes were selected based upon an examination of what the major causes of death were in 1900 and 1995. The rates are expressed in deaths per 100,000 persons and have not been adjusted or standardized for changes in age structure. As can be seen, there have been marked fluctuations in rates, with influenza and pneumonia, tuberculosis and gastritis showing significant rate decreases. While these conditions were among the five leading causes of death in 1900, they no longer contribute to overall mortality in any significant fashion. Specifically, in 1900 tuberculosis, pneumonia, and diarrhea and enteritis accounted for nearly 30% of all mortality, while in the late-1990s they accounted for less than 4%. Cancer (malignant neoplasms) and heart disease accounted for less than 12% of the deaths in the population in 1900. As the result of the growth of cancer as a leading cause of death in the United States, these two disease categories comprise about 53% of all deaths (National Center for Health Statistics 2002, table 30).

Chapter 9 on the social correlates of health status examines the factors influenced mortality in more detail.

REFERENCES

Bumpass, L., and S. McLanahan (1989). "Unmarried motherhood: Recent trends, composition, and black-white differences," *Demography* 26:279–299.

Clark, L., M. Miller, B. Vogel, K. Davis, and C. Mahan (1993). "The effectiveness of Florida's improved pregnancy outcome program," *Journal of Health Care for the Poor and Underserved*, 4:117–132.

Frisbie, P., D. Forbes, and S. Pullum (1996). "Compromised birth outcomes and infant mortality among racial and ethnic groups," *Demography* 33:469–481.

Huntington, J., and F.A. Connell (1997). "For every dollar spent—The cost savings argument for prenatal care," *New England Journal of Medicine*, 35:1303–1307.

Nathanson, C.A., and K.J. Young (1989). "Components of change in adolescent fertility, 1971–1979," *Demography* 26:85–98.

National Center for Health Statistics (2001). *Vital Statistics for the United States, 1999, Volume 1. Natality*. Hyattsville, MD: National Center for Health Statistics.

National Center for Health Statistics (2002). *Health, United States, 2002*. Hyattsville, Maryland: National Center for Health Statistics.

Rogers, M., M. Sheps-Peoples, and C. Suchindran (1996). "Impact of a social support program on teenage prenatal use and pregnancy outcomes," *Journal of Adolescent Health* 19:132–140.

Smith, H., P. Morgan and T. Koropeckyj-Cox (1996). "A decomposition of trends in the nonmarital fertility ratios of blacks and whites in the United States: 1960–1992," *Demography* 33:141–151.

Sowards, K.A. (1997). "Premature birth and the changing composition of newborn infectious disease mortality: Reconsidering 'exogenous' mortality," *Demography* 34:399 409.

Ventura, Stephanie J. and Christine A. Bachrach (2000). "Nonmarital Childbearing in the United States, 1940–99," *National Vital Statistics Reports* (October). Hyattsville, MD: National Center for Health Statistics.

ADDITIONAL RESOURCES

Centers for Disease Control and Prevention (Weekly). *Morbidity and Mortality Weekly Review*. Atlanta, GA: Centers for Disease Control and Prevention.

Kelly, Michael P., and David Field (1996). "Medical sociology, chronic illness and the body." *Sociology of Health and Illness*, 18:241–257.

Pol, Louis G., and Richard K. Thomas (2001), *The Demography of Health and Health Care*. New York: Kluwer Academic/Plenum.

Roth, Julius, and Peter Conrad (eds.) (1987). *The Experience and Management of Chronic Illness*. Newbury Park, CA: Sage.

Rushing, William (1995). *The AIDS Epidemic: Social Dimensions of an Infectious Disease*. Boulder, CO: Westview Press.

Singh, Gopal K., and Stella M. Yu (1995). "Infant mortality in the United States: Trends, differentials, and projections, 1950 through 2010," *American Journal of Public Health*, 85:957–964.

Subidi, Janardan, and Eugene B. Gallagher, eds. (1996). *Society, Health, and Disease: Transcultural Perspectives.* Upper Saddle River, NJ: Prentice Hall.

INTERNET LINKS

Centers for Disease Control and Prevention (CDC) homepage: www.cdc.gov.
National Center for Health Statistics (NCHS) homepage: www.cdc.nchs.
Office of Disease Prevention and Promotion (Department of Health and Human Services) homepage: http://odphp.osophs.dhhs.gov.
National Institutes of Health (NIH) homepage: www.nih.gov.
U.S. Census Bureau homepage: www.census.gov.

Chapter **9**

The Social Dimension of
Health Status

Much of the work of medical sociologists involves the establishment of meaningful associations between indicators of health status and various characteristics of the population under study. In recent years researchers have begun to generate the baseline information necessary to develop a true appreciation of the epidemiology of health conditions. As a result, our knowledge of the non-biological factors that contribute to health status has greatly increased. The health status of the population has now been linked to a wide range of biosocial, sociocultural and lifestyle attributes.

Despite this growing body of knowledge, caution should be exercised in reviewing the correlates of morbidity and mortality presented in this chapter. The interplay of the numerous variables that influence health status is obviously complex. Some studies have simply explored the direct effects of a particular variable on health status without controlling for the influence of other factors. When controls for additional variables are introduced, the impact of the original variable may be reduced, eliminated, or otherwise modified. For example, a strong relationship has repeatedly been found between race and health status. Virtually every indicator of health status is found to be higher for whites than for blacks, suggesting a direct correlation between race and health status and even implying causation (National Center for Health Statistics 1998a, table 70). However, when other variables (e.g., income) are taken into consideration, the relationship between race and health status is substantially reduced (Kim et al. 1998; Waidmann and Shoenbaum 1996).

This effort at isolating the factors involved in morbidity and mortality has been aided significantly by the recent work of Rogers, Hummer and Nam (2000). Their landmark analysis involved the matching of death records with data on respondents drawn from several years of federal health surveys (i.e., the National Health Interview Survey). This approach allowed the researchers to link for the first time actual mortality data with the characteristics of both survivors and decedents. Even given this additional information, however, the research results reported here should be interpreted with caution.

SOCIAL CORRELATES OF HEALTH STATUS

The social correlates of health status for the contemporary U.S. population are numerous, and their omnipresence underscores the relative insignificance of biological factors. Compositional variables such as age, sex, and race allow social epidemiologists to infer a great deal about a population's health characteristics. This chapter builds on the growing knowledge of the ways in which sociocultural variables can contribute to variations in health status between populations.

Overall Health Status

Various community surveys have utilized global indicators as a means of measuring health status based on self-reports. The major government study to take this approach is the National Health Interview Survey (NHIS) conducted by the National Center for Health Statistics. The Center's 2000 study found that most respondents (91.0%) rated their health as "good", "very good" or "excellent." Only 9.0% rated it as "poor" or "fair" (National Center for Health Statistics 2000, table 59). (Table 9–1 presents self-assessment data related to selected population characteristics.)

As can be seen in the table, health status assessment based on self-reports declines as people age. While less than two percent of those under 18 describe their health as only poor or fair, 27.0% of those 65 and over assessed their health this unfavorably (National Center for Health Statistics 2000, table 59). Interestingly, over one-third of all persons 65 and over assess

Table 9–1.   Self-Assessment of Health Status, 2000

Characteristic	Percent in poor or fair health
Age distribution	
Under 18	1.7
18–24	3.2
25–44	5.7
45–54	11.9
55–64	17.9
65–74	22.6
75 and over	32.2
Sex	
Male	8.8
Female	9.3
Race/Ethnicity	
White	8.2
Black/African American	14.6
American Indian	17.2
Asian American	17.2
Hispanic	12.9
Poverty Status	
Poor	20.9
Near poor	15.3
Nonpoor	6.3

SOURCE: National Center for Health Statistics.

their health as excellent or very good, and this proportion has actually been increasing over time (National Center for Health Statistics 1998, table 70).

The difference in the self-assessment of health status between males and females is narrow, with males more positive in their self-assessments overall. Some 8.8% of males considered themselves to be in poor or fair health, compared to 9.3% for females (National Center for Health Statistics 2000, table 59).

The discrepancy in self-assessed health status by race is substantial, with blacks being much less positive in their self-assessment. While only 8.2 of whites assessed their health as poor or fair in 2000, 14.6% of blacks report such a negative evaluation (National Center for Health Statistics 2000, table 59). Given that blacks have a younger age structure, the "true" differential in health status is probably even greater. American Indians are the most likely of the racial and ethnic groups to report poor or fair health (17.2%), while Hispanics were closer to the white pattern than most other groups (12.9%).

When self-reported health status is examined by level of affluence, a clear pattern is seen. The proportion reporting poor health declined steadily with socioeconomic status, with 20.9% of the poor reporting poor or fair health compared to 6.3% of the non-poor.

For convenience, the social characteristics to be considered below are divided into biosocial and sociocultural characteristics. Biosocial characteristics are traits that have an underlying physical basis such as age, sex and race (and, to a lesser extent, ethnicity). Biosocial traits are for the most part ascribed at birth, while sociocultural traits are acquired. The former are considered biosocial in that they reflect the social dimension of the particular status as much if not more than the biological dimension. Thus, males and females are not only different in a physical sense, but by virtue of being male or female they take on certain traits and are subjected to certain expectations by society. (Note that correlations between sociocultural characteristics and mental health status are covered in Chapter 13 on the sociology of mental illness.)

From a social epidemiological perspective there has been interest in assessing health status at the community level. One of the major challenges in healthcare over the past three decades has been the development of acceptable measures of aggregate health status. A variety of attempts have been made to quantify health status focusing on the development of a single, objective measure. Attempts to develop a single global index of health status have not been very successful, and specific measures continue to be utilized as indicators. Recent efforts to develop a single index incorporating measures of mortality and morbidity that reflects healthy life years have been more successful (Hyder et al. 1998). (Box 9-1 addresses the development of health status indices.)

Biosocial Characteristics

Age and Health Status

There has been long-standing acceptance of the notion that health status is linked closely with age. Conventional wisdom suggests that as one ages, the more numerous and more serious health problems become. While there is some truth to this assertion, research conducted in recent years indicates that the situation is much more complex than had been previously thought. Patterns of morbidity, disability, and even mortality display complicated relationships with the age structure of the population.

The prevalence of chronic conditions does in fact increase with age, and there appears to be a clear cumulative effect. However, the incidence of acute conditions actually declines with age. Thus, while the younger age cohorts are characterized by high rates of respiratory conditions, injuries, and other acute conditions, the elderly are less affected by these types of conditions. Instead, they are faced with a growing number of chronic conditions such as hypertension, arthritis, and heart problems. It has been suggested that the actual average number of conditions does not differ much from the youngest age cohorts to the oldest. The differential is primarily in the types of conditions common among various age groups (U.S. Bureau of the Census 1997).

On the other hand, the proportion of the population experiencing some level of activity limitation due to chronic conditions increases steadily with age, and the oldest age cohorts are characterized by limited-activity days several times as numerous as those for the younger age cohorts. For example, 5.8% of the 15–44 age cohort in 2000 reported some limitation of activity. The comparable figure for the 65–74 age group was 26.2% (National Center for Health Statistics 2002, table 58).

The most well established relationship has been the association between age and mortality. Beginning with the 5- to 14-year-old cohort, there is a direct and positive relationship between age and mortality in contemporary U.S. society. The mortality rate for those under one year of age is relatively high (729/100,000) but this drops rapidly after year one. The rate in 2000 of 19/100,000 for those aged 5 to 14 (the lowest risk of death) increases gradually up through age 50. After 50, the increase in the mortality rate is dramatic. The rate of 19 increases to 432/100,000 for the 45–54 age group and 5,688/100,000 for the 75–84 age group. (It is noteworthy that all of these rates have declined since 1990.) This same age-related pattern holds for all race-sex categories (Minino et al. 2002, table 5).

The increase in overall life expectancy for the U.S. population has been well documented. One of the findings derived from the analysis of life tables is the fact that longevity appears to feed on itself. (In other words, the longer one lives, the longer one lives.) In 1999 projected life expectancy at birth was 76.7 years. However, for individuals who live to age 65, life expectancy increases to 82.7 years. Similarly, individuals who survive until age 75 experience an increase in life expectancy to 86.2 years (National Center for Health Statistics, 2002, table 28).

Not only does each age cohort carry its particular risk of death, but the causes of death vary widely among the age cohorts. For example, the leading causes of death for infants (under 1 year) are birth defects, respiratory conditions, and infectious diseases. The leading causes for young adults are accidents and suicide and, for young adult blacks, homicide—and, more recently, AIDS—have been added to the list. The elderly are more likely to fall victim to the major killers: heart disease, cancer and stroke. Each age cohort, thus, has its own peculiar cause-of-death configuration.

Variations in health status by age do more than reflect the physical implications of age for health. The health status—actual and perceived—of

---

Box 9-1

The Health Status Index

One of the greatest challenges in healthcare over the years has been the development of an acceptable health status index. Beginning with the social indicators movement of the 1960s, there has been periodic interest expressed in the development of an index that could be used to represent the health status of a population or a community in either absolute or relative terms. While the interest in such an index had waned for a period, there is renewed interest in the concept today.

A health status index is a single figure that represents the health status of a population or a community. It involves an attempt to quantify health status in objective and measurable terms. A health status index is constructed by combining a number of individual health status indicators into a single index. This index can then be utilized to compare the level of need from community to community. It can be used as a basis for setting priorities and evaluating the worthiness of proposed programs. It can also serve as a basis for allocating resources and as a tool for evaluating the effectiveness of existing programs.

A number of conceptual problems surround the development of health status indices. These problems begin with the quesiton of what indicators to include. To this are added the issues of quantification and measurement.

U.S. seniors does not simply reflect the affects of the aging process but is tied up with our notions of the elderly and our perceptions of aging. It reflects perceptions of the role of the elderly in society—their own and other peoples—as well as societal expectations with regard to the health status of various age groups. (Box 9-2 describes the "new" elderly in terms of their health status.)

Sex and Health Status

One of the most important, although perplexing, correlations discussed in this context is that between sex and health status. There is perhaps no other demographic variable for which differentials in health status are so clear-cut. Yet, at the same time, there is probably none for which more questions are raised concerning the meaning of the findings and the possible explanations for the perceived differences.

Any discussion of the relationship between sex and health status must begin with what has become a maxim: Women are characterized by higher levels of morbidity than men, but men have a much higher mortality rate. Although this is a somewhat simplistic summary of a complex situation,

Further, the question of how to weight the various component indicators is also raised. There are no simple means for resolving these issues. Every analysis must address them in the best manner possible and carefully document the process that is used in developing the index.

A variety of indicators can be utilized in the creation of a health status index. Many of the indicators that might be included—e.g., death rates—are fairly obvious. Others, such as certain demographic indicators, might not be. Nevertheless, it is common to use demographic traits such as the proportion nonwhite, the dependency ratio, and educational attainment as component indicators in a health status index. Some of these are referred to as "proxy" measures of health status, in that they are not direct indicators of health conditions but can be assumed to indirectly indicate the level of health status within a population.

In addition to this type of measure, the major categories of health status indicators utilized include morbidity indicators, outcome indicators, utilization indicators, resource availability indicators, and functional status indicators. *Morbidity measures* are obvious indicators of health status, since they reflect the prevalence and/or incidence of various conditions, as well as the level of disability within a population. Thus, the extent to which a population is affected by various acute and chronic conditions constitutes an important component in any health status index. (Unfortunately, it is difficult to obtain actual data on morbidity and, although extremely important, this remains a problematic area in health status index construction.)

(*continued*)

there is a great deal of evidence to suggest that, by any measure of morbidity one might care to use, women are "sicker." On the other hand, there is no doubt that mortality rates are higher and life expectancy is considerably lower for males. In fact, the mortality rate for males is higher than that for females for every age cohort and for virtually every cause of death.

When global measures are utilized, females tend to characterize themselves as being in slightly poorer health than males (National Center for Health Statistics 2002, table 59). On symptom checklists for both physical and mental symptoms, females tend to score much higher (i.e., they report more symptoms). For reported conditions and diagnoses, females are characterized by higher incidence rates. (The one acute "condition" more common among males is injuries.) While females report an even higher level of chronic conditions than acute conditions, these tend to be conditions that are not particularly life-threatening. Comparable proportions of males and females are characterized by some level of activity limitation. Females, however, accumulate on the average more work-loss days, more school-loss days, and more bed-restricted days than males (National Center for Health Statistics 1998, table 67).

Outcome measures are so called because they ostensibly reflect the extent to which the health care system is effective. Outcome measures include such indicators as death rates, infant death rates, life expectancy, and potential years of life lost. Of these measures, the infant mortality rate is probably the most useful as a component of a health status index, since it represents far more than just the rate as which infant deaths occur; it speaks volumes about living conditions, nutritional levels, domestic violence and a number of other dimensions of socioeconomic and health status.

Utilization measures are also used as components of a health status index. This includes indicators such as the hospital admission rate, the rate of emergency room visits, the physician visit rate, and so forth. These measures tend to be among the more controversial, since it could be argued alternately that these are positive or negative indicators.

Resource availability entails another important set of indictors. These include the ratio of hospital beds to the population, the ratio of physicians to the population, and other measures of resources. The rationale for the use of such indicators is that the level of resource availability should be correlated with higher health status. Although this, too, is controversial, such indicators are frequently employed in index construction.

Measures of functional state constitute an additional category of health status indicators. These include a range of measures such as days of work lost, days of school lost, bed-restricted days, activity-restricted days, and so forth. The use of these measures reflects the notion that individuals who are limited in their functional abilities reflect poor health status (regardless of the source of the limitation).

Rogers et al. (2000) found 73% higher odds of mortality for men without controls for other factors. When demographic, social and economic factors were controlled, the odds ratio for males actually increased to 2.0. In effect, the overall mortality rate for males is nearly twice that of females, with males reporting an age-adjusted mortality rate of 1,062 per 100,000 in 1998 compared to 744 per 100,000 for females. For each of the 15 leading causes of death in 1999, males recorded a higher mortality rate, and for some causes the male/female ratio exceeds 3:1 (National Center for Health Statistics 2002, table 30).

Further, the mortality rate for males is higher at every age. At the ages 15–24 and 35–44 it is almost three times as high. Even the fetal death rate for males is higher than that for females, indicating that the greater mortality risk characterizing males predates birth. These figures, of course, are reflected in differentials in life expectancy. In 1999, life expectancy from birth for males was 73.9 years compared to 79.4 years for females (National Center for Health Statistics 2002, table 28).

Health status indices can be calculated for any level of geography for which data are available. However, the smaller the unit of geography the finer the distinction that can be made. Many health planning agencies conduct analyses down to the census tract level, while others utilize the zip code or county as the unit of analysis.

Once the indicators have been chosen, values must be assigned to each indicator for each unit of geography being analyzed. A number of different methodologies can be utilized for this process, and the important factor is to come as close to both scientific rigor and face validity as possible. Assuming that all indicators are to be equally weighted, one approach might be to score each indicator on a scale of 1 to 5 for each geographic unit. Negative characteristics would be scored closer to 1 and positive characteristics closer to 5. The scores for each indicator could be summed and then divided by the number of indicators to provide an average score for each geographic unit somewhere between 1 and 5. It should be noted that the absolute number generated through the process means little; its value is derived from the ability to compare it with other figures. This index number could be used, for example, to compare one community to another or track the health status of a particular community over time.

The current methodologies for constructing health status indices are certainly not without their critics. There are numerous conceptual, methodological, and practical issues that must be addressed in the development of a health status index. Nevertheless, the need to better understand the health characteristics of our communities mandates continued efforts toward the development of defensible health status indices.

On one hand, it can be argued that males die from different causes than females. However, for every condition except diabetes and sex-related disorders, the mortality rate is higher for males. Interestingly, the excess male mortality for each age cohort is attributable to a different cause in each case. For example, a major killer of infants is chronic respiratory disease, and this is more common among male infants. Accidents are the major cause of death for children aged 1 to 14, and males have approximately twice the risk of accidents.

One other interesting finding with regard to sex differentials in health status is the fact that, although males are sick less often, when they are sick the condition is more likely to be serious or even fatal. All things being equal, the disease acuity level for males who do become ill is higher than for females with comparable conditions.

It is beyond the scope of this book to evaluate the various explanations that are offered to account for these phenomena. Briefly, these explanations include reporting anomalies, differential exposure to environmental

---

Box 9-2

The "New Elderly" and Their Impact on Healthcare

No demographic trend has received more attention over the past decade than the aging of the U.S. population. Along with increases in life expectancy has come tremendous growth in the size of the older American population. By 2000, the median age of the U.S. population had reached 36 years and there were over 58 million Americans 55 years or older, representing 21% of the total population. By 2025 there will be 62 million citizens 65 or older, accounting for nearly 20% of the population. While all older age groups will increase significantly in numbers for the foreseeable future, the 85 and over age group will grow faster than any other cohort.

The numbers by themselves are noteworthy since the current cohort of seniors constitutes a population one-and-one-half times the total population of Canada. As this age group has grown in size, it has also increased its economic, political and market clout. "Mature Americans" are living longer and enjoying greater health, while having more money to spend than any previous generation. As with many demographic trends, however, the size of the phenomenon may not be as important as the characteristics of the population under consideration.

The attributes of this new generation of seniors are noteworthy along two dimensions. First, these new seniors have distinct characteristics that set them apart from previous cohorts of seniors. While today's oldest seniors share many characteristics with the elders of previous generations, they are also likely to be distinct from their forebears in a number of ways. While today's 80-year-olds grew up during the Depression and are likely to carry scars from that period, today's 65-year-old, on the other hand, was twelve years old when World War II ended and grew up in a much different world. In fact, this cohort as a group is unlike any previous generation, and it appears

---

conditions and social stress, cultural expectations, and outright biological differences. There is evidence that women are more sensitive to the existence of symptoms of both physical and mental illness, and that they more readily take action in response to perceived symptoms, thereby showing up more often in clinical records. On the other hand, recent research has found that men and women do not differ in their reporting of initial conditions (McIntyre et al. 1999). It is also argued that men have historically been exposed to more dangerous environmental and occupational conditions, thereby accounting for the excess mortality. But it follows that these same conditions should contribute to morbidity, which they apparently do not.

Differences in health status related to sex do more than reflect the implications of different physical characteristics for males and females.

that its behavior, including the use of health services, will be strikingly different from that of its forebears throughout the aging process. (Indeed, they are so different that the term "elderly" has been essentially taken out of use.)

The mature consumer of the 1990s represents the first cohort in history to benefit from the extraordinary advances in medicine and technology of this century. The additional 10–20 years of life expectancy gained in recent decades appears to have been added to the middle rather than to the end of the life span. This means today's 65-year-old is roughly equivalent to yesterday's 50-year-old, with all that implies for senior lifestyles. In fact, the oldest old have gained more in terms of health status than any other cohort. Their tastes, interests, and concerns are quite different from those of their parents. These seniors are interested in autonomy, self-sufficiency, personal growth, and revitalization.

Second, there is significant differentiation within the nation's older population. For almost two decades it has been realized that the senior population was not simply one homogenous cohort of individuals. Now, as more data have become available, researchers realize that American seniors are a highly differentiated population with wide variations in needs, preferences, and behaviors. In fact, it has been suggested that we are becoming less alike, rather than more, as we age. For demographic purposes, this generation of seniors has been categorized as the "young old", the "middle old", and the "old old". Other more descriptive terms ("working mature", "young retirees", and even the traditional "elderly") may also be applied. However differentiated, each subgroup has specific implications for health status and health services utilization.

Key indicators of health, social, and economic characteristics among older Americans vary considerably by race and ethnicity, for example, often mirroring disparities in wider racial and ethnic populations. In addition to

(continued)

Males and females do not simply differ in physical terms but also along a number of social and psychological dimensions. The respective sex roles of society dictate certain behaviors, attitudes and preferences on the part of males and females. In fact, the traits our society associates with masculinity are also traits that contribute to excess mortality. The social groups with which males and females interact and their respective work environments also influence their behavior and subsequent health status.

Race, Ethnicity, and Health Status

Race is a biosocial attribute, because it combines physical attributes with social connotations. Racial groups are defined based on one or more distinguishable physical attributes considered important in the particular

living longer, Americans are becoming more racially and ethnically diverse. While the number of older whites will increase 97% between 1995 and 2050, elderly African-Americans will increase by 265%, Native Americans by 294%, Hispanic-Americans by 530%, and Asian-Americans by 643%.

Of course, the nature of future seniors will be driven to a great extent by the characteristics of the baby boomers. Nearly 78 million Americans were born between 1946 and 1964, and the oldest among them were in their 50s as the 20th century ended. Boomers are determined to reinvent retirement, a process that appears to already be underway. Retirement is no longer seen as a type of "default" condition, but as a context for a new and different lifestyle. Boomers, in fact, have already influenced the health-care delivery system in significant ways. They were primarily responsible for the establishment of health maintenance organizations, birthing centers, urgent care centers, and outpatient surgery centers as components of the healthcare landscape. Now they are driving the demand for a wide range of new services such as laser eye surgery, skin rejuvenation, and menopause management.

The new generation of seniors is not likely to be nearly as docile as previous ones. Baby boomers are used to having things their way and are already much more demanding as "middle-agers" than previous cohorts. Their expectations are much higher, they are better informed, and they are used to being in charge. The stereotype of the docile grandmother happily accepting whatever Medicare metes out to her will not persist very long under the onslaught of demanding baby boomers.

The health status of the senior population will be a critical issue for the United States during the twenty-first century. Today's seniors are living longer, and they tend to suffer fewer limitations than previous generations of elderly. In fact, self-assessed health status improved significantly for seniors between 1987 and 1995, according to the National Center for Health Statistics.

society. In U.S. society and many others, skin color is the most important factor in racial categorization. The major racial categories utilized in most analyses are white, black (or African American), Asian-American/Pacific Islander, and Native American (or American Indian).

Ethnic group distinctions are based on differences in cultural heritage. Members of distinct ethnic groups have a common cultural tradition, including values and norms and perhaps even a language, that sets them apart from the larger society. While ethnic distinctions are not primarily biological, prolonged "inbreeding" often leads to the development of distinctive physical characteristics. The major ethnic groups in U.S. society include Hispanics, Jews, and certain large national groups that, in some regions at least, have been able to maintain their ethnic identity.

Recent research has found an actual generation-to-generation improvement in functional ability among those 65 and older.

Today's seniors are staying active longer as a result of being in better health than previous generations. Although there is an understandable drop in the proportion involved in outdoor recreation and more strenuous activities, the numbers of seniors involved in other types of exercise programs has increased dramatically. A new generation of health professionals is also encouraging lifelong physical activity, and sports products companies are modifying their equipment to meet the needs of seniors.

Nevertheless, an increase in chronic conditions and activity limitations is inevitable among seniors. Physical and mental deterioration can be delayed but it cannot be eliminated. This means that we can expect a growing proportion of the U.S. population to be characterized by one or more chronic conditions and one or more activity limitations in the future. Even with improved health status, the numbers alone will assure that healthcare costs for this population will increase significantly.

Despite the evidence of improving health status among the seniors, older Americans still account for the majority of federal healthcare expenditures. Over half of the federal healthcare dollar is spent on Medicare beneficiaries. While seniors account for only 12 percent of Medicaid enrollment, they account for over one-third of Medicaid expenditures (primarily for nursing home care). Americans over 50 account for 60% of healthcare spending and 80% of prescription drug spending, while representing 35% of the total population.

The good news, for seniors at least, is that over 99 percent of the elderly have healthcare coverage. Virtually all elderly are covered under Medicare, and more than two-thirds of those 65 and over have supplementary coverage. The role of the federal government in subsidizing care for American seniors will continue to be an issue to be faced as the "new elderly" begin to dominate the health care system.

When the various racial groups in the United States are examined in terms of health status, significant differences are found. The major distinction is between whites and blacks, with Asian-Americans and Native Americans manifesting less distinct health status characteristics. Whites have historically rated themselves high in terms of health status relative to blacks, with other racial/ethnic categories falling somewhere in between. Differences in global health assessment and functional limitations in daily activities by race and ethnicity persist even when income and education are controlled (Ren and Amick 1996). Differences in self-assessment should be interpreted with caution, since there are indications that members of different racial groups may use different criteria for assessing their own health status (Larsen et al. 1998).

Clear-cut differences in morbidity are found primarily between whites and nonwhites. The number of symptoms, the number of sickness episodes, and the severity of the conditions all place blacks at a health status disadvantage. Although relatively more prone to acute health conditions, blacks actually suffer higher rates of both acute and chronic conditions than whites. In the early 1990s, for example, blacks represented 12% of the population but accounted for 28% of the diagnosed hypertension (Hidreth and Saunders 1992). Further, all things being equal, blacks contracting life-threatening conditions are more at risk of death from them than are whites with the same conditions.

Differences in cause-specific morbidity exist between various racial and ethnic groups, with the epidemiology of cancer being a good example. Whites in the United States are more likely to suffer from colon/rectal cancer, breast cancer, and bladder cancer, to name a few, than are blacks. However, the incidence rate for several other types of cancer are higher for blacks. These include lung, prostate, stomach, and esophageal cancer.

Specific ethnic groups are likely to display unique morbidity and mortality profiles. Polish-Americans suffer from relatively high levels of lung and esophageal cancer, for example, while among Italian-Americans bladder, intestinal, and pharyngeal cancer are more common. Japanese-Americans suffer from stomach cancer at rates many times higher than Japanese nationals, while cervical cancer is almost unknown among Jewish women. Hispanics report by far the highest incidence of AIDS among the various ethnic groups (National Center for Health Statistics 2002, table 54).

When racial differences in the level of disability are examined, it is found that the proportion of blacks reporting some level of activity limitation is nearly half again as high as that for the white population. The proportion with activity limitation is 18% for blacks compared to 14% for whites.

Mortality rates for the black population are considerably higher than those for the white population. When the 1999 mortality rate is examined, the overall age-adjusted mortality rate is 882 per 100,000 population. The mortality rate for the white population as a whole was 661 deaths per 100,000 population, compared to a rate of 1,147 per 100,000 population for blacks (National Center for Health Statistics 2002, table 30). African-Americans are characterized by higher mortality risks at nearly all ages and for nearly all causes (Rogers et al. 2000). The gap in mortality rates for whites and African-Americans has actually increased since 1990.

In 2000 American Indians actually recorded a mortality rate lower than that for African Americans (716/100,000). Asian-Americans recorded a rate of 518 and Hispanics 601, indicating relatively good health for these two groups (National Center for Health Statistics, 2002, table 30).

This mortality differential is reflected in life expectancy for the two racial categories. In 1999, life expectancy at birth for whites was 77.3 years compared to 71.4 years for blacks. The greatest differential in life expectancy is between white females (79.2 years) and black males (67.8). Overall Hispanic mortality rates compare favorably to those for both whites and blacks (National Center for Health Statistics 2002, table 28).

Important differences exist between blacks and whites in terms of the common causes of death. To a great extent these differentials reflect the differences in morbidity characteristics discussed above. Whites in the United States are more likely to be characterized by chronic conditions, especially those associated with aging. Blacks and certain ethnic groups are more likely to be characterized by acute conditions. Further, nonwhites are more likely to be affected by environmentally caused health problems and life-threatening problems associated with lifestyles (such as homicide and accidents). Consequently, the dominant causes of death among the white population are heart disease, cancer, and stroke. While these are important among various other racial and ethnic groups, blacks in particular are more likely to die as a result of infectious conditions, respiratory and digestive systems conditions, and the lifestyle-associated problems noted above.

Another important cause of death for African Americans is infant mortality. Although infant mortality has been dramatically reduced as a cause of death in the United States in this century, it continues to be a serious health threat for many groups of nonwhites. The infant mortality rate for blacks in 1999 was more than twice that for whites, or 14.0 per 1,000 live births versus 5.8 (National Center for Health Statistics 2002, table 29). The rates for both groups has declined since the late 1980s, with the percentage point gap between the two narrowing somewhat in recent years.

Other racial and ethnic groups recorded quite disparate rates of infant death. Certain Asian groups, for example, report much lower than average infant mortality, while Hispanics as a group record infant mortality rates between those of whites and blacks. Native Americans and native Alaskans historically have recorded very high infant mortality rates; however, since the 1950s, their rates have come to resemble the U.S. average. The infant mortality rates recorded in 1999 for various racial and ethnic groups were diverse. In addition to the figures for whites and blacks noted above, we find an infant mortality rate of 5.7 for Hispanics, 2.9 for Chinese-Americans, and 3.4 for Japanese-Americans (National Center for Health Statistics 2002, table 20). This is clearly a situation in which sociocultural factors play a greater role than biological factors.

Indicators of disability are also found to be higher among blacks than whites. Data from the 2000 National Health Interview Survey indicated that 11.5% of the white population had some limitation due to chronic conditions, compared to 14.3% of the black population (National Center for

Health Statistics 2000, table 58). American Indians had by far the greatest degree of limitation, with 20.1% of that group reporting limitation of activity. The Hispanic population was the least limited, only 10.3% reporting limitations due to chronic conditions.

This significant variation in health status by race is less a reflection of biological differences than it is of sociocultural factors. There are few conditions that are peculiar to a particular racial or ethnic group. Thus, most of the variation in health status must be due to some other factor. The fact that various racial and ethnic groups are characterized by differences in types and levels of conditions reflects the social dimension that accompanies the racial and ethnic groups. These groups may differ in terms of marital status, type of employment and environmental context. They are likely to vary in terms of income and education which, for most researchers, override the importance of race and ethnicity. They may be characterized by differing lifestyles which encourage healthy behavior or condone risky health behavior. While certain ethnic groups may have lifestyles that help or hinder health status, many of the differences found between racial and ethnic groups wash out when socioeconomic status is controlled for. (See Box 9-3 for a discussion of the use of "race" as a statistical category.)

SOCIOCULTURAL CHARACTERISTICS

Sociocultural characteristics refer to those traits that characterize individuals related to their position or status in society. While biosocial traits are ascribed essentially at birth, sociocultural traits are typically acquired through the actions of the individual. Sociocultural traits are important not only because they indicate one's place in society, but also because of their correlation with health status.

Marital Status and Health Status

Although Durkheim's study of suicide in the 1890s (Durkheim 1951) found marital status to be a factor in differential suicide rates, it is only recently that the association between marital status and both physical and mental illness has been fully appreciated. Today, many consider marital status to be one of the best predictors of both health status and health behavior, although, as will be shown, the relationship is actually a very complex one. The categories of marital status for the discussion below include: never married, married, divorced, and widowed. (The term "single" has generally been eliminated from research terminology, since it can be interpreted to mean never married, widowed, or divorced.)

The relative health status of members of these three groups actually depends on the measure that is being utilized. In general, it is held that health status, both physical and mental, is higher for the married in U.S. society than for those of any other marital status. Married individuals are found to have lower levels of morbidity and mortality, to have lower levels of disability and restriction of activity, and to perceive themselves as being in much better health.

Married persons have a higher level of physical and psychological well-being than their unmarried counterparts (Mookherjee 1997). It has also been found that married individuals, when affected with a health problem, suffer less serious problems, face a more favorable prognosis, and report a more favorable outcome. Although never-married, divorced, and widowed individuals have poorer health status overall than the married, there is no clear-cut ranking among these three groups.

With regard to disability, only 15% of married men and 14% of married women were found to be restricted in the performance of their normal activities in the 1995 NHIS survey, compared to 20% or more of both men and women in other marital status categories. This same pattern is found with regard to other indicators of disability. The NHIS found that married men are restricted in their work, home, or school activities an average of 10 days per year; the figure is 12 days for married women. Only never-married males, with 9 days of restrictions, fared better; all other categories were substantially worse off. The same was true for bed-restriction days. Married and never-married men and women were similar in the number of days they were restricted to bed annually, but divorcees and widows were clearly worse off.

The exception to these patterns relates to the incidence of acute conditions. Married men and women report slightly more acute conditions than never-married men and women. However, the married are still better off than the divorced and widowed on this indicator of morbidity. It has been suggested, as in the case with sex differentials, that the never married may suffer fewer episodes of acute conditions but are affected by more serious and prolonged conditions. The incidence of injuries also represents something of an exception; while married people are less prone to injuries than never-married and divorced individuals, they are more at risk for injuries than are the widowed. Although the never married are better off on some measures of morbidity, they are more likely to commit suicide or die as a result of homicide or an accident.

It is sometimes argued that there are other factors that actually explain these differences in morbidity and mortality, and some of these factors are discussed below. However, evidence for the importance of marital status as a predictor of health status can be drawn from data on changes in health status that accompany changes in marital status. When individuals shift from one status to another, changes in health status are frequently seen. The change is probably the most extreme when the shift is from the married

---

Box 9-3

The Use of Race as a Statistical Category

In the implementation of health services research projects, race is often used as an independent variable in the testing of hypotheses. However, the routine use of race as a category in health services research is not without its critics. The invalidity of the very notion of "race" aside, there are several arguments against the continued use of race in this manner.

For one thing, in studies of health status and health behavior "race" is seldom defined. Even when the researchers define the concept, the use of standard indicators of racial status is problematic. In studies involving primary research, race is likely to be determined through self-reports by the respondent or by visual identification on the part of the researcher. In studies using aggregate data, race is typically based on self-reports obtained from census data or some other large-scale data collection process. In either case, there is the opportunity for a great deal of "slippage" in allocation of the study population to racial categories. Respondents may misreport their race or misunderstand the meaning of the categories from which they must chose, and bi- and multi-racial individuals are becoming increasingly common in the U.S. population. Interviewers may vary in their criteria for assigning individuals a racial classification.

A more serious criticism of the use of race in such research has been generated by studies that examined the impact of race on health disparities along with other independent variables. These studies have found that most racially based disparities in health status are eliminated when socioeconomic status is controlled for. That is, individuals in comparable positions within the status hierarchy are likely to exhibit comparable levels of health status *regardless* of their race. Despite the findings, researchers persist in attributing variations in health status to variations in racial characteristics.

---

status to the divorced or widowed category. Increases in both morbidity and mortality have been documented for individuals undergoing such a transition (Waldron et al. 1997). In addition, poor health status has been shown to increase the probability that divorce will occur (Joung et al. 1998).

Limited research has been conducted on the mortality implications of marital status and household characteristics. However, recent work by Rogers et al. (2000) found that married individuals living with their spouses and children are at the lowest risk of mortality of any marital status/living arrangement combination. Situations that are characterized by high mortality levels include unmarried individuals who live with their parents, members of particularly large families, and single parents with three or more children living in the household.

Not only does the use of race in this manner present a potentially misleading picture of disparities in health status in the U.S., but it has "political" implications as well. Attributing disparities to racial characteristics serves to place the "blame" on the racial group rather than on other "external" factors. Thus, one would conclude that African Americans suffer from relatively poor health status because of something about African Americans themselves. The assumption becomes that something(s) that African Americans are doing (or not doing) is responsible for their condition. Further, linking disparities to race implies that there is little that can be done about the disparities, since they could almost be considered inherent to the various racial groups.

Critics of this the use of race contend that placing the blame on racial differences rather than socioeconomic differences deflects attention (and action) away from the economic system. If, indeed, the root causes of disparities in health status are found in the existing stratification system, the obvious solution is to modify the stratification system. This line of reasoning, of course, represents a threat to those who have a vested interest in the existing system and people who would be opposed to the potential redistribution of wealth that might be involved in any such attempt to address these disparities. While it is doubtful that many individuals involved in health services research feel a vested interest in the status quo, the continued use of race as an independent variable in the study of health status disparities inadvertently contributes to the deflection of attention away from the social, economic and political implications of the use of race in health services research.

Sources: David R. Williams and Chiquita Collins (1996). "U.S. Socioeconomic and Racial Differences in Health: Patterns and Explanations," in P. Brown (ed.), *Perspectives in Medical Sociology* (2nd edition). Prospect Heights, IL: Waveland Press.

Marital status and living arrangements are both considered good predictors of health status, and various explanations are provided for their operation in this regard. The primary contention is that the presence of a significant other in some type of stable relationships has both a prophylactic and therapeutic benefit. The social and emotional support available from a spouse or significant other is thought to help prevent the onset of health problems and, should they occur, limit the impact of the condition and shorten its duration. Thus, the presumed better social integration of married individuals compared to the never married, the divorced and the widowed appears to have a salutary effect. In addition, such individuals have someone available in the household to assure that they follow proper health practices and utilize the system appropriately.

On the other side of the coin, we find that unmarried individuals not only do not have someone to support them, but they tend to pursue less healthy lifestyles and are more likely to participate in risky health behavior. Without family responsibilities, the unmarried are likely to get less sleep, eat erratically, drink and smoke more, and otherwise participate in behaviors that do not contribute to enhanced health status.

Socioeconomic Status and Health Status

During the 1960s and 1970s, when poverty in the United States was being rediscovered, an appreciation of the relationship between socioeconomic status and health status emerged. This relationship had not been fully explored heretofore, despite episodic reporting of surprisingly poor health status within pockets of disadvantaged populations such as Native Americans and Appalachian residents. Only in the 1970s was the extent of the health-social class relationship recognized.

Social scientists generally see U.S. society as being divided into three to six social classes. The three major divisions are the upper, middle, and lower classes. When more divisions are utilized, the categories are typically subdivisions of the three major groupings. A common variation involves the carving out of a "working class" category out of the lower-middle and upper-lower classes. (See Chapter 11 for a more detailed discussion of social stratification in the United States.)

One of sociology's most enduring contributions to the health field is the documentation that social class position is a key determinant of variations in the distribution of disease (Williams and Collins, 1996). Researchers in diverse disciplines recognize that socioeconomic status is so strongly linked to h᠆alth that they must statistically control for it in order to study their phenomena of interest.

Socioeconomic status is often defined in terms of income, education or occupational status. Since income is the measure of social class most easily quantified, it has been the socioeconomic variable most frequently linked to health status. It has been found that no matter what indicator of health status is utilized, there is generally an inverse relationship between income and health status. As income increases, the prevalence of both acute and chronic conditions decreases. When symptom checklists are utilized, the lower the income, the larger the number of symptoms identified. Not surprisingly, members of lower-income groups assess themselves as being in poorer health than do the more affluent.

Not only are there more episodes of both acute and chronic conditions recorded as income decreases, but the severity of the conditions is likely to be greater when income is lower. When afflicted by acute conditions, the poor tend to have more prolonged episodes characterized by greater severity. In a society that has become characterized by chronic health conditions, acute disorders remain surprisingly common among the lower-income groups. There is a direct and monotonic inverse relationship between income level and activity limitation. The level of activity limitation due to chronic conditions was 23.2% for the "poor" in 2000, compared to 9.5% for the "non-poor" (National Center for Health Statistics, 2002, table 58).

The relationship between income and health status persists when mortality is examined. The mortality rate for the lowest income levels may be twice that of the most affluent in some communities, even after adjusting for age. The poor are also characterized by relatively high levels of infant mortality and even maternal mortality.

The relationship between income level and health status has been explained in a number of ways. The most obvious has to do with the ability to pay for health services and, thus, with the affluent presumably able to ameliorate many health problems that the unaffluent may not. This ability to pay may extend to the acquisition of preventive services and lifestyle factors such as good nutrition. It has also been suggested that the correlation of educational levels with income levels is the underlying explanation for the observed relationships.

While other socioeconomic indicators are useful for predicting a population's health status, education is thought by some to be the single most important indicator in this regard (Cockerham 2001). Those at higher educational levels are likely to rate themselves as being in better health than those with less education (National Center for Health Statistics 1998, table 70). Typically, the higher the educational level, the lower the morbidity level. This is true for both acute and chronic physical conditions, with a clear inverse relationship demonstrated between educational levels and major health threats such as cardiovascular disease (Wamala et al. 1999). These relationships also hold for indicators of disability.

The pattern with regard to mortality resembles that for income. The death rate for the poorly educated is much higher than that for those with higher educational achievement, with age-adjusted death rate for those with less than 12 years of education of 599/100,000 compared to 255/100,000 for those with 13 years or more (Minino, 2002, table 36). Infant mortality, in fact, has been virtually eliminated from the groups with the highest educational levels. The poorly educated, however, account for the bulk of infant deaths. Like the poor, the causes of death for the poorly educated are more likely to be the acute problems typically associated with less developed countries than the chronic conditions characterizing much of American society. Also like the poor, the less educated are more likely to be characterized by lifestyle-related deaths such as homicides and accidents.

Various explanations have been offered to explain the close relationship between educational level and health status. The explanation most frequently posited has to do with the greater knowledge that better education brings with regard to health practices. This includes an acceptance of preventive practices, awareness of various symptoms and disease states, access to information on sources of care and how to utilized them. The fact that the better educated typically have higher incomes also means that they have the resources available to obtain preventive services and otherwise "purchase" health.

The relationship between occupation and health status is somewhat more complex than that for other measures of socioeconomic status. Occupation can be examined in terms of occupational status (e.g., blue-collar, white-collar, professional) or in terms of specific occupations. In the first case, there is a relatively direct and positive relationship between the occupation one holds and health status. In general, the higher the occupational prestige, the better the health status. Those at lower occupational levels tend to be characterized by higher rates of morbidity and disability. Like the poor and the uneducated, they tend to be characterized both by more conditions and by more serious conditions.

At the same time, mortality rates and longevity vary directly with occupational status. Past research has consistently found a clear link between mortality and occupational status, with age-adjusted death rates for the lowest occupational group (unskilled laborers) being considerably higher than those of the highest (professionals). The recent research by Rogers et al. (2000) has reaffirmed this finding, showing mortality rates for those with the lowest occupational status to be considerably higher than those for the highest.

A second approach to examining the relationship between the conditions of employment and health status involves an analysis of health status in terms of specific industries and occupations. Although this is a highly complex process, it is found that certain industries tend to be characterized by inordinately high levels of both morbidity and mortality. Among the standard industry categories utilized by the Department of Labor, the industry with the highest rate of injuries involving work loss is the transportation/communications/utilities industry. A similar pattern is displayed with regard to work-related deaths. In 2000, the mining industry reported the highest rates or occupational injuries, followed closely by the manufacturing and construction industries. This contrasts vividly with the "safest" industry (finance, insurance and real estate) that reported an occupational injury rate of less than one per 100,000 workers (National Center for Health Statistics, 2002, table 50).

A similar pattern was found for occupation-related deaths. In 2000 the highest rate of occupational injury deaths was recorded for mining, with

30 deaths per 100,000 workers. This was followed by agriculture, forestry and fishing with a rate of 21 per 100,000. This compares to the finance, insurance and real estate industry which recorded an occupational injury death rate of less than one per 100,000.

One other consideration when examining occupational categories is the issue of employment status. This issue may, in fact, be more significant than occupational differentials. When the employed are compared to the unemployed, clear-cut differences surface in terms of physical and mental illness. The unemployed appear to be sicker in terms of most health status indicators; they have higher levels of morbidity and higher levels of disability than the employed. While it could be argued that poor health leads to unemployment, it has been found that otherwise healthy individuals who have undergone loss of employment often develop symptoms of health problems (Catalano, 1991).

Apart from evidence linking unemployment to high suicide rates, little research has been conducted on the relationship between the lack of employment and mortality. However, the recent work by Rogers et al. (2000) has demonstrated that the employed tend to have a lower risk of mortality than the unemployed. Interestingly, the analysis also found that individuals who were not in the labor force (i.e., neither employed nor looking for employment) were at the greatest risk of mortality of all employment statuses.

Individuals with various socioeconomic characteristics are likely to be characterized by differing lifestyles. These lifestyles are likely to be major contributors to health status.

Religion and Health Status

Perhaps the least well-documented relationship between a social variable and health status is the link between religion and health conditions. Religion is relatively poorly studied in U.S. society, and information linking religious affiliation or religiosity with health status is fragmented. However, a growing body of empirical evidence suggests that religious involvement has beneficial effects on health status and mortality rates (Oman and Reed 1998).

Ecological studies have found a correlation between overall health status and religious affiliation. In addition, specific conditions have been linked to the degree of religious commitment (Jarvis and Northcott 1987). A recent study (Dwyer et al. 1990) found that religious "concentrations" are associated with lower rates of digestive cancer, respiratory cancer, and overall morbidity. Even more recently, Hummer et al. (1999) found a clear relationship between church attendance and mortality rates. People who never attend church services exhibit a risk of death 1.87 times that for those who attend services two or more times per week. This calculates out to a seven-year difference in life expectancy (at age 20) between non-attenders and frequent attenders. These studies have also associated higher frequency of church attendance with lower blood pressure, lower mortality from cardiovascular disease, and less physical disability (Oman and Reed 1998). The lifestyles of strict religious groups such as Mormons and Seventh Day Adventists have been found to contribute to their higher health status.

Some religion-specific differentials in morbidity that have been found are typically not in terms of overall prevalence, but in regard to group-specific conditions. For example, the Jewish population in the United States is characterized by higher levels of some conditions and lower levels of others. However, it is usually argued that these differences reflect cultural variations rather than religious differences.

Of all of the relationships discussed in this section, the link between religion and health status is perhaps the most difficult to explain. There is evidence that having a "faith" provides one a sense of security or a sense of coherence that things are going to eventually work out. This "peace of mind" may serve as a buffer with regard to the onset of various health problems. At the same time, as illustrated by certain religious denominations, the dictates of the religion restrict the types of behavior that often contribute to ill health. Finally, the integrative nature of social group affiliation, along with its social support function, may reduce stress and otherwise serve as a deterrent to ill health.

Notwithstanding the numerous disparities in health status found in U.S. society related to sociocultural factors, the question should still be raised: Are health status disparities inevitable? (Box 9-4 discusses the issue of the inevitability of disparities in health status.)

Lifestyles and Health Status

Perhaps the most significant finding over the past quarter-century by medical sociologists relates to the impact of lifestyles on health status and health behavior. Americans are characterized by a wide diversity in lifestyles and this diversity has important implications for the distribution of health problems. The behaviors associated with lifestyles can have either positive or negative consequences for health. These activities typically consists of choices and practices that range from brushing one's teeth and using automobile seat belts to relaxing at health spas. For most people, health lifestyles involve decisions about food, exercise, relaxation, personal hygiene, risk of accidents, coping with stress, smoking, alcohol and drug use, and having physical checkups.

Although lifestyle choices may appear to involve individual behaviors, it should be remembered that few behaviors are really based on individual volition. While we may think we are acting as individuals, our cultural background, our status within society, and our social group affiliations determine a large part of how we behave.

The federal government has become increasingly concerned with the impact of unhealthy lifestyles on the nation's health status. In an attempt to monitor unhealthy behavior the Centers for Disease Control and Prevention introduced the Behavioral Risk Factor Surveillance System (BRFSS) in the 1980s. This national survey attempts to track trends in unhealthy behavior around the country and is a major source of information on healthy and unhealthy behaviors. Some of the more important findings are discussed below.

Tobacco Use.   Cigarette smoking is the single most preventable cause of disease and death in the United States. Smoking results in more deaths each year in the United States than AIDS, alcohol, cocaine, heroin, homicide, suicide, motor vehicle crashes, and fires combined. In the late 1990s, 35 percent of adolescents were current cigarette smokers. In 1998, 24 percent of adults were current cigarette smokers. Tobacco-related deaths number more than 430,000 per year among U.S. adults, representing more than 5 million years of potential life lost. Direct medical costs attributable to smoking total at least $50 billion per year.

Smoking is a major risk factor for heart disease, stroke, lung cancer, and chronic lung diseases—all leading causes of death. Smoking during pregnancy can result in miscarriages, premature delivery, and sudden infant death syndrome. Other health effects of smoking result from injuries and environmental damage caused by fires. Environmental tobacco smoke (ETS) increases the risk of heart disease and significant lung conditions, especially asthma and bronchitis in children.

Following years of steady decline, rates of smoking among adults appear to have leveled off in the 1990s. However, every day, an estimated 3,000 young persons start smoking. These trends are disturbing because the vast majority of adult smokers tried their first cigarette before age 18 years; more than half of adult smokers became daily smokers before this same age. Almost half of adolescents who continue smoking regularly will die eventually from a smoking-related illness.

American Indians and Alaska Natives, blue-collar workers, and military personnel have the highest rates of smoking in adults. Men have only somewhat higher rates of smoking than women within the total U.S. population. Low-income adults are more likely to smoke than are high-income adults. The percentage of people aged 25 years and older with less than 12 years of education who are current smokers is nearly three times that for persons with 16 or more years of education.

Box 9-4

Are Disparities in Health Status Inevitable?

One of the most significant findings from recent research on health status involves the persistent existence of disparities in health status among various segments of U.S. society. Given the evidence for disparities in health status in the United States, the question arises as to the inevitability of these disparities. One way to address this issue would be to examine health status disparities in international and historical perspective. Comparisons of inequality in health status and trends in social equalities over time provide valuable insights into this issue.

The statistics indicate that national mortality rates are not strongly related to a country's overall economic status. On the other hand, they are closely linked to the level of inequality within each country. Countries with the least inequality have the best health profiles. Differences in income distribution alone account for two-thirds of the variation in national mortality rates for the 23 countries belonging to the Organization for Economic Cooperation and Development. Trends in income inequality are also related to variations in health status by socioeconomic status over time within a given country. An analysis of socioeconomic differences in mortality in England and Wales between 1921 and 1981 revealed that the gap in mortality rate between different social classes widened or narrowed to correspond with increases or decreases in relative poverty.

A study of the relationship between education and mortality in nine industrialized countries also suggests that a country's level of egalitarian social and economic policy is linked to the nature of socioeconomic differentials in health within that country. Inequalities in mortality were twice as large in the United States, France, and Italy as in the Netherlands, Sweden, Denmark, and Norway. Most statistics also show that the lowest social classes in Sweden have lower mortality than the highest social classes in Great Britain. Thus, the benefits of income redistribution within a society may affect the health status of the majority of the population.

A clear illustration of the link between economic inequality and health is found in the comparison of the trends in life expectancy and income for Japan and Great Britain over the past two decades. In 1970, Japan and Great Britain were similar in average life expectancy and income distribution. During the 1970s and 1980s socioeconomic differentials in Japan became the narrowest in the world, while the income distribution gap widened in Great Britain. During this same period, Japan's life expectancy rapidly increased to become the highest in the world, while Britain's relative international ranking on

---

Substance Abuse. Alcohol and illicit drug use are associated with many of this country's most serious problems, including violence, injury, and HIV infection. Use of these substances is associated with child and spousal abuse, sexually transmitted diseases (including HIV infection),

life expectancy declined. Changes in Japanese nutrition, health services, or prevention policies do not account for these differences.

Further evidence that the health status disadvantage of low socioeconomic status is not driven by an absolute standard of economic well-being comes from comparisons of the African-American population in the United States with their counterparts in the Caribbean. Although the average annual income in Barbados was under US$3,000 in 1988, life expectancy among black men in Barbados was 71 years, while it was 65 years for black men in the United States. Infant mortality in Barbados was similar to that of U.S. blacks.

The evidence is fairly clear that reductions in inequalities in health are closely linked to reductions in social inequality. Factors such as medical care, even if equally provided to all, are unlikely to diminish socioeconomic differentials. Improved access to health-enhancing resources may improve health for both high and low social status groups without reducing the health disparity between them. Reducing the socioeconomic gradient in health will require more fundamental changes. Conditions such as substandard housing, low educational levels, poor social support and unemployment, as well as insufficient access to preventive health services, contribute to the disparities in health status that exist in the U.S.

Income is probably the component of socioeconomic status that is most amenable to change through redistributive policies such as tax credits or direct income supplementation. Research has documented that changes in household income can enhance health status. In a study of expanded income support, researchers found that the birth weight of infants of mothers in the experimental income group was higher than those of mothers in the control group, although neither group experienced any experimental manipulation of health services. Improved nutrition, probably as a result of income manipulation, appeared to have been the key intervening factor. Similarly, an analysis of mortality over a ten-year period found that changes in the proportion of workers with low earnings in specific occupational categories were significantly associated with changes in occupational mortality.

To answer the initial question, it appears that disparities in health status among different socioeconomic groups in society do not have to be inevitable. However, to the extent that relative deprivation exists in society, disparities in health status can be expected to persist.

Sources: David R. Williams and Chiquita Collins (1996). "U.S. Socioeconomic and Racial Differences in Health: Patterns and Explanations," in P. Brown (ed.), *Perspectives in Medical Sociology* (2nd edition). Prospect Heights, IL: Waveland Press.

teen pregnancy, school failure, motor vehicle crashes, low worker productivity, and homelessness. Alcohol abuse alone is associated with motor vehicle crashes, homicides, suicides, and drowning—leading causes of death among youth. Long-term heavy drinking can lead to heart disease, cancer, alcohol-related liver disease, and pancreatitis. The annual economic costs to the United States from alcohol abuse were estimated to be $167 billion in 1995, and the costs from drug abuse were estimated to be $110 billion.

In 1998, 79 percent of adolescents aged 12 to 17 years reported that they used alcohol or illicit drugs in the past month. In the same year, 6 percent of adults aged 18 years and older reported using illicit drugs in the past month; 17 percent reported binge drinking in the past month, which is defined as consuming five or more drinks on one occasion. Excessive alcohol consumption can cause fetal alcohol syndrome, a leading cause of preventable mental retardation.

Although the trend from 1994 to 1998 has shown some fluctuations, about 77% of adolescents aged 12 to 17 years admitted to the use of alcohol and/or illicit drugs at some time. Alcohol is the drug most frequently used by adolescents aged 12 to 17 years. Eight percent of this age group reported binge drinking, and 3 percent were heavy drinkers. Drug use among youth today, however, is well below the high rates of the 1970s.

Risky Sexual Behavior.   Risky sexual behavior has numerous serious consequences for health. Unintended pregnancies and sexually transmitted diseases (STDs), including HIV infection, can result from unprotected sexual behavior.

Sexually transmitted diseases are common in the United States, with an estimated 15 million new cases of STDs reported each year. STDs are an exception to the general decline in infectious diseases during this century. Four million of the new cases of STDs each year occur in adolescents. Women generally suffer more serious STD complications than men, including pelvic inflammatory disease, ectopic pregnancy, infertility, chronic pelvic pain, and cervical cancer from the human papilloma virus. African Americans and Hispanics have higher rates of STDs than whites. The total cost of the most common STDs and their complications is conservatively estimated at $17 billion annually.

The latest estimates indicate that 800,000 to 900,000 people in the United States currently are infected with HIV. About one-half of all new HIV infections in the United States are among people under age 25 years, and the majority are infected through sexual behavior. HIV infection is the leading cause of death for African-American men aged 25 to 44 years. Compelling worldwide evidence indicates that the presence of other STDs increases the likelihood of both transmitting and acquiring HIV infection.

Half of all pregnancies in the United States are unintended, although unintended pregnancy rates in the United States have been declining. The rates remain highest among teenagers, women aged 40 years or older, and low-income African-American women. Approximately one million teenage girls each year in the United States have unintended pregnancies. Nearly half of all unintended pregnancies end in abortion. The cost to U.S. taxpayers for adolescent pregnancy is estimated at between $7 billion and $15 billion a year.

Injury and Violence.   More than 400 Americans die each day from injuries due primarily to motor vehicle crashes, firearms, poisonings, suffocation, falls, fires, and drowning. The risk of injury is so great that most persons sustain a significant injury at some time during their lives. Motor vehicle crashes are the most common cause of serious injury. In 2000, there were 1.5 deaths from motor vehicle crashes per 100,000 persons (National Center for Health Statistics, 2002, table 11). In 1995, the cost of injury and violence in the United States was estimated at more than $224 billion per year. These costs include direct medical care and rehabilitation expenses as well as productivity losses to the nation's workforce. The total societal cost of motor vehicle crashes alone exceeds $150 billion annually.

Motor vehicle crashes are often predictable and preventable. Increased use of safety belts and reductions in driving while impaired are two of the most effective means to reduce the risk of death and serious injury of occupants in motor vehicle crashes.

Death rates associated with motor vehicle-traffic injuries are highest in the age group 15 to 24 years. In 1996, teenagers accounted for only 10 percent of the U.S. population but 15 percent of the deaths from motor vehicle crashes. Those aged 75 years and older had the second highest rate of motor vehicle-related deaths.

Nearly 40 percent of traffic fatalities in 1997 were alcohol related. Each year in the United States it is estimated that more than 120 million episodes of impaired driving occur among adults. In 1996, 21 percent of traffic fatalities for children aged 14 years and under involved alcohol; 60 percent of the time the driver of the car in which the child was a passenger was impaired. The highest intoxication rates in fatal crashes in 1995 were recorded for drivers aged 21 to 24 years. Young drivers who have been arrested for driving while impaired are more than four times as likely to die in future alcohol-related crashes.

In 1997, 32,436 individuals died from firearm injuries; of this number, 42 percent were victims of homicide. In 1997, homicide was the third leading cause of death for children aged 5 to 14 years, an increasing trend in childhood violent deaths. In 1996, more than 80 percent of infant homicides were considered to be fatal child abuse.

Many factors that contribute to injuries also are closely associated with violent and abusive behavior, such as low income, discrimination, lack of education, and lack of employment opportunities. Males are most often the victims and the perpetrators of homicides. African Americans are more than five times as likely as whites to be murdered. Because no other crime is measured as accurately and precisely, homicide is a reliable indicator of all violent crime.

In 1998, the murder rate in the United States fell to its lowest level in three decades—6.5 homicides per 100,000 persons. There has been a decline in the homicide of intimates, including spouses, partners, boyfriends, and girlfriends, over the past decade, but this problem remains significant and the U.S. still reports one of the highest homicide rates in the world.

Obesity.   Obesity is a major contributor to many preventable causes of death. On average, higher body weights are associated with higher death rates. The number of overweight children, adolescents, and adults has risen over the past four decades. During 1988–94, 11 percent of children and adolescents aged 6 to 19 years were overweight or obese. During the same years, 23 percent of adults aged 20 years and older were considered obese. Total costs (medical costs and lost productivity) attributable to obesity alone amounted to an estimated $99 billion in 1995.

Overweight and obesity substantially raise the risk of illness from high blood pressure, high cholesterol, type II diabetes, heart disease and stroke, gallbladder disease, arthritis, sleep disturbances and problem breathing, and certain types of cancers. Obese individuals also may suffer from social stigmatization, discrimination, and lowered self-esteem.

More than half of adults in the United States are estimated to be overweight or obese. The proportion of adolescents from poor households who are overweight or obese is twice that of adolescents from middle- and high-income households. Obesity is especially prevalent among women with lower incomes and is more common among African-American and Mexican-American women than among white women. Among African Americans, the proportion of women who are obese is 80 percent higher than the proportion of men who are obese. This gender difference also is seen among Mexican-American women and men, but the percentage of white, non-Hispanic women and men who are obese is about the same.

Obesity is a result of a complex variety of social, behavioral, cultural, environmental, physiological, and genetic factors. Efforts to maintain a healthy weight should start early in childhood and continue throughout adulthood, as this is likely to be more successful than efforts to lose substantial amounts of weight and maintain weight loss once obesity is established. The behavioral changes—a healthy diet and regular exercise—typically require only minor lifestyle adjustments on the part of obese individuals.

Neverthless, various social and cultural factors often mitigate against the adoption of healthier lifestyles.

REFERENCES

Catalano, Ralph (1991). "The health effects of economic insecurity," *American Journal of Public Health* 81(9): 1148–1152.

Cockerham, William C., (2001). *Medical Sociology* (8th ed.) Upper Saddle Creek, NJ: Prentice Hall.

Durkheim, Emile (1951). *Suicide*. New York: The Free Press.

Hidreth, Carolyn J., and Elijah Saunders (1992). "Heart disease, stroke, and hypertension in blacks," pp. 90–105 in R. Braithwaite and S. Taylor, eds., *Health Issues in the Black Community*. San Francisco: Jossey-Bass.

Hummer, Robert A. (1993). "Racial differences in infant mortality in the United States: An examination of social and health determinants,"*Social Forces*, 72:529–554.

Hummer, Robert A., Richard G. Rogers, and Charles B. Nam (1999). "Religious involvement and U.S. adult mortality," *Demography* 36:273–285.

Hyder, A.A., G. Rotlant, and R.H. Morrow (1998), "Measuring the burden of disease: Healthy life years," *American Journal of Public Health* 88:196–202.

Jarvis, George K., and Herbert C. Northcott (1987). "Religion and differences in morbidity and mortality," *Social Science and Medicine* 25:813–814.

Joung, I.M., H.D. Van de Mheen, K. Stronks, F. Van Poppel, and J.P. Mackenbach (1998). "A longitudinal study of health selection in marital transition," *Social Science and Medicine* 46:425–435.

Kim, J.S., M.H. Bramlett, L.K. Wright, and L.W. Poon (1998). "Racial differences in health status and health behaviors of older adults," *Nursing Research* 47:243–250.

Larsen, C.O., M. Colangelo, and K. Goods (1998). "African-American-white differences in health perceptions among the indigent," *Journal of Ambulatory Care Management* 21:35–43.

McIntyre, S., G. Ford, and K. Hunt (1999). "Do women 'over-report' morbidity? Men and women's responses to structure prompting on a standard question on long standing illness," *Social Science and Medicine* 48:89–98.

Minino, Arialdi, Arias, Elizabeth, Kochanek, Kenneth D., Murphy, Sherry L., and Betty L. Smith (2002). "Deaths: Final Data for 2000," *National Vital Statistics Reports* 50(15).

Mookherjee, H.N. (1997). "Marital status, gender and perception of well-being," *Journal of Child Psychology* 137:95–105.

National Center for Health Statistics (1997). *Health, United States, 1997*. Hyattsville, MD: National Center for Health Statistics.

National Center for Health Statistics (1998). *Health, United States, 1998*. Hyattsville, MD: National Center for Health Statistics.

National Center for Health Statistics (2002). *Health, United States, 2002*. Hyattsville, MD: National Center for Health Statistics.

Oman, D., and D. Reed (1998). "Religion and mortality among the community-dwelling elderly," *American Journal of Public Health* 88:1469–1475.

Proctor, S.P., T. Heeren, R.F. Wolfe, M.S. Borgos, J.D. David, L. Pepper, R. Clapp, P.B. Sutker, J.J. Vasaterling, and D. Ozonoff (1998). "Self-reported symptoms, environmental exposure and the effect of stress," *International Journal of Epidemiology* 27:1000–1010.

Ren, X.S., and B.C. Amick (1996). "Racial and ethnic disparities in self-assessed health status: Evidence from the national survey of families and households," *Ethnic Health* 1:293–303.

Rogers, Richard G., Robert A. Hummer, and Charles B. Nam (2000). *Living and Dying in the USA: Behavioral, Health, and Social Differentials in Mortality.* New York: Academic Press.

U.S. Bureau of the Census (1997). *Statistical Abstract of the United States.* Washington, DC: U.S. Government Printing Office.

Waidmann, T., Bound, J. and M. Schoenbaum (1995). "The illusion of failure: Trends in the self-reported health status of the U.S. elderly," *The Milbank Quarterly* 73(2):253–287.

Wamala, S.P., M.A. Mittleman, K. Schenck-Gustafson, and K. Orth-Gomer (1999). "Potential explanations for the educational gradient in coronary heart disease: A population-based case-control study of Swedish women," *American Journal of Public Health* 89:315–321.

Williams, David R., and Chiquita Collins (1996). "U.S. Socioeconomic and Racial Differences in Health: Patterns and Explanations," in P. Brown (ed.), *Perspectives in Medical Sociology* (2nd edition). Prospect Heights, IL: Waveland Press.

ADDITIONAL RESOURCES

Bird, Chloe E., and Patricia P. Rieker (1999). "Gender matters: An integrated model for understanding men and women's health." *Social Science and Medicine.* 48:745–755.

Ellison, Christopher G. (1991). "Religious involvement and subjective well-being." *Journal of Health and Social Behavior*, 32:80–99.

Evans, Robert G., M. Barer, and T. Marmor (eds.) (1994). *Why are some people healthy and others not? The determinants the health of populations.* New York: Aldine de Gruyter.

Hummer, Robert A. (1993). "Racial differences in infant mortality in the U.S.: An examination of social and health determinants." *Social Forces*, 72:529–554.

LaClede, Felicia B. (1998). "Neighborhood social context and racial differences in women's heart disease mortality." *Journal of Health and Social Behavior*, 39:91–107.

Lorber, Judith (1997). *Gender and the Social Construction of Illness.* Thousand Oaks, CA: Sage.

Otten, Mac W., Steven M. Teutsch, David F. Williamson, and James S. Marks (1990). "The effect of known risk factors on the excess mortality of black adults in the United States," *Journal of the American Medical Association*, 268:845–850.

Pappas, Gregory, Susan Queen, Wilbur Hadden, and Gail Fisher (1993). "The increasing disparity in mortality between socioeconomic groups in the United States, 1960 and 1986," *New England Journal of Medicine*, 329:103–109.

Robert, Stephanie A. (1998). "Community-level socioeconomic status effects on adult health," *Journal of Health and Social Behavior*, 39:18–37.

Rogers, Richard G. (1996). "The effects of family composition, health, and social support linkages on mortality," *Journal of Health and Social Behavior*, 37:326–338.

Ross, Catherine E., and Chia-Ling Wu (1995). "The link between education and health," *American Sociological Review*, 60:719–745.

Verbrugge, Lois M. (1985). "Gender and health: An update on hypotheses and evidence," *Journal of Health and Social Behavior*, 26:156–182.

INTERNET LINKS

Centers for Disease Control and Prevention (CDC) homepage: www.cdc.gov.
HealthyPeople 2010 homepage: www.health.gov/healthypeople/
National Center for Health Statistics (NCHS) homepage: www.cdc.nchs.
National Institutes of Health (NIH) homepage: www.nih.gov.
Office of Disease Prevention and Promotion (Department of Health and Human Services) homepage: http://odphp.osophs.dhhs.gov.
Office of Minority Health (DHHS) homepage: http://www.omhrc.gov/omhhome.htm.

Chapter 10

The Social Dimension of Sickness Behavior

Sickness behavior might be broadly defined to include the utilization of formal health services, as well as the informal health behavior characterizing a population, in response to some acknowledged symptom or symptoms. Sickness behavior is a complicated process and typically involves much more than meets the eye. In fact, there is an enormous, and generally unrecognized, chasm between the medical model of illness and the concepts used by laypersons to develop an understanding of their conditions and to make decisions about their health. This gap is built into the structure of professionalized medicine, where—by definition—the layperson does not share the specialized body of knowledge used by the professional (Freidson, 1970: 278–279).

Sickness behavior is often more broadly defined as "help-seeking behavior", and a wide variety of responses to symptoms are included. According to Cockerham and Richey (1997) "help-seeking behavior" is "that part of the illness process that involves efforts to access formal medical service providers, especially physicians, when one is ill or otherwise has been defined as sick. Help-seeking may also involve turning to more informal sources of care."

The concept of sickness behavior is a relatively new one in both social science and medical circles. The earliest discussions singling out a pattern of behavior in response to health threats are found in the literature of the 1950s. Many consider Parsons' (1951) early work on the "sick role" as the first scientific treatment of sickness behavior. Since then, a considerable amount of research has been accumulated on the responses of individuals and groups to ill health. The significance of the concept of health behavior cannot be overemphasized in a society that is as highly "medicalized" as the United States.

The importance of sickness behavior in this context lies in the fact that variations in sickness behavior reflect variations in social characteristics. The variations in sickness behavior are infinite and are very much influenced by social characteristics. While it is true that there is something of a correlation between health status and use of at least the most sophisticated types of services, most sickness behavior ultimately involves a number of decisions on the part of the affected party.

Individuals sometimes choose to utilize health services because these services are ordered; however, if all dimensions of sickness behavior are considered, it is obvious that a great deal of volition is involved in the use of such services. This is clearly demonstrated by the fact that there are three health status/health utilization combinations found in U.S. society: those with "real" illnesses who utilize health services; those with "real" illnesses who do not utilize health services; and those without "real" illnesses who utilize health services.

The discussion below focuses primarily on the social correlates of formal measures of health services utilization, although some attention will first be given informal sickness behavior. This approach reflects both conventional usage and the fact that data on formal participation in the healthcare system are more readily available than are data on informal types of health behavior. (Box 10-1 describes approaches to measuring health services demand.)

INFORMAL SICKNESS BEHAVIOR

The historical emphasis of researchers on formal medical care has masked the fact that a large portion of sickness behavior is informal in nature. Much of this behavior would be considered self-care. According to Cockerham and Richey (1997), "self-care" refers to the actions on a layperson's part to prevent, detect, and treat his or her own health problems. Self-care is self-initiated and self-managed and is the most common response to symptoms of illness by people throughout the world. Self-care has been encouraged in recent years in the U.S. due to the increase in chronic conditions with their accompanying emphasis on management rather than cure, a growing dissatisfaction with depersonalized medical care, and a recognition of the limitations of modern medicine. This trend also reflects a desire on the part of individuals to exercise greater personal responsibility in health-related matters.

Contrary to common misconception, health seeking is largely not a process of getting professional medical care. Most help-seeking measures are non-medical, and only a very small portion of ailments are ever brought to a physician's attention. In fact, the vast majority of actions people take to prevent illness or to treat everyday health problems are done without expert help, either medical or nonmedical. This observation is corroborated by recent studies documenting the "iceberg of morbidity"—referring to the vast majority of physical problems that are neither brought to medical attention (Verbrugge, 1986) nor show up in formal health statistics.

Research has verified the fact that, although individuals frequently suffer from various symptoms, formal healthcare is generally not the first response considered. It is not that individuals fail to respond to their symptoms but that, for most common symptoms, people elect to do something on their own without medical help (Verbrugge and Ascione, 1987). Rather than turning to formal medical care, affected individuals reported self-dosing with prescription or nonprescription drugs as the most common response. Self-imposed restriction of activities (such as cutting down on errands and chores) was also common, used on nearly 24 percent of the days on which symptoms were noticed.

The Verbrugge and Ascione study also found that about half the time people responded to their health problems by talking with family or friends. This response is both therapeutic in its own right and also a way of consulting with other laypersons about what action to take vis-à-vis specific symptoms. Laypeople rely upon their own networks of contact for advice, including suggestions about where to seek further help. Family, friends, neighbors, and colleagues at work or school, religious groups, and social clubs all constitute potential sources of advice. There is growing evidence that these lay advice networks rely especially upon women as knowledgeable sources of referrals and as the seekers of health advice both for themselves and for members of their families (Graham, 1985).

Not all lay advice comes form existing networks, however. Sometimes people seek out new sources of advice or create a new network of lay advisors. A person with an uncommon disease may seek out a group of fellow sufferers (perhaps formalized as a "support group"), whose advice on such matters may be more valued than that of longtime friends or even doctors who have not experienced the disease themselves. The Internet has

---

Box 10-1

The Demand for Health Services

The demand for health services on the part of the U.S. population ultimately determines the type and volume of health services provided by the healthcare delivery system. Most decisions on whether or not to offer a service will be predicated upon presumed levels of demand. Once a service is offered, virtually all decisions related to the provision of that service should be a function of the level of demand demonstrated by the population of the market area. For these reasons, health services planners spend a great deal of their time and effort trying to determine current and future levels of demand for overall health services or for the specified services offered by the organization involved in the planning process.

Despite the importance of the level of demand for the system, the concept of "demand" is seldom defined. "Demand" is an imprecise concept as applied to health services and the term is often used interchangeably with other terms. In fact, there is technically no one definition of demand in common usage. The concept is sufficiently vague and is used in so many different ways that it is difficult to provide an operational definition.

Perhaps the best way to approach the concept of demand is by examining its component parts. For analysis purposes, demand can be conceptualized as the ultimate result of the combined effect of: 1) healthcare needs; 2) healthcare wants; 3) recommended standards for healthcare; and 4) actual utilization patterns.

Healthcare Needs

Healthcare *needs* can be defined in terms of the number of conditions that require medical treatment found within a population. These are the health conditions that an objective evaluation—e.g., physical examinations—would uncover within a population. These might be thought of as the *absolute* needs that exist in "nature" without the influence of any other factors. All things being equal, the absolute level of need should not vary much from population to population. These are the epidemiologically based needs that a team of health professionals would identify in a "sweep" through a community and could be considered to represent the "true" prevalence of illness within the population.

A population with certain characteristics can be expected to manifest a specified level of various health conditions. However, these absolute needs, at least in contemporary societies, do not translate directly into demand. In fact, the mismatch between these baseline needs and ultimate utilization of services is substantial. There are many conditions that go untreated (indeed, even undiagnosed) for various reasons. There are many other conditions for which treatment is obtained that would not be identified among the absolute needs of the population.

Healthcare Wants

Health care *wants* can be conceptualized as wishes or desires for health services on the part of the population. Unlike needs, wants would not necessarily be uncovered by a sweep of clinicians through the community. Wants are shaped less by the absolute needs of the population than by the variety of factors that influence the consumption of other goods and services besides healthcare. In fact, many health services that are consumed are considered medically unnecessary or elective, reflecting the operation of wants rather than needs. Examples of these services include cosmetic surgery and laser eye surgery. The U.S. healthcare system has adapted itself to the existence of wants as well as needs, and important components of the system cater to those desiring elective services.

Recommended Standards for Healthcare

The third component involves recommended *standards* for the provision of health care. As health professionals have become more attuned to prevention and early detection, the number of established standards has grown. This component of demand involves primarily diagnostic procedures, the administration of which can typically be linked to fairly clear-cut indications. Thus, a wide range of diagnostic procedures are now recommended for certain age groups and other population segments at risk of various health conditions.

There are standards that call for diagnostic tests at a certain frequency, the performance of certain medical procedures at specified times, and the carrying out of various treatment plans on the part of patients. For example, an annual mammogram is recommended for all women over 50, an annual prostate exam for all men over 40, and regular cholesterol measurement for individuals at risk of certain conditions.

Health Services Utilization

The fourth component of demand involves the actual *utilization* of services. This is frequently used as a proxy measure for demand, in that utilization rates can be calculated for virtually any type of health service or product. More data are available related to health services utilization than for the other components of demand, primarily because utilization data are routinely collected for administrative purposes whenever a health service is provided. More so than any other measures discussed here, utilization rates indicate the level of activity within the healthcare system.

Because of the perceived relationship between demand and utilization, researchers may work backward from utilization levels and use them as a proxy for demand. However, utilization does not equal demand and, depending on the circumstances, the level of demand may exceed actual

(continued)

utilization or, conversely, utilization levels may exceed reasonable demand for services. For example, there may be less utilization than expected because of limited access to health services. On the other hand, some services may be overutilized for various reasons (e.g., insurance coverage, physician practice patterns) unrelated to the actual level of demand.

A determination of the demand for health services is critical to an understanding of the healthcare delivery system. Such a determination, however, is problematic given the factors that must be taken into consideration in estimating the demand for services. Data on the utilization of health services

become an increasingly common source of information outside the existing lay network and also a means of access to support groups.

Through lay referrals, the individual learns of various treatment options and obtains recommendations with regard to physicians, alternative therapists, and non-clinical options such as prayer groups and meditation centers. Thus, it is not unusual for sick persons with effective networks of family and friends to receive concrete assistance in selecting and negotiating entry to both institutional health resources (e.g., prenatal care programs) and noninstitutional help (e.g., spiritual healers). These kin networks serve a health education function because of their role in teaching members where to seek help, how to select among available help resources, and how to deal with barriers to getting help (Schensul and Schensul, 1982).

FORMAL SICKNESS BEHAVIOR: THE SICK ROLE

One of the most important contributions made by sociologists to our understanding of sickness behavior has been the conceptualization of the sick role. The sick role was first described by Talcott Parsons (1951) and further explicated by other sociologists beginning in the 1950s. Working within the structural/functional perspective, Parsons viewed illness as a symptom of dysfunction within the system. Not only did illness create dysfunction for the individual, it also had negative implications for the social system. Since a certain of amount of sickness is unavoidable, every society must come up with some way of institutionalizing the sickness episode. No negative connotation is placed on the sick person by sociologists, although it is realized that from a societal perspective the sick individual is problematic. If large numbers of people adopted the sick role, it is argued, this phenomenon could have dire consequences for society.

From a structural/functional perspective, one's "health" is determined by his ability to carry out his social roles. As long as one can

may be more readily attained than other measures of demand and these data may be used as a proxy. Yet, utilization rates represent a measure of the *use* of services and this may not equate to demand. Indeed, it is often argued that past or current utilization of health services cannot be assumed to reflect future utilization of services in a rapidly changing industry. The researcher must thus consider the existence of healthcare needs, the desires of the target population with regard to healthcare wants, and the necessity of providing for recommended services. All four components must be considered in developing a true picture of health services demand.

continue to work, maintain family life and otherwise maintain social interaction, the individual is not considered "sick" from this perspective. However, to the extent that sickness threatens role performance and, hence, the achieving of societal goals, it becomes a social issue rather than a personal issue.

The American value system emphasizes economic productivity, the work ethic, and activism, all values that cannot be effectively pursued by someone who is sick. Thus, society tends to discourage unnecessary participation in the sick role and, if resorting to the sick role is necessary, a rapid return to productivity is encouraged. Because of the particular American ethos, there appears to be more urgency in this regard in the U.S. than elsewhere.

As with any role, the sick role involves a set of rights and obligations that attend the status of "patient". Although the sick role, unlike many other roles, is a role open to virtually every one in society, society members still must learn how to perform this role just as any other role.

The rights associated with the sick role include the right to obtain relief from one's duties. That is, the sick role occupant can be excused from work, from school, from carrying out family obligations, and so forth. Further, the sick person can demand assistance and care (either formal or informal) from others in the social group. The fact that the individual is not in a position to carry out his normal social functions is recognized, as well as the right to expect supportive care that would not be appropriate under other circumstances.

At the same time, there are important obligations associated with the sick role. The role occupant must make every possible effort toward recovery. This includes informal means such as resting and otherwise attempting to restore health, as well as formal means involving the healthcare delivery system. The appropriate use of physicians, hospitals and other health facilities and personnel is mandatory, and compliance with doctor's orders is also an obligation. The sick role occupant is also discouraged from abusing the privilege by not pursuing a rapid recovery or by demanding too much in the way of personal care. Otherwise, some of the rights may be removed from those who do not meet the obligations of the sick role.

One other aspect of the sick role involves the issue of disease causation. Thus, the sick role is based on the assumptions that the health condition is not self-inflicted, that it does not involve a choice made by the individual, and that it is not something that the individual was able to take care of himself. Thus, we are ambivalent as a society and as health professionals when someone with HIV or other sexually transmitted diseases, chronic alcoholism or drug abuse, or smoking-caused emphysema seeks to occupy the sick role. While medical ethics demand that all afflicted persons be given appropriate treatment, there is likely to be less than wholehearted enthusiasm for allowing such individuals to benefit from the sick role.

Beyond the institutionalization of sickness behavior, the sick role performs numerous functions relative to both individuals and society. Its functions vis-à-vis the individual and the social group include: promoting restoration of health and social functioning; clarifying the patient/provider relationship; and lessening the disruption caused by the sickness episode by clarifying the nature of the status. The sick role also provides a motivation for others to remain well and, at the same time, serves as an escape route for those unable to perform their social roles.

There are also some other functions that the sick role performs vis-à-vis the social system. These include: managing dysfunction within the system and contributing to system readjustment; preventing infection of others (in both biological and social senses); and preventing the sick from forming a deviant subculture. While the individual is concerned with recovery, the social system is concerned with the reintegration of the patient, renewed productivity, and a return to system equilibrium.

Although the sick role is open to virtually every member of society, it is one of the few roles that requires "official" certification prior to both entry and exit. A symptomatic individual cannot enter the sick role unless he is certified by a physician as having a clinically diagnosed condition. The condition constitutes "illness" until a physician declares it to be "sickness." While family and members of one's social groups may provide provisional authentication of the sickness, this will not get the individual excused from work or school, nor will it allow the affected individual access to medical therapy, hospital admission, or drug prescriptions.

At the same time, the individual remains in the sick role until formally dismissed by the physician. Thus, employees must have medical "clearance" to go back to work or athletes to return to the field of play. Patients technically cannot leave a hospital unless a doctor dismisses them, and this applies particularly to mental hospitals. While the individual, family and friends may feel like the patient is "cured" and capable of carrying out some of his responsibilities, the patient is not *officially* cured until the doctor says so. (This becomes somewhat problematic when we are dealing with conditions like diabetes, arthritis, and various mental disorders for which no actual cure is available.)

While the concept of the sick role provides insights into the behavior of the patient and the relationship between the sick person and society, some limitations to its application have been noted. Like all roles, the sick role is a little fuzzy around the edges. Role prescriptions and proscriptions are not always clearly delineated, and the individual's social group or the circumstances may influence the patient's interpretation of the role requirements. The application of the sick role makes certain assumptions concerning the traditional doctor/patient relationship and might be considered to reflect a middle-class bias with regard to appropriate role performance.

Today, perhaps the greatest limitation of the sick role is its lack of applicability for many increasingly common health conditions. The application of the concept to individuals with chronic conditions, mental illness and symptoms of aging is problematic and requires a rethinking of the concept in the face of contemporary health problems.

Sociologists have identified an additional, but thankfully less frequent, role that a patient might play, the "death role". The death role refers to the pattern of obligations, responsibilities, and privileges perceived as appropriate for someone who is identified as terminally ill. A terminally ill patient is expected to restrict demands on physicians, keep complaints to a minimum, accept palliative treatments in place of curative ones, and rely more heavily on personal and family resources to deal with emotional issues surrounding an oftentimes protracted dying process. With terminally ill patients, the physician's role changes also, as he or she tends to follow a pattern of decreasing involvement.

Except for those clinicians specifically trained to care for terminally ill patients, most healthcare practitioners—and especially physicians—are very uncomfortable dealing with dying patients. The total thrust of medical training and practice involves treatment and cure. Thus, the physician has expectations of a cure, and a dying patient represents failure. Since the treatment of the terminal patient is so antithetical to the thrust of medical practice, scant attention is given to this aspect of care in the training of physicians. Ultimately, the terminal patient does not make a good candidate for the sick role, thereby creating tension within the system.

BECOMING A PATIENT

As useful as the sick role is, some feel that it focuses on only a limited segment of the "patient career." Influenced by the medical model, the sick role considers only that portion of the patient career that involves formal medical care. As researchers have broadened the notions of health and sickness, we have become aware of the range of health and sickness behavior that may occur outside the patient care component. Indeed, it can be argued that most of what happens with regard to the health-to-sickness-to-health progression takes place outside of formal medical care. When one considers the numerous decisions that are involved in becoming a "certified" patient, it is obvious that the sick role represents only one segment of a sometimes-complicated process.

Assuming that the individual in the typical case starts out in a state of wellness or health and is essentially symptom free, the first step in the process of becoming a patient involves *symptom recognition*. This would involve noting the sensation of pain, stuffiness in the head, dizziness, or any of dozens of other possible symptoms. Symptom recognition is not an automatic process and many individuals continue to function without being consciously aware of sensations that would immediately alarm others. Thus, from the very outset "external" factors influence the process of becoming a patient. The likelihood of noting the existence of a particular sensation or condition and recognizing it as a symptom is influenced by sociocultural characteristics, past experiences, and group affiliation. Thus, when a women defines, premenstrual cramps as a "symptom," this reflects social influences as much as the actual physical sensation.

Once sensations have been recognized as symptoms, a process of *symptom evaluation* takes place. The individual considers the symptom in the light of past experience, medical knowledge and psychosocial implications. For example, is this something that one should be concerned about? Is this a natural consequence of aging? Is this something that requires medical attention? As with symptom evaluation, this phase is influenced by a range of social factors. Women in the U.S., for example, are much more likely to express concern over the existence of symptoms than are men. Members of different ethnic groups are likely to interpret the presence of pain (and its potential consequences) in different ways. Members of various religious groups may attribute moral connotations to the symptoms. In any case, the symptoms do not exist solely in an objective sense, but significance and meaning comes to be attached to them, with this significance and meaning reflecting the social background and context of the affected individual.

Somewhere in this process, perhaps after the symptoms are accorded a certain level of significance, a process of *information search* is carried out by the affected individual (or his significant others). Part of this process involves an "internal" search on the part of the individual with regard to past experiences, similar experiences related by others, and/or information read in the past. This process is also likely to involve an "external" search as well. This would include obtaining written materials related to the symptoms (today facilitated by access to the Internet) and/or asking relatives or friends about the condition. The method utilized in the search for information reflects the individual's social background and social context.

The next step in the process typically involves some type of *informal help-seeking*. At this point the individual takes some overt action related to addressing the symptoms. Informal help-seeking is likely to involve some form of "self care", wherein the individual seeks to self medicate with over-the-counter drugs and/or change behavior patterns (e.g., diet, sleep) in order to control or eliminate the symptoms. Informal help-seeking behavior also involves turning to those within the social group for some form of treatment. Thus, we often hear people asking of relatives, friends or associates, "Do you have something for (insert appropriate symptom)?" The form that informal help-seeking takes reflects the social milieu of the individual and is influenced by the input of those in the social group. Whether one turns to the pharmacy, a "folk healer" in the family, or a clergyman in response to symptoms depends on one's social background and context.

Assuming that the condition is not adequately addressed by informal means, the next step typically involves *formal help-seeking*. This is the point at which the individual turns to the healthcare institution, and the formal process of becoming a patient commences. However, the decisions on the part of the individual do not end with the decision to seek formal help. This decision itself is influenced by one's social context. For example, members of certain groups would automatically think of availing themselves to the services of a psychiatrist at this point in response to emotional symptoms; others would never under any circumstances willingly go to a "shrink" for the same symptoms.

Once the decision has been made to seek formal help, a choice must be made with regard to the source of care. In many cases, insurance plans dictate the process that must be followed for obtaining *any* care. However, in most cases choices are presented and decisions must be made. For an individual with back pain, for example, an orthopedic surgeon or neurologist might be considered. At the same time, a chiropractor or even an acupuncturist might be considered in view of the symptoms. Health plan dictates aside, the choice of practitioner reflects the individual's sociocultural characteristics, social history, and current group affiliations. This is borne out by the fact that individuals who turn to chiropractors in the face of back pain are socially different from those who turn to orthopedic surgeons.

Once a source of formal care has been selected and, assuming that clinically identifiable symptoms exist, the individual will be officially declared "sick" and *sick role adoption* will occur. However, this is not automatic and another decision might be made at this point. The individual may accept the patient label or reject it. He may not agree with the assessment of sickness, or he may disagree with the diagnosis. The individual may want a second opinion or, as often is the case, choose to defer acceptance of the sick role pending the availability of other information or new developments with regard to the symptoms. The decision to accept the sick role, like those preceding it, will depend upon the social background of the individual, his experiences, and his group affiliations.

Once the individual has agreed to occupy the sick role, the next decision relates to *medical compliance*, or the following of "doctor's orders." Many of the orders of the physician are straightforward and leave little room for discussion. While the patient is in the physician's office, he may be given injections or other treatments that would be difficult to refuse. Similarly, the scheduling of hospital admission or a surgical procedure is straightforward, and there is a lot of pressure for the patient to comply with these orders. To the extent that the patient is directly under the control of the physician or other agents of the healthcare delivery system, there is often little latitude for decision making.

However, many aspects of healthcare transpire outside the view of the physician and rely upon the patient for their implementation. The most common example would be the prescribing of drugs for the treatment of a condition. Other examples would include obtaining physical therapy, changing one's diet, and following an exercise program. These are aspects of the medical regimen over which the individual has substantial control and for which there is limited oversight by health professionals. For that reason, there is a considerable amount of "slippage" with regard to the following of doctor's orders. The rate of compliance is far from satisfactory and research has indicated that a surprising proportion of patients do not comply, fully or at all, with doctor's orders. The reoccurrence of health problems and, in some cases, death are often consequences of a failure to follow a prescribed course of medical care.

The decisions made by the patient with regard to compliance, as above, will be influenced by his sociodemographic and sociocultural characteristics, past experiences, and social group influences. Indeed, the lack of support among friends and relatives and/or negative influences of those within the affected individual's social group are critical factors in compliance. (See the section on compliance below for more detail.)

Once an individual is cured (or, more likely, stabilized given the nature of contemporary conditions), the former patient often is admonished to perform certain behaviors or avoid other behaviors lest the condition return or become exacerbated. Here, as above, the likelihood of the individual behaving in a health-inducing manner depends on a variety of social factors. It is for this reason that discharge planners and social workers often voice concern about returning an individual to a social environment that spawned the condition in the first place. The environment may be a dysfunctional family or a social context that encourages poor health habits and/or risky health behavior. These agents of the healthcare system are cognizant of the significance of the social milieu in shaping behavior and, to the extent possible, encourage appropriate behavior after discharge. To see the importance of this for the healthcare system, one can consider the case of an alcoholic who has received an expensive liver transplant, only to return to a pattern of alcohol abuse once released from the hospital.

There are other aspects of the process of becoming a patient that could be considered from this perspective, but the point would be the same. The process of becoming a patient and subsequently returning to some level of health is as much a social process as a clinical process. In fact, the component that is under the control of the healthcare system, except in the case of very severe or emergency conditions, is less important than the components of the process that are under the control of the affected individual. (See Box 10-2 for a discussion of perceptions of "good" and "bad" patients.)

THE SOCIAL CORRELATES OF SICKNESS BEHAVIOR

There are a number of indicators of sickness behavior that display correlations with social characteristics. These indicators include hospital admissions, patient days, average length of stay, physician utilization, and drug utilization, among others. While each of these indicators merits explication in its own right, space does not allow that here. The glossary can be consulted for more information on the various indicators of formal sickness behavior.

Medical sociologists and other researchers have extensively studied the factors that are associated with sickness behavior. Given the variation found in help-seeking among different populations, the ability to explain this variation has become one of the primary goals of health services researchers. The focus of this section is on sickness behavior and, as in previous chapters, these relationships are discussed in terms of biosocial and sociocultural characteristics.

Biosocial Characteristics

Age and Sickness Behavior

Age is considered by many to be the single best predictor of formal help-seeking behavior. Age is related not only to levels of service utilization but to the type of services used and the circumstances under which they are received. This is true whether the indicator is for inpatient care, outpatient care, tests and procedures performed, or virtually any other measure of utilization.

Box 10-2

Good Patient/Bad Patient: What's the Difference?

Since the rise of modern American medicine during the period follow-ing World War II, medical practitioners have developed images of "good" and "bad" patients. The socialization process for doctors inevitably leads to the development of patient stereotypes. The use of such stereotypes varies according to the institutional setting; doctors in private practice are less likely than doctors on hospital staff to use pejoratives openly to re-fer to patients, although they may hold some of the same negative at-titudes. Nevertheless, the values reflected in these attitudes toward pa-tients are encouraged in both the self-selection of doctors and their medical education.

In a U.S. study, 439 family practitioners reacted negatively not only to various social and personal traits of their patients but also to certain med-ical conditions, especially those for which medical treatment offered little or no likelihood of cure or clear alleviation. The physicians particularly dis-liked situations, such as emphysema, senility, diabetes, arthritis, psychiatric conditions, and obesity, that challenge their faith in the curative powers of bioscientific medicine. They also dislike conditions, such as back pain, vague chronic pains, headaches, and chronic fatigue, that offer little probability of cure while bringing their competence or diagnostic skills into question. Fur-thermore, they dislike conditions for which they believe the patient or others are responsible, such as sexual behavior, auto accidents, suicide attempts, and other self-inflicted injuries.

One study found the leading common characteristics of patients that doctors label as "gomers" (or "get outta my emergency room") were illnesses and/or personal characteristics that created management difficulties for the hospital staff. Many patients were identified as "gomers" because their con-ditions defied solution by modern medical intervention. Their deterioration under treatment was thus a source of frustration and ideological doubts for doctors, especially the fledging doctors who typically staffed emergency rooms and clinics.

Many of the other derogatory terms used for patients reflect similar values. A widespread distinction in doctors' stereotyping of patients is be-tween "sick people" and "trolls". The latter term is applied to patients whom doctors believe lack a "real" disease and to those held culpable for the cause of and/or the failure to control their condition. Other derogatory

Although it has become a truism in U.S. society that the consump-tion of health services increases with age, this primarily reflects the heavy weight accorded to hospital care. The rate of hospitalization for individuals under 45 is very low, with the lowest admission rate in 2000 being recorded

terms for undesirable patients include "albatross", "turkey", and "crock". Such negative stereotypes often supercede even the medical model itself in informing the doctor's understanding of a case, thus leading to failed empathy.

Hospital staff generally admit that they often treat undesirable patients less thoroughly. Sometimes the stereotypes lead to misdiagnoses and other medical mistakes. For example, a homeless person brought unconscious to the emergency room may be treated as a "gomer" under the assumption that the condition was alcohol-induced, whereas a thorough treatment might discover that the symptoms resulted from a serious neurological problem.

Doctors' negative stereotypes of patients are also based upon social and personal characteristics. Doctors tended to consider "undesirable" those patients whose behavior violated the physicians' personal norms, even those with little or no relevance to health. The largest category of social characteristics eliciting negative responses from doctors included such violations as being dirty, smelly, vulgar, chronically unemployed, promiscuous, homosexual, malingering, or on welfare, Medicaid, or workers' compensation. Doctors' expectations of patients are based largely upon white, middle-class values that are accentuated by the self-selection and professional training processes. Social class differences also appear to figure into some negative stereotypes.

In the final analysis, "good" patients show up on time, don't ask annoying questions, follow doctors' orders, and pay their bills. Thus, doctors encourage the inclusion of good patients among their clientele and discourage those they consider to be "bad" patients.

"Good" and "bad" are relative descriptors and the perception of goodness or badness is influenced by a variety of factors that have little to do with the biological state of patient. Much has to do with the context within which transactions occur and the perceptions of the practitioner. The conceptualization of the "good" patient reflects a complex interplay of social and economic factors, as well as the clinical issues involved. Ultimately, the notion of good and bad patients reflects the extent to which those who present themselves with health problems correspond to the expectations of the institution and its practitioners.

Source: Peter Freund and Meredith B. McGuire (1999). *Health, Illness and the Social Body*, 3rd ed. Englewood Cliffs, NJ: Prentice Hall.

---

by the 6-to-17 age cohort at 26.5 per 1,000 population. The only exception to low rates at the younger ages, of course, is for women during their childbearing years. After 45, however, admission rates begin increasing dramatically, with the rate more than doubling from the 15-to-44 age cohort to the 45-to-64 cohort. Those 65 and over recorded an admission rate of 286.0 per 1,000 in 2000, a rate ten times that for the least hospitalized cohort (National Center for Health Statistics, 2002, table 90).

Historically, the greatest jump in admissions has been at the 60 to 65 age break; however, with the improved health status of the elderly in U.S. society, by the late 1980s, around 70 years had become the breakpoint at which hospital utilization soars (National Center for Health Statistics 2002, table 90). The average length of hospital stay increases significantly from the under-18 age group to the 65-and-over cohort, with the former recording 3.8 days and the latter 6.4 days in 2000.

Within this framework of overall high rates for the elderly and generally low rates for the non-elderly, there are some important variations. To the extent that health problems are age specific, there are conditions that have a very different configuration from that above. Childbirth has already been mentioned as one example; those admitted for tonsillectomies or myringotomies (ear tubes) are virtually all children, while those admitted for alcoholism and drug abuse treatment are more likely to be in the 20 to 35 age range. The most frequent reasons for hospitalization for those under 15 are acute conditions associated with respiratory and digestive systems.

For those aged 15 to 44, childbirth and related conditions account for nearly half of the female hospitalizations, while injuries and mental disorders are common admitting diagnoses among males. For the 45 to 64 and 65-and-over cohorts, heart disease and cancer predominate (National Center for Health Statistics, 1998, table 90). In terms of emergency room utilization (for true emergencies), teens and those in their early twenties (particularly males) account for a disproportionate share due to injuries and accidents. The discrepancy between the elderly and the non-elderly in terms of admissions is magnified with respect to patient days, with elderly patients accounting for a disproportionate share of the hospital days logged.

The relationship between nursing home utilization and age is predictable. Few nursing home residents are under 65. However, within the nursing home population itself, there are significant differences in age distribution. Overall, fewer than 5% of those aged 65 and older resided in nursing homes in 1999, a figure that has changed little in two or more decades. However, of those aged 85 and over 18.5% were institutionalized. Looked at another way, the age distribution of nursing home residents is around 13% aged 65 to 74, nearly 35% aged 75 to 84, and over 50% aged 85 or older (National Center for Health Statistics, 2002, table 97). Thus, as the American population has aged, the average age of nursing home residents has actually increased. Similarly, those 65 and over account for 70.5% of home health patients, with clients for home health services concentrated in the 75–84 age group. A similar pattern exists with regard to the use of hospice services (National Center for Health Statistics 2002, tables 88 and 89).

Age differences are also found in the use of other types of facilities. Among the older population, there is a preference for inpatient rather than outpatient care. The ingrained notion of better care and a more secure environment among older age cohorts tends to favor hospitalization. On the other hand, tendencies toward utilization of outpatient facilities among the younger age cohorts have developed. (This preference appears to be increasingly a function of changing reimbursement patterns and the influence of aging baby boomers.) The primary users of freestanding urgent care clinics, for example, are in the 25 to 40 age group. The under-45 population is also more likely to utilize other outpatient settings, such as freestanding diagnostic centers or surgicenters. These differences are partly a reflection of age-generated differences in perceptions. But they also reflect the fact that younger age cohorts are more likely to be enrolled in some alternative delivery system that mandates outpatient care and to have physicians with more "contemporary" practice patterns than those of the older age groups.

Age differences do exist in the utilization of physician services, although they are not as dramatic as those for hospital and nursing home services. With the exception of the youngest age cohorts, there is a direct relationship between age and number of physician office visits. The elderly overall visit physicians one and one-half times as often as all nonelderly taken as a group. Thus, in 2000, 60.3% of those aged 65 and over reported four or more office visits, compared to 30.0% for the 18 to 24 age group. Looked at differently, in 2000 those under 18 were nearly twice as likely to report no healthcare visit during the previous year as those 65 and over (12.2% compared to 7.6%) This difference reflects the fact that a large proportion of visits for the elderly are for regular checkups and the monitoring of chronic conditions and not for acute problems (National Center for Health Statistics 2002, table 72).

A significant difference exists in the utilization of specialists by the age of the patient. With increases in age, the utilization rate for primary care physicians decreases and that for specialists increases. For example, in 2000 over half (53.5%) of the elderly reported visiting a non-primary care specialist, compared to 20.3% of those under 18 (National Center for Health Statistics, 2002, table 85).

Age is probably the best predictor of the types of procedures that will be performed. Although some diagnostic tests and therapeutic procedures may be performed throughout the age spectrum, most clinical procedures carry a particular age configuration. For example, some tests and procedures are typically performed only on children. Women of child-bearing age tend to be virtually the only utilizers of certain other tests and procedures. In general, diagnostic procedures are less frequently performed on those under age 45 than they are on those over 45.

Although there are some exceptions, the amount of drugs prescribed by physicians tends to increase with the age of the patient. This reflects the use of drugs for the management of chronic health problems, which tend to accumulate with age. Those aged 65 and older in 1992 constituted the age cohort with by far the highest rate of prescription drug use (National Center for Health Statistics, 1997, table 1). In fact, frequent assertions of overuse of drugs by the elderly population are made.

Sex and Sickness Behavior

In U.S. society, females are more active than men in terms of formal health behavior and are much heavier users of the healthcare system. Women are heavier consumers of health services, in fact, regardless of the indicator used. They tend to visit physicians more often, take more prescription drugs, and use other facilities and personnel in general more often.

Part of the heavier utilization attributed to females in U.S. society in the 1990s can be explained by the higher reported levels of morbidity for women. Women report more symptoms and more illness episodes than men. The relative complexity of their reproductive systems also necessitates more healthcare utilization. It also should be noted that women are more conscious of the health services that are available and are more willing to utilize them. It appears that sex role differentiation in U.S. society has encouraged use of health services by females and discouraged their use by males.

Hospital utilization was significantly greater for females than males in 2000, with reported discharge rates of 116.7 and 74.3 per thousand, respectively. On the other hand, when hospitalized, males tended to remained hospitalized one and one-third times as long as females on the average, or 4.6 days versus 3.4 days (National Center for Health Statistics, 2002, table 90).

When tertiary care is examined, males tend to be particularly predominant. Although males become sick less often than females, they are more likely to contract serious conditions. For example, the 1995 the male admission rate for heart disease was considerably higher than that for females. Females averaged 5.3 days per hospital stay in 1995, compared to 6.0 days for males. Males—particularly adolescents and young adults—are more likely to utilize hospital emergency rooms for true emergencies, primarily due to the large number injuries and accidents occurring among this subpopulation.

The average number of annual physician encounters (for all physicians) for females in 1995 was 6.1, compared to 4.9 for males (National Center for Health Statistics 1998, table 74). The average number of office visits in 1995 for females was 3.7 compared to 2.7 for males. In 2000, it was reported that only 11.8% of females failed to record a healthcare visit in the previous year, compared to 21.3% of males (National Center for Health Statistics, 2002, table 72). Obviously, the rate of utilization for the range of specialties varies by sex. OB-GYNs are utilized almost exclusively by females, while men are overrepresented among the patients of urologists. Similar rate differentials are found for other healthcare practitioners. For example, females utilize dentists at a rate 1.25 times that of males.

Despite comparable hospital admission rates, females tend to be subjected to twice as many procedures on the average, once admitted. This differential primarily reflects the heavy use of services by obstetrical patients. When the older age cohorts are examined, it is found that, among those 65 and older, males are subjected to a greater number of procedures.

Females comprise the majority of nursing home admissions, and the nation's nursing home population is nearly 75% female. For the 85-and-over cohort, the female proportion is over 80% (National Center for Health Statistics 2002, table 97). This reflects the preponderance of females at the older age levels. The higher mortality rate for males, coupled with the lower survival rate for males who do become ill, means that there are more female candidates for nursing home admission. Further, males surviving into the older age cohorts are more likely to have a wife to care for them. Women also account for nearly two-thirds of home health patients.

Females are more likely to be prescribed drugs by physicians than are males (National Center for Health Statistics, 1997, table 1). This partly reflects the greater participation of females in the healthcare system and their more assertive behavior in seeking out cures. However, if calculations are made eliminating those who have received no prescriptions, females still retain an edge. One explanation offered for this has been the historical practice patterns of physicians. A tendency for physicians (typically male) to prescribe more drugs for females than for males, all other things being equal, has been documented.

Race, Ethnicity, and Sickness Behavior

A correlation has been found between racial and ethnic characteristics and the utilization of certain types of health services. The most clear cut differences have been identified between the sickness behavior of African Americans and whites. Certain Asian populations and ethnic groups also display somewhat distinctive utilization patterns. To a limited extent, differences in utilization may be traced to differences in the types of health problems experienced. However, many of the differences in sickness behavior reflect variations in lifestyle patterns and cultural preferences. For some racial and ethnic groups, in fact, differences in healthcare utilization patterns may have little relationship to differences in health status.

The hospital discharge rate for whites tends to be around 20% lower than that for African Americans, despite the older age structure of the white population. In 2000, the hospital discharge rate for whites was 92.6 per 1,000 population. This compares to a rate of 122.3 per 1,000 blacks. Discharge rates for Asian-Americans and Hispanics were much lower than those for whites, while those for American Indians were in between the white and black rates (National Center for Health Statistics, 2002, table 90).

Although whites generate a greater number of patient days per 1,000 population than African Americans, their average number of patient days per hospital episode is not that different from the figure for African Americans. In fact, when blacks are hospitalized they tend to record longer lengths of stay, presumably because they have more serious conditions on the average at the time of hospitalization. As with admissions, there is no consistent pattern with regard to patient days and length of stay for other racial and ethnic groups.

Whites are overrepresented among the nursing home population. While whites account for approximately 83% of the U.S. population, in 1999 they accounted for over 90% of the nursing home population (National Center for Health Statistics, 2002, table 97). African Americans and other racial and ethnic groups tend to be underrepresented, although Hispanics increasingly report a pattern similar to that of non-Hispanic whites. The underrepresentation among African Americans is particularly telling in view of the heavy burden of chronic disease and disability affecting this population.

In general, whites tend to utilize physicians at a higher rate than the rest of the population. In 1995, whites in the United States averaged 3.4 physician office visits, compared to 2.6 for African Americans. Thus, while African Americans constitute 12.6% of the U.S. population, they account for only 10.5% of the physician office visits despite higher rates of both acute and chronic conditions (National Center for Health Statistics 1998). Looked at differently, in 2000 16.0% of whites reported no healthcare visits, compared to 17.3% of African Americans. Interestingly, larger proportions of American Indians (21.2%), Asian-Americans (20.2%), and Hispanics (26.5%) reported no healthcare visits of any type (National Center for Health Statistics, 2002, table 72).

Whites are particularly overrepresented among the patients of specialists. On the other hand, African Americans are overrepresented among the patients of obstetricians (primary care), but underrepresented among the clients of ophthalmologists and orthopedic surgeons (specialty care). As with hospital admissions, there is little correspondence between the existence of health problems within racial and ethnic groups and their use of physician services.

Differences in utilization patterns reflect differences in lifestyle, income, education, access to care, and cultural preferences. This is also reflected in the fact that blacks are significantly more likely to utilize emergency room services than are whites. The rate of emergency room use for Hispanics is similar to that for whites, while American Indians have the highest emergency room use rates of any group. Asian-Americans are the least likely to use emergency room services of any group (National Center for Health Statistics, 2002, table 79).

Some ethnic group members (Hispanics, for example) utilize alternative types of care in the form of "traditional" healers. Thus, their physician utilization rate does not provide a full picture of their healthcare utilization. In fact, recent research into the use of alternative therapies by Americans suggests that the whole notion of the utilization of clinic services be reviewed (Eisenberg and Kessler, 1993).

There are certain differences in the types of tests and procedures performed on members of various racial and ethnic groups. Some of these differences may reflect the perceptions and practice patterns of providers in their management of members of various groups. It has been found, for example, that African Americans are likely to be subjected to more invasive forms of treatment than whites, all things being equal. At the same time, African Americans are less likely to receive major diagnostic and treatment procedures compared to whites with the same problem. It is believed, however, that this is more a reflection of socioeconomic status and the conditions under which care is received than a function of racial differences (Harris et al. 1997). While the proportion of the older female population receiving mammograms had equalized between whites and African Americans by 1995, Hispanic woman remained much less likely to receive this type of diagnostic test (National Center for Health Statistics 1998, table 80). Whites are also one and a half times more likely to obtain regular dental services than are African Americans or Hispanics.

African Americans are prescribed drugs by physicians at a higher rate than white patients, averaging approximately 1.4 prescriptions per visit compared to 1.2 for whites (National Center for Health Statistics, 1997, table 1). This is despite the fact that whites constitute a higher proportion of the elderly than they do of the general population. Members of most other racial and ethnic groups tend to use prescription drugs at a much lower rate than whites.

Sociocultural Characteristics

Marital Status and Sickness Behavior

Marital status is a relatively effective predictor of sickness behavior and the utilization of health services, just as it is of health status. Marital status is related not only to levels of service utilization but to the type of services utilized and the circumstances under which they are received. This is true whether the indicator is for inpatient care, outpatient care, tests and procedures performed, or virtually any other measure of utilization. The categories of marital status for the discussion below will be never married, married, divorced, and widowed.

In general, the married require fewer services because they are healthier. Yet, they utilize more of certain types of services because they are more aware of the need for preventive care, more likely to have insurance, and, it is argued, more likely to have a "significant other" to encourage them to use the healthcare system.

The social support provided by marriage works in two ways. First, it serves to forestall the need for intensive care by providing an environment that retards the progression of disorders. Second, social support serves to encourage individuals in the use of preventive care. The latter is particularly important in the case of informal health behavior. The married are more likely to be characterized by healthy lifestyles, and to a certain extent this reflects the presence of social support agents that encourage this behavior. The never married, divorced, and widowed, on the other hand, are more likely to be characterized by negative health behaviors.

The age-adjusted rate of hospitalization for married individuals is relatively low. Admission rates for the never married also tend to be relatively low, while those for the widowed and divorced are high by comparison. If rates of admission for various conditions are considered, the variation among marital statuses is even more pronounced. The pattern identified for the various marital statuses in terms of patient-days is similar to that for admissions. Observed differences in length of stay, however, probably reflect factors other than marital status.

The relationship between nursing home utilization and marital status is one of the most clear-cut to be discussed in this section. Few nursing home residents are married. The bulk of nursing home residents are widowed, although there are small numbers who are divorced or never married. Married individuals requiring nursing care are often maintained in the home and cared for by a spouse.

Some differences related to marital status do exist in the utilization of physician services, although they are not as dramatic as those for hospital and nursing home services. Federal surveys have found that married women "see" a doctor (i.e., via visit or telephone) an average of seven times a year. The rate of contact for divorced and widowed women is slightly higher. This may be one of the few cases in this chapter in which utilization corresponds to health status. The rate of physician contact for males is lower than that for females in every marital status category, although little difference exists from one marital status to another for men. Some differences exist in the utilization of specialists by the marital status of the patient, but these are not great.

The patterns of utilization of dentists and other health professionals are similar to physician utilization patterns for the various marital statuses. While the married have fewer dental problems, they are more regular utilizers of dentists than are those in the other marital status categories. Otherwise, no clear-cut marital status differences are found for the use of podiatrists, chiropractors, and physical therapists.

Although there are some exceptions, utilization of prescription drugs tends to be higher for the married. This may reflect more knowledge of available therapies on the part of the married. Those in the unmarried categories are found to have higher rates of utilization of nonprescription drugs.

There are several reasons for the close association between marital status and sickness behavior in its various forms. The level of health status within the population is closely related to marital status. Different levels of morbidity are associated with each marital status category, resulting in demands for differing levels and types of services. Further, lifestyle characteristics vary with marital status, and this includes not only the behavioral aspects of lifestyle but the attitudes/perceptions/preferences component as well. These factors, along with the values associated with various marital statuses, probably have more of an impact on health behavior than do actual differentials in morbidity.

Income and Sickness Behavior

Sickness behavior has been demonstrated to be highly correlated with socioeconomic status. Income, for example, is probably one of the better predictors of sickness behavior and the utilization of health services. Income is related not only to levels of service utilization but to the types of services utilized and the circumstances under which they are received. This is true whether the indicator is for inpatient care, outpatient care, tests and procedures performed, or virtually any other measure of utilization.

Hospitalization rates tend to decrease directly with income and, in fact, greater discrepancies exist among the various income groups than for any of the other social variables examined. The rate of hospitalization for the lowest income group in the U.S. is the highest of any income group, reflecting the higher incidence of health problems. The "poor" recorded a hospital discharge rate of 171.5 per 1,000 in 2000, compared to 70.8 for the "non-poor.) Further, after admission, the length of hospital stay is longer on the average for members of the lowest income group, 4.7 days for the "poor" compared to 3.4 days for the "non-poor" (National Center for Health Statistics, 2002, table 90).

The differences noted for admissions and length of stay reflect the types of conditions for which members of different income categories are admitted. The higher fertility levels of the lower income groups result in a higher rate of admissions for childbirth and related problems. The relatively unhealthy and unsafe environments in which the lower-income groups are likely to live result in a higher rate of emergency admissions, especially for children. The pattern of longer stays for the less affluent is complicated somewhat by unexpected cases of shorter lengths of stay for lower income patients because of their limited ability to pay for services.

Lower income groups are heavier users of hospital emergency room care, especially for non-emergency conditions. On the other hand, lower-income populations are less likely to utilize freestanding emergency clinics or urgent care clinics. This is presumably due to a lack of knowledge of their availability (they are often located in suburban areas) and the fact that payment is typically demanded when care is rendered.

In the past, significant differences have existed in the utilization of physicians in relation to income. Historically, the number of annual physician visits per capita increased with income, although the highest income groups always represent something of an anomaly. The lowest income groups tended to be infrequent users of physician services. This reflects a lack of family physicians and the use of alternative sources of care such as public health clinics. This situation has improved somewhat since the 1960s due to the availability of government-sponsored insurance programs and programs that subsidize physician services in underserved communities.

By the 1980s, the rate of physician utilization by income had essentially equalized, and by the mid-1990s the low-income groups reported utilization rates comparable to or greater than those for the high-income groups (National Center for Health Statistics 1998). However, the lower income groups continue to be underrepresented among the patients of private-practice physicians and overrepresented among emergency department users. For example, in 2000 30.2% of the "poor" and 25.1% of the "near-poor" reported emergency room visits during the previous year, compared to 18.6% of the "non-poor" (National Center for Health Statistics, 2002, table 79). Evidence of continued underutilization of the healthcare system by the poor is found in the fact that in 2000 21.9% of the "poor" and 22.2% of the "near-poor" reported no healthcare visits for the previous year, compared to 13.7% for the "non-poor" (National Center for Health Statistics, 2002, table 72).

As income increases, the utilization rate of primary care physicians decreases and that of specialists increases. For example, in 2000 21.5% of non-poor compared to 12.7% of poor reported visiting a non-primary care specialist (National Center for Health Statistics, 2002, table 85). There is also a direct and inverse relationship between income and dental care utilization. The more affluent see dental care as a preventive service, while the less affluent see it as an expensive service only to be used in emergencies.

Although diagnostic tests and therapeutic procedures are typically performed as necessary in the eyes of the physician, many clinical procedures have a particular income configuration. For example, the non-poor report a mammography rate one and a half times that of the poor (National Center for Health Statistics 1998, table 80). Not surprisingly, elective surgery is much more likely to be performed on the affluent. An obvious example is cosmetic surgery for which the majority of procedures performed to improve the appearance of the affluent are almost never performed on the poor.

Although there are some exceptions, utilization of prescription drugs tends to increase with income. This reflects the fact that the affluent visit private physicians more frequently than the non-affluent.

Education and Sickness Behavior

The relationship between education and sickness behavior resembles that of income, although some of the relationships are even stronger. In fact, some have suggested that utilization differentials linked to income actually reflect educational differences. Educational level is probably one of the better predictors of health behavior and the utilization of health services. Education is related not only to levels of service utilization but to the types of services utilized and the circumstances under which they are received. Educational attainment demonstrates a particularly close association with sickness behavior in its various forms.

The rate of hospitalization for the least educated segments of the U.S. population is very low, despite the fact that the incidence of health problems is greater for the poorly educated than for any other group. The better educated, although less affected by health problems, have much higher rates of hospitalization. This is thought to be a function of a greater appreciation of the benefits of healthcare and more insurance coverage on the part of the better educated. (The pattern for education contrasts with that for income in this regard.)

The relationship between nursing home utilization and education is not very clear-cut. Educational differences are found, however, in the use of other types of facilities. Less-educated groups are heavier users of hospital emergency room care, especially for non-emergency conditions. On the other hand, better-educated populations are more likely to utilize freestanding emergency clinics or urgent care centers. The better educated are also more likely to utilize other outpatient settings, such as freestanding diagnostic centers or surgicenters.

Physician utilization is considerably higher for the best educated than for the least. In general, the number of annual physician visits per capita increases with education. The lowest educational groups record the lowest rates of physician visits. As education increases, the utilization rate for primary care physicians decreases and that of specialists increases. This partly reflects the prestige dimension of medical specialists and the knowledge required to select a specialist. The presumed greater expertise of specialists makes them appealing to the well educated.

There is a direct relationship between education and dental care utilization. The better educated see dental care as a preventive service, while the least educated are less likely to appreciate its benefits.

Although diagnostic tests and therapeutic procedures are typically performed as necessary in the eyes of the physician, certain clinical procedures that have a correlation with income also are differentiated on the basis of education. This is reflected in the high proportion of elective surgery, for example, performed on the better educated.

Although there are some exceptions, utilization of prescription drugs tends to increase with education. This reflects the fact that the better educated visit the physician more frequently than the poorly educated. They are also more likely to comply with medical regimens. (See Box 10-3 for a discussion of issues surrounding compliance with doctor's orders.)

Occupation, Employment, Status, and Sickness Behavior

Occupational status is related not only to levels of service utilization but to the types of services utilized and the circumstances under which they are received. This is true whether the indicator is for inpatient care, outpatient care, tests and procedures performed, or virtually any other measure of utilization.

To a limited extent, the use of health services by members of the various occupational status categories corresponds with the differentials in health status identified. In general, those in higher occupational categories require less services because they are healthier. Yet, they utilize more of certain types of services because they are more aware of the need for preventive care and tend to have better insurance coverage.

The higher occupational groups have somewhat higher admission rates. The pattern identified for the various occupational statuses for patient days is comparable to that for admissions. The lower-status occupational categories make up for any differences in admissions by recording more patient days.

Some differences are found in the use of other types of facilities on the basis of occupational status. Income and educational levels no doubt play a role here, and the type of insurance coverage available (which is primarily a function of employment status) is important in determining the type of service utilized. Some differences related to occupational status do exist in the utilization of physician services.

Although there are some exceptions, utilization of prescription drugs tends to be higher for those at higher occupational levels. This partially reflects the higher use of physician services on the part of these groups. Those in the lower occupational categories are found to have higher rates of utilization of nonprescription drugs.

Differences in sickness behavior based on employment status are probably greater than those among the various occupational categories. When the employed and unemployed are compared, the employed have significantly higher admission rates, despite the greater level of morbidity identified for the unemployed. The unemployed, in fact, use less of all types of health services. The only exceptions might be higher use of hospital emergency rooms and public health facilities. The unemployed are also likely to be characterized by informal health behavior that contributes to the poor health status.

There are several reasons for the close association between occupation and sickness behavior in its various forms. Different levels of morbidity are associated with each occupational status category, resulting in demands for differing levels and types of services. An important factor related to occupational status is its implications for lifestyle and (Box 10-4 discusses lifestyle segmentation and health behavior.)

Religion, Religiosity, and Sickness Behavior

Associations between religious affiliation and/or degree of religiosity with sickness behavior are probably the most idiosyncratic of those discussed in this chapter. These relationships have been subjected to limited research and clear patterns are difficult to discern. Further, in contemporary U.S. society, religious affiliation and participation tend to be associated with so many other variables that it is difficult to break out the influence of these variables per se.

There appears to be little difference in the rate of hospitalization for the major religious groups in the United States. Rates of admission for

---

Box 10-3

Compliance with Medical Regimens

The extent to which patients follow doctors orders or otherwise follow a prescribed medical regimen is referred to as "adherence" or "compliance". Compliance refers to the degree to which a medical patient complies with "doctors orders". Compliance is typically measured in terms of the percentage of patients who purchase and use prescribed medicines and/or return for scheduled clinic visits. Under a broader definition of healthcare, compliance may refer to the extent to which individuals follow a diet or exercise regimen. A medical doctor's recommendations may not be the only course of action to which a sick person would adhere; the advice of a lay consultant, an herbalist, a massage therapist, or spiritual healer might also be considered. Some sick persons deliberately seek several opinions—medical or otherwise—and therefore obtain several therapeutic recommendations. Compliance thus implies actively choosing which advice to follow.

Some formulations of the sick role have included following the doctor's orders as a role expectation. Many doctors, likewise, consider it a patient's duty to comply with his therapeutic regimen. The very notion of patient compliance implies a power relationship: The doctor is treated as authoritative and powerful, the patients as powerless and appropriately obedient.

A number of studies show that healthcare professionals greatly underestimate the amount of patients' non-compliance to medical regimens. One estimate suggests that some 20 percent of prescriptions are never filled; 30 to 50 percent of medications are taken incorrectly. When doctors' "orders" involve major lifestyle changes (such as modifying eating or exercise patterns), compliance is even less frequent. Doctors often experience patient non-compliance to their recommendations as an affront to their authority; they consider the patients to be irresponsible.

There are many other reasons, however, why patients do not adhere to recommended therapies. Many patients, especially those dealing with chronic illnesses, develop their own strategies for managing their illness. Such strategies include the selective use of biomedical approaches, but often also involve other therapeutic approaches, advice from more than one doctor, and/or their tailoring of the doctor's advice. From the patient's point of view, such noncompliant health-seeking behavior is rational, and it preserves for them some element of control.

The patient is engaged in an ongoing process of evaluation of recommended therapies; whether the recommendation is medically correct is only one criterion in this evaluation. Other criteria include: the extent to which the doctor appears to understand the condition; the extent to which the doctor's approach and attitude meet patient expectations; the apparent effectiveness of the therapy; and the availability of more desirable options from the patient's perspective. When dissatisfied, patients may try to modify the treatment either by negotiating with their doctor or by modifying the plan themselves.

Much patient non-compliance can be traced to difficulties in understanding and communication in the doctor-patient interaction, especially when there are differences in the perspectives and goals of doctors and their patients. The doctor's focus is typically on curing or managing the specific disease presented by the patient. Laypersons, by contrast, are more likely to have a broader notion of health and illness and to be concerned with all aspects of their life, not merely one health problem, no matter how serious. For example, a patient may feel that the depression experienced as a side effect of blood pressure medicine is so debilitating that continuing the medication is not worth the price.

Often the decision not to follow a doctor's recommended course of action (or not to seek professional help in the first place) is due to a discrepancy between the layperson's and the professional's understandings of the sickness. If there is no cure for the condition and disease management involves repeated ineffective yet costly visits, compliance is unlikely. If the doctor doesn't seem to appreciate the social implications of the recommended therapy, compliance is similarly unlikely. Given the fact that practitioners do not, in the majority of cases, understand the condition from the patient's perspective, the low level of compliance is not surprising. This lack of shared understanding of the nature of illness is likely to lead to considerable non-compliance with doctors' orders and to dissatisfaction on the part of both medical professionals and their patients.

Adherence to any therapeutic regimen is likely to require some effort. The sheer logistics of putting all recommendations into effect are enormous, especially for chronic illness, for which the therapeutic regimen must last a lifetime and is likely to become more demanding as the condition deteriorates. Health seeking is an active process throughout, but the active participation of the sick person is especially evident when it comes to choosing and putting some or all therapeutic advice into effect.

Ultimately, the likelihood of compliance extends beyond any characteristics of the affected individual. The patient's demographic, economic and sociocultural characteristics are likely to contribute to the degree of compliance with doctor's orders. After all, compliance with medical regimens represents a form of social behavior, with all that that implies.

Source: Peter Freund and Meredith B. McGuire (1999). *Health, Illness and the Social Body,* 3rd ed. Englewood Cliffs, NJ: Prentice Hall.

Box 10-4

Lifestyle Segmentation Systems and Health Behavior

Lifestyle segmentation systems have been used for decades in other industries but have never received wide acceptance in health care. For the most part, healthcare provider organizations depended on physicians or health plans to channel patients to them. They, in fact, had little interest in the characteristics of their patients. In the new healthcare environment, however, there is growing interest in customer segmentation. The market has become much more consumer driven and individuals are taking a much more active role in healthcare decision making. Today, growing numbers of health plans, health services providers and other organizations are expressing an interest in customer segmentation and target marketing.

Lifestyle segmentation is also of interest to medical sociologists and others who are interested in the distribution of healthcare phenomena within a population. Although variations in demographic and sociocultural characteristics serve to explain a lot of the differences found in health status and health behavior among various groups, there is growing evidence that lifestyle characteristics may actually transcend these standard dimensions for segmentation. Among the elderly, for example, it was customary to classify those over 65 into one monolithic category or at best three categories based on age breaks (e.g., 65–74, 75–84, and 85 and over). Lifestyle analysis indicates, however, that the 65–74 age cohort actually contains two or more lifestyle clusters that may have similar demographic traits but be different in terms of the lifestyles. For this reason, medical sociologists must consider the lifestyle clusters that characterize the population under study.

The first lifestyle segmentation systems—also referred to as psychographic segmentation systems—were developed in the 1970s. This new approach to segmenting the population was developed in response to some of the perceived deficiencies in demographic profiling. Marketers had come to realize that people in the same demographic category may fall into different groupings based on lifestyle despite being very similar on paper. Lifestyle research discovered that within a demographic category there could be various lifestyle categories that had a greater impact on consumer behavior than, say, age did.

The best-known early lifestyle segmentation system was developed by Stanford Research International (SRI) in the 1970s. It was called VALS for "values and lifestyle system" and inspired a variety of subsequent lifestyle segmentation systems. The VALS system never benefited from widespread use but three subsequent systems are widely used today. These are lifestyle segmentation systems developed by Claritas (PRIZM), Experian (Mosaic) and CACI Marketing Systems (ACORN). While the various systems are built using similar methodologies, they differ in terms of the specific procedures utilized to create the categories.

The concept behind all segmentation systems is the use of geodemographic data in conjunction with data on consumer behavior, attitudes and preferences in establishing distinct lifestyle clusters that cover the entire population. This allows researchers to classify consumers into distinct categories, each with its peculiar characteristics. Once the lifestyle segments have been identified for a population, it is possible to attach a broad range of characteristics to the respective categories.

The PRIZM system developed by Claritas may be the best known system, primarily due to the clever names it has given its lifestyle categories. Individuals may be classified as, for example, "Patios and Pools", "Shotguns and Pickups", or "Executive Suites" among the 62 PRIZM clusters. The PRIZM system is the only one that has been used extensively to date to link health characteristics to lifestyle clusters. This information, however, is proprietary and can only be obtained by becoming a client of a Claritas value-added reseller.

U.S. Mosiac is the latest version of the Experian lifestyle classification system. This system also includes 62 lifestyle clusters grouped into 12 major categories. The naming scheme is somewhat more straightforward than for the PRIZM system, with the "Upscale Singles Category" including such clusters as "High-income urban singles in apartments" and "Urban, upper-mid-income seniors in apartments".

CACI's ACORN is an acronym for "A Classification of Residential Neighborhoods". A number of multivariate statistical methods were applied to create this system. CACI analyzed and sorted the country's 226,000 neighborhoods by 61 unique lifestyle characteristics, such as income, age, household type, home value, occupation, education, and other key determinants of consumer behavior. Next, market segments were created by a combination of cluster analytic techniques. The techniques were selected to produce statistically reliable solutions and to handle an immense amount of information. This process results in the assignment of over 220,000 neighborhoods to 43 lifestyle segments.

Medical sociologists and other researchers are increasingly emphasizing the importance lifestyles for both health status and health behavior. It is only natural to begin to link various health characteristics to the respective lifestyle clusters. As the value of lifestyle segmentation becomes more obvious to health services researchers, the range of health-related characteristics that are likely to be associated with the various lifestyle segments can be expected to grow.

Catholics, Jews, and Protestants overall have not been found to vary much. There are some patterns specific to particular religions. Jews, for example, are found to have higher rates of psychiatric treatment—particularly outpatient—than other religious groups. (This, incidentally, is in contrast to the finding that Jews have the lowest rate of psychiatric impairment of the three groups.) Catholics and Baptists were found in another study to have higher rates of admission to public mental hospitals than other denominations. Differences in usage rates of physicians by religious affiliation are probably related to other factors than religion. Jews report higher usage of medical specialists, and this is thought to be attributable to both cultural preferences and higher socioeconomic status.

Limited research has been conducted on the relationship between religiosity and health behavior. There is too little information available to make concrete distinctions between the healthcare utilization patterns and informal health behaviors of those with various degrees of religious commitment. There have been some studies that link religiosity with choice of hospital when there are different religion-affiliated facilities available. The most that can be concluded, however, is that, for some religiously committed individuals, hospitals supported by their denomination are preferred over other hospitals.

REFERENCES

Cockerham, William C., and Ferris J. Richey (1997). *The Dictionary of Medical Sociology*. Westport, CT: Greenwood.

Eisenberg, D., and R.C. Kessler (1993). "Unconventional medicine in the United States," *New England Journal of Medicine* 328:246–252.

Freidson, Eliot (1970). *Profession of Medicine*. New York: Dodd, Mead.

Graham, Hilary (1985). "Providers, negotiators, and mediators: Women as the hidden careers," pp. 25–52 in E. Lewis and V. Oleson, eds., *Women, Health, and Healing: Toward a New Perspective*. New York: Tavistock.

Harris, R., R. Andrews, and A. Elixhauser (1997). "Racial and gender differences in the use of procedures for black and white hospitalized adults," *Ethnicity and Disease* 7:91–105.

Klein, David, Najman, Jackob, Kohrman, Arthur, and Clarke Munro (1982). "Patient characteristics that elicit negative responses from family physicians," *Journal of Family Practice* 14(5):881–888.

National Center for Health Statistics (1998). *Health, United States, 1998*. Hyattsville, MD: National Center for Health Statistics.

National Center for Health Statistics (2002). *Health, United States, 2002*. Hyattsville, MD: National Center for Health Statistics.

Parsons, Talcott (1951). *The Social System*. Glencoe, IL: The Free Press.

Schensul, Stephen L., and Jean J. Schensul (1982). "Healing resource use in a Puerto Rican community," *Urban Anthropology* 11:59–79.

Verbrugge, Lois M. (1986). "From sneezes to adieux: Stages of health for American men and women," *Social Science and Medicine*, 1195–1212.

Verbrugge, Lois M., and Frank J. Ascione (1987). "Exploring the iceberg: Common symptoms and how people care for them," *Medical Care* 25:539–569.

ADDITIONAL RESOURCES

Gochman, D.S. (1997). *Handbook of Health Behavior*, vol. 1–4. New York: Plenum Press.

INTERNET LINKS

Centers for Disease Control and Prevention (CDC) homepage: www.cdc.gov.
National Center for Health Statistics (NCHS) homepage: www.cdc.nchs.
National Institutes of Health (NIH) homepage: www.nih.gov.

Chapter **11**

Social Stratification in Society and Healthcare

THE NATURE OF SOCIAL STRATIFICATION

Every society divides itself into subgroups based on the attributes considered important by that society. Societies formalize these divisions by developing social stratification systems. This process inevitably results in the formalization of inequality among social groups in that society, with some people having more of the things (tangible and intangible) that society considers valuable and others less. Thus, social stratification refers to a system by which a society ranks categories of people in a hierarchy, in effect creating "strata" or social layers within society.

Social stratification is a creation of society, not simply a natural grouping of individuals or a reflection of individual differences. Because we emphasize individual achievement in the U.S. we tend to think of social standing in terms of personal talent and effort, exaggerating the extent to which we control our own destinies. However, the differences we see among individuals do not reflect their personal differences as much as their position in the social stratification system.

Some form of social stratification exists in every society—large or small, traditional or modern. However, the basis for stratification varies from one society to another. Stratification based on sex and age is found in virtually every society, and, in societies with multiple racial and/or ethnic groups, distinctions related to physical features or cultural heritage are likely to provide the basis for differentiation among society members. While variations in socioeconomic status may provide a basis for stratification in some societies, modern societies place special emphasis on income, education, and occupation as bases for differentiation.

The stratification system that evolves reflects the needs of the particular society. As the things that society considers important change, the bases for social stratification change as well. This has clearly been seen in the United States as the society has progressed through various stages of development, from an agrarian society to an industrial society to a post-industrial society. In colonial times social stratification was based on land ownership. With the industrial revolution it shifted to the ownership of capital, and with the post-industrial period to the control of information.

There are four basic steps in the process of creating a stratification system: 1) differentiation; 2) evaluation; 3) ranking; and 4) differential rewards. *Differentiation* refers to the process of identifying distinctions among members of society. Clearly, society members differ from each other in terms of sex and age. They may also differ based on physical characteristics or subcultural traits. Distinctions may be made based on family membership or participation in some other social group. Whatever the basis for distinction, every society develops ways of "seeing" its members in terms of such traits.

Evaluation involves applying some meaning to the distinctions that are identified in the first step. Society may place significance on what it means to be male rather than female, old rather than young, or white rather than non-white. Thus, the identified social traits are not simply objective identifiers but convey subjective meaning. When someone is identified in terms of their sex, age or race, this immediately conjures up notions of the attributes of this person. Thus, some characteristics carry a favorable connotation and others an unfavorable one. The meaning that society attaches to various attributes ultimately impacts individuals' health status and their relationships with the healthcare delivery system.

Ranking takes the process a step further and places the individuals that have undergone differentiation and evaluation in some type of "order". This is where the status hierarchy begins to take form as, for example, men are ranked higher than women, the elders are ranked higher than the youth, and members of some racial or ethnic groups are ranked higher than members of others. Each society subsequently develops an ideology that explains and justifies the dominance of individuals with certain characteristics and the subordination of others.

The final step in the creation of a stratification system is the provision of *differential rewards*. Now that individuals have been categorized, evaluated and ranked, the system provides differential benefits in the form of both rewards for those occupying various positions in the social hierarchy and incentives for those who are being recruited for specific statuses. Thus, it is argued, physicians play such an important role in the welfare of modern societies that they deserve inordinate rewards for their role performance. Looked at differently, high rewards must be offered to encourage individuals to make the sacrifices necessary to complete the lengthy training required to become a physician.

Social stratification involves not only the existence of inequality but a system of beliefs that support the system. In order for the system to work—that is, be accepted by the members of society—it must be supported by an underlying ideology. Every system of inequality not only gives some people more than others, it provides justification for these disparities. This ideology should be logical and plausible enough to be widely accepted. Just as what is unequal differs from society to society, so do the explanations for why people *should* be unequal.

Once a social stratification system is established, is transcends individual characteristics. Thus, inequality persists from generation to generation as parents pass their social positions on to their children. Even in industrial societies, where some individuals do experience social mobility, the position of most people within the stratification system remains much the same over their lifetimes.

In analyzing the social stratification process, sociologists pay attention to the manner in which individuals attain their statuses. There are, in essence, two ways in which one can attain a status—through ascription and achievement. An ascribed status is a social position a person receives at birth or assumes involuntarily later in life. Examples of ascribed statuses are being a daughter, a Cuban, a teenager, or a widower. Ascribed statuses are matters about which people have little or no choice.

By contrast, an achieved status refers to a social position that a person assumes voluntarily and that reflects personal ability and choice. Examples of achieved statuses include the positions of graduate student, registered nurse, health plan enrollee, and any number of other achieved statuses within the healthcare institution.

In practice, of course, most statuses in contemporary U.S. society involve a combination of ascription and achievement. That is, people's ascribed statuses influence the statuses they achieve. People who achieve the status of physician, for example, are likely to share the ascribed trait of being born into relatively privileged families. By the same token, many less desirable statuses, such as criminal, drug addict, or unemployed workers, are more easily "achieved" by people born into poverty. Many individuals "achieve" the status of "disabled" by virtue of risky health practices that result in chronic conditions.

THE DIMENSIONS OF STRATIFICATION

Sociologists identify three dimensions of stratification or, looked at differently, three types of rewards meted out within the system. Wealth, power, and prestige, offered in various combinations, are the three legs of the stratification stool. In modern societies, *wealth* is typically measured in terms of money income or control of financial resources. It could also be measured in terms of land ownership or ownership of other resources. Wealth is often used as a proxy for other measures of social status because it is relatively easy to quantify.

Power refers to the amount of influence that an individual (or group) has over other individuals (or groups) in society. Although some individuals may have power by virtue of their personal influence (e.g., a journalist or star athlete), this typically refers to the power that is derived from the "office" the individual holds. Thus, individuals occupying such disparate statuses as corporate CEO, hospital administrator, director of a government agency, or a minister of a large church hold power of different types. This power, for the most part, is derived from the position held and not from any characteristics of the individual.

Prestige refers to the amount of esteem provided the individual by society. Many of the same individuals noted above may be accorded a significant measure of prestige, within their particular field or throughout the entire society. Deference is typically accorded to individuals because of the status they occupy or because of occupational skills. Thus, university professors are often accorded significant prestige by virtue of their erudition in their chosen field and their association with a prestigious organization. Physicians are accorded significant prestige due to their presumed skills in the healing arts.

THE CONSEQUENCES OF STRATIFICATION

The consequences of stratification for any society are numerous, and particularly so in a society as complex as the United States. The two primary categories of consequences are lifestyles and life chances. "Lifestyles" refers to the way of living characterizing the members of a social stratum. Lifestyles are acquired through the socialization process in the context of the family and, later, through other social groups with which one comes in contact. These influences convey the beliefs, values and behaviors of that social stratum to the new society member. In this sense, the socialization process teaches individuals their "station" in life and the characteristics appropriate for one's place in the status hierarchy. If an acceptable ideology is in place, new society members are appropriately socialized into their proper status.

The lifestyle component of social class involves not only notions of normative behavior and values, but attitudes, perceptions, and opinions. While the objective measures are the easiest to operationalize and thereby to use as a basis for dividing the population into measurable groups, less tangible aspects of lifestyles have important implications for health status and health behavior.

"Life chances" include a variety of factors that reflect the operation of the stratification system. These include the chances of growing up in a stable, nurturing family, the opportunity to attend certain schools, the likelihood of obtaining a well-paying job, and so forth. Of particular importance are life chances related to health and, as will be seen below, one's chance of surviving infancy, avoiding various deadly diseases, and generally living a long, healthy life are a function of one's position in the stratification system.

White, native-born Americans do not live longer than African-Americans, Hispanics and Native Americans because they are smarter, more responsible, or luckier. They live longer because they are born with certain advantages and have access to certain opportunities that members of minority groups do not have. This situation results in significant disparities in life chances among various groups in society. Children born into affluent families are more likely than children born into poverty to enjoy good health, be successful at school, succeed in a career, and live long lives. While neither rich nor poor are responsible for the existence of social stratification, the system influences the life chances of all members of society.

THE SIGNIFICANCE OF STRATIFICATION FOR SOCIETY

Sociologists who support a structural-functional approach to the understanding of society would contend that social stratification plays a vital role in the operation of society. How else, it is asked, can one explain the fact that all known societies have displayed some form of stratification? One justification for the existence of the stratification system is that different jobs (or roles) make differing contributions to the functioning of society. From this perspective, the greater the functional importance of a position, the more value a society attaches to it. Thus, the role of the "hospital administrator" is considered to be more important to the functioning of the hospital than the role of "orderly" and, consequently, the administrator is likely to be compensated at a rate several times that of the orderly. This strategy is intended to promote productivity, since rewarding important work with income, prestige, and/or power encourages society members to perform the roles that society considers most important. Differential rewards, then, are the key to more effective institutions whether they be in the political, educational or healthcare realms.

While this view of social stratification makes logical sense, it oversimplifies the reality of stratification in societies such as the United States. Many counterexamples can be found of individuals who are provided inordinate rewards but are performing roles that make a limited contribution to society. Also, there is no logic that can justify the fact that physicians on the average make six times the income of the average worker or that top executives in Fortune 500 companies earn as much as 600 times the salary of the average employee in that company. Some of the wealthiest individuals, in fact, arguably make *no* active contribution to society, drawing their income and wealth from investments (perhaps made by their forefathers). Such examples indicate that this is, indeed, an imperfect system of stratification.

Critics of the structural-functional approach argue that this explanation amounts to a justification for the status quo. From this critical perspective, the existence of inequality in terms of wealth, power, and prestige does not reflect the relative contributions to society of different roles. It serves primarily to rationalize the fact that many roles in society carry greater rewards than others and to preserve the unequal distribution of wealth that exists. This approach is supported by those who take a social-conflict approach to society.

Social-conflict theorists site numerous statistics to support their assertions. First, wealth remains highly concentrated in U.S. society, with about half of all privately controlled corporate stock owned by one percent of the population. Second, many of today's white-collar jobs offer no more income, security, or satisfaction than factory work did a century ago. Third, many benefits enjoyed by today's workers came about through "class conflict" in the form of union-management conflict and not through the rational application of differential rewards. Fourth, while workers have gained legal protections, the law has not helped ordinary people use the legal system as effectively as the rich use it.

The United States is a dynamic society marked by significant social mobility. Adequate opportunity exists for individuals (and groups) to change their position within the stratification system, particularly by improving their standing on the wealth dimension. At the same time, downward mobility is not at all rare, as individuals, either through personal circumstances or through the vagaries of the economy, find themselves relegated to a lower level of the hierarchy. The millions of personal bankruptcies filed every year attests to the possibility of dropping down in the stratification system.

Over the long term, social mobility is less a function of individual actions then it is of changes in society itself. During the first half of the twentieth century, for example, industrialization expanded the U.S. economy and pushed up living standards. Since a rising tide raises all boats, many prospered during this period. During the early 1990s, the boom in technology, particularly in computerization, made millionaires out of thousands of individuals. Their success was not so much due to the fact that they were smarter or more talented than other workers, but due to their fortunate positioning within a burgeoning industry. During the late 1990s, on the other hand, economic setbacks generated substantial downward mobility, again regardless of one's individual situation.

STRATIFICATION IN COMPARATIVE PERSPECTIVE

In examining stratification systems across different societies, sociologists have identified a number of factors that can be used for comparison purposes. For example, one might consider the relative degree of inequality characterizing the systems in question. Considering the sharpness of distinction between the various strata, one might ask: Are people in different social strata markedly different from each, and can someone's position in the stratification system be identified by looking at them or listening to them? One might also speak of the rigidity of the lines between the various strata. Are the lines separating the strata clearly marked? How difficult is it to cross these lines? Further, one might consider the degree of legal support for the system. Are the various strata set (or at least reinforced) by law? Are there theocratically enacted rules (taking the force of law) that prescribe the strata in society? Finally, one might consider the "span" of the system. That is, what is the "distance" from the top to the bottom? Is the system relatively flat, with most strata grouped closely together? Or is the span from the richest to the poorest wide? How much of society's resources are controlled by the various strata of society?

Stratification systems can be classified as "open" or "closed" systems. Most traditional systems are considered relatively closed. These would include the caste system of India and the feudal systems of medieval Europe, as well as the less complex systems characterizing smaller traditional societies. Closed systems are highly structured with clear-cut distinctions between the strata, a strong ideological basis for the system, legal and/or religious support for the system, and virtually no opportunity for social mobility. Such systems emphasize the status quo and are relatively impervious to change.

Open systems, such as those that characterize the United States and most modernized societies, are "informal" compared to closed systems. They tend not to be formally structured but evolve out of the interaction of groups in society. They tend to be relatively flexible, with unclear lines of demarcation, often openly encouraging social mobility. Older European societies tend to be open while retaining some of the traits of closed systems (such as the hereditary English monarchy).

A more open class system allows individuals who obtain education and skills to become socially mobile in relation to their parents or siblings. Such mobility, in turn, blurs class distinctions so that even family members may have different social status. Categorizing people according to their color, sex, or social background gradually comes to be seen as both inappropriate and counterproductive.

The industrial production characteristic of modern societies requires a relatively open system for its operation. Compared to agrarian societies where a rigid "caste" system is the rule, industrial societies move in the direction of meritocracy, a system in which social position is based entirely on personal merit. Thus, there is considerable reliance on credentials, degrees, and other objective indicators of "merit" in modern, industrial societies. Class systems in industrial societies move toward meritocracy to promote productivity and efficiency but retain some traditional elements of stratification in order to maintain order and social cohesion.

One other measure for comparing stratification systems not discussed above involves the degree to which society members relate to their social strata. Are individuals constantly aware of their position in the stratification system, or is this only something that comes up occasionally if someone attempts to cross a line? In a class system, sociologists speak of "class consciousness" and, indeed, earlier social observers felt that class consciousness in capitalist societies would ultimately bring the system down, as entrenched class differences pitted one class against another.

In actuality, class consciousness has never developed to any extent in the U.S. Most Americans would, in fact, deny the existence of a class system. While most society members have some vague notion of where they fit into the overall stratification system, they typically do not feel constantly aware of their positions nor do they feel a particular kinship with others in their social stratum.

This lack of class consciousness within the U.S. stratification system reflects a number of factors. For one thing, there are numerous laws that seek to guarantee equality of opportunity, and society members are constantly reminded that everyone is equal. For another, there are many other dimensions that traverse class lines so that strata distinctions become blurred. Religious and ethnic affiliations, for example, cut across class lines and create vertical divisions within society that cut across the horizontal layers of the stratification system. In addition, there is a significant amount of status inconsistency within U.S. society. College professors may be at the highest level of educational prestige but have moderate incomes. Truck drivers may make an upper middle class income, but be relatively low in the system in terms of power and prestige. Further, there is ample opportunity for social mobility within the U.S. class system, with individuals frequently crossing class lines through upward mobility (and occasionally through downward mobility).

THE U.S. CLASS SYSTEM

The social stratification system in the United States is considered a "class system." Although the existence of this system is not formally recognized by society, an informal status hierarchy exists within the United States. More implicit than explicit, the U.S. stratification system nevertheless impinges on every individual in U.S. society every day.

Defining the stratification system in the United States is difficult, and the challenge can be demonstrated by the application of the criteria noted above. Whatever class distinctions exist in U.S. society are not very clear. Individuals can identify different strata in only the most general terms (e.g., the "rich", the "working class", the "poor") and even scholars cannot agree on how many classes there are and how to distinguish them. Even if some consensus could be reached on the U.S. class structure, the distinctions would be difficult to operationalize since the lines between the strata are so indistinct. While it may be possible to distinguish in general terms between members of the middle class and the upper class, it is difficult to determine where, for example, the upper-middle class ends and the lower-upper class begins. These distinctions are further blurred by the constant movement of individuals between strata—through upward or downward mobility— and by virtue of the status inconsistency common in U.S. society.

In addition, not only is there no legal support for the stratification system in the U.S., there are proscriptions against any type of formal stratification. While it is true that laws exist to preserve the property rights of individuals thereby supporting the status quo, the U.S. legal system guarantees that all individuals are equal before the law. The capitalist ideology implicitly supporting the system is contradictory in that it justifies the status quo while, at the same time, assuring society members that anyone can rise up in the status hierarchy. The one aspect of stratification in the U.S. that suggests the existence of a formal stratification system relates to the "span" that exists from the top to the bottom of the system. The gap between the very rich and the very poor is quite wide and, after decades of narrowing, has once again widened.

Box 11-1

Major U.S. Class Divisions

Descriptions of the major divisions within the U.S. stratification system are presented below. Since no formal distinctions exist with regard to class divisions in the U.S., these divisions represent the conclusions of social scientists who study such phenomena.

Upper Class

Upper-class households constitute about 5 percent of the United States population. These households may have incomes of $150,000 or more annually, although most earn considerably more. Many of those in the upper class come from families with "old money", or fortunes that were accumulated by their ancestors. Much of their income may come from investments rather than wages. Others work as top executives in large corporations, as leading professionals (such as physicians or scientists). or as senior government officials.

The upper-upper class includes less than one percent of the U.S. population and is an exclusive "club" that one can only be born into. The lower-upper class might be referred to as the "working rich" in that most of these individuals have high incomes as a result of the wages they earn rather than through inheritance. These "nouveau riche" seldom achieve acceptance by the "old money" crowd.

Middle Class

The U.S. middle class constitutes 40 to 45 percent of the U.S. population and, as such, exerts a great deal of influence on American culture. These representatives of "mainstream" America are the typical subjects of television shows and movies, and advertisers view consumers from this stratum as the "average" American. While the upper class is restricted primarily to white Anglo-Saxon Protestants, the middle class is more representative of the overall U.S. population.

Because of the fluidity within the U.S. system, "status inconsistency" is an inherent aspect of U.S. stratification. Traditional stratification systems are characterized by little social mobility and high status consistency, so that the typical person has the same relative standing with regard to wealth, power and prestige. The greater mobility of class systems, however, generates considerable status inconsistency. Low status consistency reflects the fact that classes are less well defined than they are in traditional systems.

Social scientists generally see U.S. society as being divided into three to six social classes. The three major divisions are the upper, middle, and lower classes. When more divisions are utilized, the categories are typically subdivisions of the three major groupings. A common variation involves

Upper-middle class households have above average household incomes and may accumulate considerable property or other wealth. Members of this group typically have highly paying professional or executive positions and many are business owners. This stratum is highly educated and exerts a dominant influence in national and local cultures.

The middle-middle class represents perhaps the stratum closest to the middle of the U.S. class system. Members of this class generally have a moderate amount of education and hold lower-level white-collar jobs or upper-level blue-collar jobs.

The lower-middle class, sometimes referred to as the "working class", includes the third of the U.S. population that works for "average" wages from primarily blue-collar and low-paying service jobs that place the households above subsistence level but not in the comfort zone of the middle-middle class. Members of this class are generally poorly educated and do not display the ambitions of higher social classes. The lowest segments of this class may be thought to overlap with the upper segments of the lower class.

Lower Class

The lower class includes the 20 percent of the U.S. population at the bottom of the stratification system. This includes the poor and the near-poor who barely have enough resources to put them beyond the poverty level. Members of this class may hold low-paying jobs in manual labor or service occupations that are often temporary and unstable and do not provide the benefits associated with most employment in the U.S. Many are unemployed or underemployed and participation on the welfare roles is common. Racial and ethnic minorities are overrepresented in this segment of the class system and this class is disproportionately affected by illness and disability.

Source: John J. Macionis (2000). *Society: The Basics.* Upper Saddle River, NJ: Prentice Hall.

the carving out of a "working class" category out of the lower-middle and upper-lower classes. (See Box 11-1 for a description of the major "classes" in U.S. society.)

Social scientists often emphasize the objective measures of class such as income, education, and occupation. While these are the demographic dimensions that will be utilized in the discussion below, it should be noted that the subjective component can not be ignored. This "lifestyle" component of social class involves not only notions of normative behavior and values, but attitudes, perceptions, and opinions. While the objective measures are the easiest to operationalize and thereby to use as a basis for dividing the population into measurable groups, these groups' lifestyles

---

Box 11-2

Time Horizons and Their Implications

Although the class distinctions in U.S. society are not very clear-cut, there are certain traits that are consistently associated with various class levels. Thinking in terms of what are typically considered the three major classes in U.S. society—the lower class, middle class and upper class—it can be argue that distinct differences exist with regard to the "time horizons" associated with each of these classes. The time horizon refers to the time dimension—past, present or future—to which one's perceptions and behavior are oriented. For the most part, the lower class is oriented to the present, the middle class to the future, and upper class to the past.

The time horizon is particularly important in a society such as the U.S. because of its influence on the individual's worldview and his subsequent behavior. Whether one is oriented toward the past, the present, or the future provides an important clue to the values and norms characterizing the group to which the individual belongs. In general terms, an orientation to the past tends to be relatively conservative, emphasizing tradition and the status quo and resisting change. An orientation to the future, on the other hand, disdains tradition, supports orderly change, and encourages investment in hopes of future benefits. An orientation to the present implies no ties to the past and limited confidence in the future, creating a mindset that involves living for today and an emphasis on immediate gratification.

The orientation to the past characteristic of the upper income groups in U.S. society places emphasis on family lineage, tradition and an attachment to place. Its orientation reflects the fact that its wealth may have been accumulated in the past, encouraging an emphasis on preserving the status quo and deemphasizing the importance of future endeavors. This group's pride rests with the ancestors that established their position in society, and children are valued for their role in perpetuating the glories of the past rather than their usefulness in forging new paths.

---

have important implications for health status and health behavior. (One important aspect of the class system is the different time horizons that members of different classes observe and the implications of these time horizons for health and health care. Box 11-2 illustrates the different time horizons characterizing the various social classes.)

SOCIAL STRATIFICATION WITHIN THE HEALTHCARE INSTITUTION

The occupational structure of healthcare is often depicted as a microcosm of the larger social system, particularly in terms of social stratification. The

The upper income group is relatively small and, while no doubt exerting more influence than its numbers would warrant, does not reflect the dominant view in U.S. society. Thus, an orientation to the past is not common among the majority of society.

The orientation to the present characteristic of lower income groups in U.S. society impinges dramatically on the everyday lives of lower-income individuals. Members of this class are concerned about the immediate needs of survival and, of necessity, live day to day. There is nothing glorious about the past to be honored and, indeed, the "sins of the fathers" may account for the current state of poverty. There is limited hope for the future, given that there are barely enough resources for survival in the present. There are certainly no resources for investing in the future.

The lower income group, although numerically larger than the upper income group, does not represent a dominant influence in U.S. society. In fact, the values often spawned by a present time orientation are antithetical to the dominant values of U.S. society. Thus, the values and behavior of members of the lower class members of society are held in disdain by the other groups and, indeed, for members of this group to attain upward mobility, they must typically exchange a present time orientation with all that implies for a future time orientation.

The orientation to the future characteristic of middle class America is considered the dominant ethos of U.S. society. By far the largest of the three classes, middle class values are thought to reflect the basic tenets of the American culture and exert much more influence than the past or present time horizons. The middle class holds the next higher class as a reference group and aspires to reach that level in the future, if not for themselves for their children. This class values children because they embody the future and are considered worth "investing" in. A major trait of this class is deferred gratification, in which individuals forego benefits in the present for presumed greater benefits in the future. This class invests heavily in insurance and retirement programs that will serve them in the future even if it means short-term hardship.

(continued)

healthcare occupational structure replicates the patterns of discrimination in society. The racism, sexism and class discrimination that exists in U.S. society are reflected, if not magnified, within the healthcare system.

As noted in the chapter on occupations and professions, women and non-whites have historically held the lowest status positions in healthcare and white males have held the highest. The medical staff and hospital administration have been dominated by white males with little opportunity for women or minority group members to break in. However, this situation has been undergoing a dramatic shift. Females are beginning to become a numerical majority in medical school and their numbers among practicing physicians have increased dramatically over the past two decades.

The particular time orientation has numerous implications for both health status and health behavior. This is particularly true for the lower and middle classes whose perspectives are diametrically opposed. The upper classes display rather idiosyncratic tendencies with regard to health behavior and are less easily characterized in this regard. One thing is clear, however, and that is the upper class's ability to pay for healthcare. Regardless of their health practices, they do not face the same concerns as the lower-income groups and some of the members of the middle-income group.

Because of the present orientation of members of the lower class, health is only considered a value to the extent that ill-health is an expensive inconvenience. There is little striving for higher health status, on the assumption that sickness is an inherent part of (lower-class) life. When symptoms do appear, there is a tendency to ignore them or delay treatment as long as possible. And treatment that does occur is likely to be aimed at eliminating the immediate problem (e.g., pain or impairment) with little concern for the future implications of the actions.

Because of the emphasis on immediate gratification within the lower class, little thought is given to preventive care or investment in insurance.

The number of women also has increased significantly among the rolls of healthcare administrators. African Americans, Hispanics and Asian-Americans have achieved more than "token" status among both medical staffs and hospital administrators.

The stratification system in healthcare has historically been perpetuated through the recruitment processes of the various occupations and professions in healthcare. While medical students are no longer drawn almost exclusively from the upper strata of society, they still reflect an upper-middle class ancestry. Nurses continue to be drawn from working class or middle class segments of society, and lower-level personnel are drawn from the working class and lowest income groups. Low SES individuals may escape the neighborhood to become hospital orderlies but few make it as hospital administrators. Few people from upper-middle-class backgrounds are recruited for the low level positions in health care.

All of this has contributed to a rigid occupational structure within the healthcare institution. In fact, the occupational structure of healthcare resembles more of a caste system than a class system in most respects. There is a tremendous span from the top to the bottom of the system, with physicians ranking as the highest paid occupation in society and those at the bottom often making minimum wage. The distinctions between the levels are quite clear and there is no mistaking the position of a nurse with that of a physician or of an intake clerk with that of a hospital administrator. These boundaries are clearly demarcated and often use symbols to assure awareness of these distinctions.

The demands of the present, coupled with a general discounting of the future, do not make preventive measures like tooth-brushing, appropriate diet, and well-child checkups very important. The notion of spending limited resources on something like insurance that *might* have some future value is a concept that has no resonance with this population. In fact, the present orientation encourages a passivity that is very uncharacteristic of the American ethos.

The future orientation of the middle class fosters quite different characteristics. There is a great deal of emphasize on a proactive approach to health conditions. This means not only addressing them promptly and aggressively when they occur, but utilizing whatever means necessary to prevent the conditions in the first place. Members of the middle class are quick to recognize symptoms and, if anything, tend to overutilize the healthcare system in their desire to be proactive. The middle class (particularly the upper-middle class) has set the tone with regard to healthy lifestyles and has led the movement toward fitness and healthy diets. The middle class tends to be highly insured and considers health insurance a high priority. Such an investment in the future is an inherent trait associated with a future orientation.

The system is also caste-like in that there is virtually no upward mobility. In fact, healthcare is unique among U.S. industries in terms of the existence of rigid horizontal strata that remain impermeable to penetration. An occasional hospital administrator may work himself up from the mailroom, but that is rare given the professionalization of hospital administration. On the clinical side, there is virtually no opportunity for crossing stratum boundaries and, even within a stratum such as nursing, there are likely to be rigid lines between, say registered nurses and nursing assistants. Essentially the only opportunity for advancement requires that the worker leave the structure, obtain additional training or credentials, and then reenter the system at a different stratum.

The implications of stratification for the operation of the healthcare system and the consequences of the system for various groups in society are discussed in a later section.

IMPLICATIONS OF STRATIFICATION FOR HEALTH AND HEALTH BEHAVIOR

There are many aspects of social stratification that have implications for health and healthcare. The most clear-cut of these relate to the impact of socioeconomic status on both health status and health behavior. Although the discussion below focuses on the implications of income and education stratification on healthcare, other dimensions of stratification also have implications for the system. These include the impact of differences based on sex, age, and race among other factors.

Socioeconomic Status and Health Status

Income and Health

It has been found that no matter what indicator of health status is utilized, there is generally an inverse relationship between income and health status. There is a strong inverse relationship between income level and morbidity for both physical and mental disorders. As income increases, the prevalence of both acute and chronic conditions decreases. Not surprisingly, members of lower-income groups assess themselves as being in poorer health than do the more affluent.

Not only are there more episodes of both acute and chronic conditions recorded as income decreases, but the severity of the conditions is likely to be greater when income is lower. When afflicted by acute conditions, the poor tend to have more prolonged episodes characterized by greater severity. Interestingly, in a society that has become characterized by chronic health conditions, acute disorders remain surprisingly common among the lower-income groups. In fact, the disease profiles of many low-income communities more closely resemble those of developing countries than they do the United States.

There is a direct monotonic neonotomic and inverse relationship between income level and activity limitation. The lower the income, the greater the number of bed-disability days, work-loss days, school-loss days, and restricted-activity days. The mortality rate for the lowest income levels may be twice that of the most affluent in some communities, even after adjusting for age. Virtually all infant mortality in the United States today is accounted for by the lowest income groups, and maternal mortality (which has been virtually eliminated society-wide) is still disturbingly frequent among the poor.

The highest overall rates of mental disorder are found in the lower class, including schizophrenia—the most severely disabling form of mental illness (Cocker 2000b). Anxiety and mood disorders, however, tend to be more prevalent among the upper and middle classes, although the lower class suffers from these problems as well. Research on the epidemiology of mental disorders has uncovered an inverse relationship for three major disorders—schizophrenia, alcohol abuse, and major depression (Dohrenwend 1990). Socioeconomic status here was measured by a combination of income, education, and occupational characteristics. (See the chapter on the sociology of mental illness for more detail on the relationship between mental disorders and various social factors.)

The relationship between income level and health status has been explained in a number of ways. The most obvious has to do with the ability to pay for health services. The affluent are able to ameliorate many health problems that the unaffluent cannot. This ability to pay may extend to the acquisition of preventive services and lifestyle factors such as good nutrition.

Income is probably one of the better predictors of sickness behavior and the utilization of health services. Income is related not only to levels of service utilization but to the types of services utilized and the circumstances under which they are received. This is true whether the indicator is for inpatient care, outpatient care, tests and procedures performed, or virtually any other measure of utilization. It is also true for measures of informal health behavior.

Hospitalization rates tend to decrease directly with income and, in fact, greater discrepancies exist among the various income groups than for any of the other social variables examined. The rate of hospitalization for the lowest income population in the U.S. is the highest of any income group, reflecting the higher incidence of health problems. The differences noted for admissions and length of stay reflect the types of conditions for which members of different income categories are admitted. The relatively unhealthy and unsafe environments in which the lower-income groups are likely to live result in a higher rate of emergency admissions, especially for children. Admission rates for psychotic conditions and substance-abuse problems tend to be higher for the least affluent. The pattern of longer stays for the less affluent is complicated somewhat by unexpected cases of shorter lengths of stay for lower income patients because of their limited ability to pay for services.

Lower income groups are heavier users of hospital emergency room care, for nonemergency conditions. This phenomenon is explained by the lack of family physicians among lower-income patients, their lack of accessible services other than emergency rooms in inner city areas, the hospital emergency room's obligation to provide treatment, and the now well-established cultural preference for emergency room care. On the other hand, lower-income populations are less likely to utilize freestanding emergency clinics or urgent care clinics. This is presumably due to a lack of knowledge of their availability (they are often located in suburban areas) and the fact that payment is typically demanded when care is rendered.

Income also has usefulness as a predictor of the types of clinical services that will be utilized. Although diagnostic tests and therapeutic procedures are typically performed as necessary in the eyes of the physician, many clinical procedures have a particular income configuration. For example, the non-poor report a mammography rate one and a half times that of the poor. This also reflects the high proportion of elective surgery performed on the affluent. The majority of such procedures performed to improve the appearance of the affluent are almost never performed on the poor.

Education and Health

While other socioeconomic indicators are useful for predicting a population's health status, education appears to be the single most important indicator in this regard (Cockerham 1997). Typically, the higher the educational level, the lower the morbidity level. This is true for both acute and chronic physical conditions, with a clear inverse relationship demonstrated between educational levels and major health threats such as cardiovascular disease (Wamala et al. 1999).

The pattern with regard to mortality resembles that for income. The death rate for the poorly educated is much higher than that for those with higher educational achievement (National Center for Health Statistics 1998, table 36). The age-adjusted death rate for those with less than twelve years of education is three times that for those with thirteen or more years of schooling. Infant mortality, in fact, has been virtually eliminated from the groups with the highest educational levels. The poorly educated, however, account for the bulk of infant deaths. Like the poor, the causes of death for the poorly educated are more likely to be the acute problems typically associated with less developed countries than the chronic conditions characterizing much of American society. Also like the poor, the less educated are likely to be characterized by lifestyle-related deaths such as homicides and accidents. Education, it fact, has been recently shown to demonstrate a stronger influence on mortality than income (Rogers et al. 2000).

The relationship between educational level and mental illness, like that for physical illness, appears fairly clear-cut. In fact, some researchers have suggested that the social class differentials noted above are a function of differing levels of education. As the level of education increases, there appears to be an increase in the prevalence, but a decrease in the severity, of disorders. The better educated appear to be more characterized by anxiety disorders, while the less educated appear to be more frequently psychotic. Ironically, the rate of suicide is much higher among the better educated, but this is generally attributed to the differing means of coping characterizing various educational levels.

As with income, the relationship does not necessarily reflect the level of education per se but the differential consequences of varying education levels. Those with less education are also likely to have more financial problems, poor housing conditions, and unsafe environments, all contributing to an unhealthy situation (Schrijvers et al. 1999).

The relationship between education and sickness behavior resembles that for income, although some of the relationships are even stronger. In fact, some have suggested that utilization differentials linked to income actually reflect educational differences. Education is related not only to levels of service utilization but to the types of services utilized and the circumstances under which they are received.

Ironically, the rate of hospitalization for the least educated segments of the U.S. population is very low, despite the fact that the incidence of health problems is greater for the poorly educated than for any other group. The better educated, although less affected by health problems, have much higher rates of hospitalization. This is thought to be a function of a greater appreciation of the benefits of healthcare and more insurance coverage on the part of the better educated. Physician utilization is considerably higher for the best educated than for the least. Less-educated groups are heavier users of hospital emergency room care, especially for non-emergency conditions. On the other hand, better-educated populations are more likely to utilize freestanding emergency clinics or urgent care clinics. The better educated are also more likely to utilize other outpatient settings, such as freestanding diagnostic centers or surgicenters. Those with higher educational levels are likely to be highly mobile and to be supportive of innovative and/or cost-effective forms of care.

There is direct and inverse relationships between education and dental care utilization. The better educated see dental care as a preventive service, while the least educated are less likely to appreciate its benefits. The use of various types of mental health counselors tends to increase with education.

Although diagnostic tests and therapeutic procedures are typically performed when deemed medically necessary, certain clinical procedures that have a correlation with income also are differentiated on the basis of education. This is reflected in the high proportion of elective surgery performed on the better educated.

Sexual Stratification and Healthcare

Sex-based discrimination is prevalent throughout American society and affects every aspect of women's lives, including their health, both physical and mental. Clearly, economic status, membership in a minority group, and gender are all overlapping and interacting factors in determining both access to health services and the content of healthcare research (Reed, 1999). "Sexism" involves the notion that one sex is innately superior to the other. Every society assigns different meanings to "masculinity" and "femininity" and develops notions concerning positive and negative sex role behavior. Sexism is not just a matter of individual attitudes, it is built into the institutions of our society. Institutional sexism pervades the economy, for example, with women highly concentrated in low-paying jobs. Similarly, the legal system has long excused violence against women, especially on the part of boyfriends, husbands, and fathers. In healthcare, women have historically been deemed unfit to practice medicine, excluded as subjects from clinical research, and told by physicians that their symptoms were "all in their head".

According to the Institute of Medicine (1997), the medical enterprise, both in scientific research and in clinical practice, has traditionally viewed female lives and bodies through a lens of masculine experience and assumptions. A common medical view has been that the female reproductive organs occupy a special realm, distinct from the body at large, and one that just happens to define their owner's essential nature. Under this model, the male body and male behavior were viewed as normative, while the female body was viewed as "other," with particular emphasis on the reproductive tract as setting women apart from men.

At the same time, many male physicians denigrate the female-dominated care-giving professions and asserted their role as the "experts" on the provision of women's health care. Despite this so-called expertise, women patients are frequently ignored, mistreated, not taken seriously, or denied access to needed services. Historically, it was common for gynecologists to "treat" women for symptoms such as nymphomania, epilepsy, and nervous and psychological problems, such as hysteria, by removing the ovaries and/or amputating the clitoris. As recently as the 1970s, a popular gynecology text advised gynecologists that the greatest diagnostic aid to use when listening to women's health complaints is the ability to distinguish "fact from fancy," implying that women were not to be taken seriously.

Despite the progress made by the women's health movement, the health status of men and women is still not equal in terms of access to care, treatment, and the quality of services received. When it comes to screening, detection and treatment, women are frequently short-changed. For example, battering is a major factor in illness and injury among women, but is often overlooked by medical professionals. Men with AIDS are four times more likely to receive the "therapy of choice" than women, even when controlling for other factors, and treatment programs for alcoholics are usually based on the model of the male alcoholic, even though women alcoholics have very different needs and responses to treatment.

It has been suggested that the disparities found in the health status of men and women stem from three sources: different biologies and physiologies; divergent life courses; and unequal social statuses. Women have remarkably dissimilar experiences in growing up, during maturity, and as they age. Despite the rapid social change of the last generation, they still play different roles in society and face different pressures and expectations.

Perhaps the most important factor influencing health status is economic and, when economic considerations are interfaced with gender traits, females are especially vulnerable. As a group, women are far less able than men to pay for all of the health services they need, primarily because they are paid less than men. Although a greater percentage of women are covered by some form of health plan, women more often depend on public sources of coverage than do men. Women in the childbearing years face the highest risk of inadequate coverage, at a time in their lives when the need is most acute (Benderly, 1997). For low-income women, the lack of child care, adequate transportation, a dearth of providers willing to accept public insurance, and shortages of providers in rural and inner-city areas compound the problem of access.

These disparities in health status between men and women are further reinforced by the disparities in the area of clinical research. A major concern of the women's health movement has been that women have historically been excluded from clinical trials. This exclusion has been based on fears among researchers that women's menstrual cycles and their potential for becoming pregnant might skew the results and/or harm the mother/fetus. Consequently, many conditions that disproportionately affect women have been understudied. Despite current mandates on the inclusion of women in clinical trials, there are lingering concerns that women's health needs are not being appropriately addressed.

Age Stratification and Healthcare

Virtually all societies include age as a component of their stratification system and the United States, albeit in subtle ways, is no exception. "Ageism" involves the differential treatment of individuals based on their age, and in the U.S. this primarily involves discriminatory treatment of older Americans. Despite the size of the elderly population, the youth-oriented culture of the U.S. predisposes society members to develop negative attitudes toward aging and the elderly.

Despite the disproportionate use of the healthcare system by the American elderly, the system has never been very comfortable treating this segment of the population. The youth-oriented values of society are reflected in the attitudes of healthcare providers. The medical enterprise is oriented toward treatment and cure, and the conditions of most elderly patients defy this approach. Patients characterized by chronic conditions that can only be managed and not cured do not make attractive patients for physicians. They are not "interesting" and their inability to be cured makes them fall outside the normal scope of healthcare operations. Further, healthcare providers expect patients to be able to understand the information they receive and to act in a responsible manner with regard to doctors' orders. The inability of many elderly patients to act in this manner puts them into the "bad patient" category in the eyes of many practitioners.

This discomfort with the elderly on the part of healthcare providers has at least three major implications. First, the elderly may not be taken seriously as patients and may thus be rendered less care than a younger patient. Older patients are not expected to be knowledgeable concerning their conditions and are criticized for both providing too much information and not providing enough. There is a preconceived notion that many are hyperchondriacs.

Practitioners are often inclined to "write off" elderly patients, feeling that they deserve less attention than younger patients. This involves providing them less time and attention and assuming that they are not going to be responsive to therapy. There are plenty of other patients who can benefit from the doctor's skills, so elderly patients who are not likely to get better anyway may be considered "in the way."

Second, when care is provided it is likely to be different from that provided to younger patients. Elderly patients may not be offered the same treatment as younger patients, and there is a tendency to "maintain" older patients on drugs rather than aggressively treating them. Further, symptoms of disease that would warrant immediate concern among younger patients are assumed to be natural accompaniments of aging and are often ignored. "Do not resuscitate" instructions may be readily complied with for elderly patients, when their functioning could be restored through simple medical procedures.

Third, medical practitioners have a tendency to generalize the traits of the elderly and, in the absence of any incentive to determine otherwise, see most elderly patients as essentially the same. Social scientists and policy makers dealing with older Americans long ago realized that the elderly category includes a wide variation in the characteristics of its members. Yet, physicians are used to thinking in terms of clinical categories. If clinicians are apt to refer to "the gall bladder in Room 305," they are even more likely to refer to "the 'geri' in Room 306".

The antipathy of the system toward the elderly (gerontophobia) is reflected in the lack of attention paid to geriatric medicine during medical education. Medical students receive little training in and few are attracted into geriatrics. As a result there are not many more geriatricians available to this population than there were two decades ago. It is ironic that a relative handful of the nation's 126 medical schools require separate courses in geriatric medicine. Even in 2002, there were only about 4,000 board-certified geriatricians in the United States, a figure that has remained fairly stable for several years.

Reasons for such shortages include the lack of recognition accorded geriatric medicine among the specialties, the lower pay and lack of glamour associated with geriatric medicine, the lack of professional reinforcement for those involved in geriatric care, the irreversible physical declines and inevitable death associated with geriatric care, and complicated paperwork and poor reimbursement through government-funded programs for the elderly. Physicians are just as susceptible to negative stereotypes of the elderly as the general population and have been found to be especially reticent to deal with death.

The resulting mistreatment of elderly patients has been well documented. A recent study by the Rand Corporation (Brook et al. 1991) found that, among other things, improper medical care could be blamed for perhaps 27% of the deaths from common illnesses among the elderly; older persons are either over- or under-prescribed with medications (Alliance for Aging Research, 2000), and comprise more than one-half of all deaths from drug reactions. People over 75 are less likely to receive prescriptions that reduce heart attacks and receive clot-busting drugs only one-sixth as often as younger patients. While women over 65 are twice as likely to develop breast cancer as younger women, those with the disease are one-half as likely to be treated appropriately for it even though they are just as likely to benefit from treatment. On the other hand, between 25 and 40 percent of all acute hospital procedures performed on older patients were found to be unnecessary

Ironically, the lack of interest in geriatric care on the part of health professionals has spawned a major market for products for the elderly. The neglect on the part of clinicians is offset by the eagerness with which providers of related services and products target the older population cohorts.

Racial/Ethnic Stratification and Healthcare

The growing significance of race and ethnicity in the United States has numerous implications for health and healthcare. Racial and ethnic attributes are linked with the disparities that exist in health status and influence the health behavior for large segments of the U.S. population. Further, the healthcare system treats members of different racial and ethnic groups differently, with the likelihood of diagnosis and treatment differing based on the racial or ethnic characteristics of the patient.

A "race" is a category of people who share biologically transmitted traits that society deems significant. Racial groups are defined based on one or more distinguishable physical attributes considered important in the particular society. In U.S. society, as in many others, skin color is the most important factor in racial categorization. Although race is not a recognized biological concept but a social construct, the existence of perceptions of racial distinctions makes racial classification real in its consequences.

Ethnic group classification, or ethnicity, is based on differences in cultural heritage. Members of an ethnic category may have common ancestors, language, and religion that contribute to a distinctive social identity. They have a common cultural tradition, including values and norms and perhaps even a language that sets them apart from the larger society. While sociologists distinguish between race and ethnicity, the two may go hand in hand. Japanese Americans, for example, have distinctive physical traits and—for those who maintain a traditional way of life—a distinctive culture as well. Both race and ethnicity can be grounds for minority status.

The federal government is the primary agency in the "official" recognition of racial and ethnic groups in the U.S. Categories are established for statistical purposes and scholars generally utilize the Census Bureau's classifications for their research. Although increasingly blurred by intermarriage, the four major racial categories in the United States are whites (Caucasians), blacks (African Americans), Asian Americans, and Native Americans. (These categorizations of racial and ethnic groups should not be thought of as "real"—i.e., scientifically accurate—groupings, and some of the problems associated with racial and ethnic classification have already been noted.)

Due to the heterogeneity of the U.S. population and continued high rates of immigration, ethnic groups of various types abound in American society. Some of these groups are highly distinct and strive to maintain their cultural identity in the face of overwhelming majority forces. Others are less visible, with their existence a function of perceptions held by the majority population and the majority's reaction to them. In the latter case, it may not even be appropriate to use the term "group" since these groupings of individuals with similar cultural backgrounds may not have the characteristics of a true group. (Box 11-3 discusses the implications of foreign immigration for healthcare.)

When the various racial groups in the United States are examined in terms of health status and health behavior, significant differences are found. The current state of knowledge on the relationship between race and ethnicity and health is summarized here, with more detail provided in the chapters on health status and sickness behavior. The major distinction is between whites and blacks, with Asian-Americans and Native Americans manifesting less distinct health status characteristics.

Significant disparities exist with regard to both health status and health behavior. With regard to health status, clear-cut differences in morbidity are found primarily between whites and African-Americans. The number of symptoms, the number of episodes, and the severity of the conditions all place blacks at a health status disadvantage. Blacks suffer higher rates of both acute and chronic conditions compared to whites. Further, all things being equal, blacks contracting life-threatening conditions are more at risk of death from them than are whites with the same conditions. Specific ethnic groups are also likely to display unique morbidity and mortality profiles.

Mortality rates for the black population are considerably higher than those for the white population. African-Americans are characterized by higher mortality risks at nearly all ages and for nearly all causes (Rogers et al. 2000). The gap in mortality rates for whites and African-Americans has actually increased since 1990. Overall Hispanic mortality rates compare favorably to those for both whites and blacks. This advantage is particularly apparent for the major killers like heart disease and certain forms of cancer (National Center for Health Statistics 2002, table 28). The mortality rate for Asian populations in the United States generally falls in between the rates for blacks and whites. Native Americans record the lowest mortality rate for cancer for any group but by far the highest mortality rates for diabetes, suicide, and accidents.

Although infant mortality has been dramatically reduced as a cause of death in the United States in this century, it continues to be a serious health threat for certain segments of society (Hummer 1993). The infant mortality rate for blacks in 1999 was more than twice that for whites, 14.0 per 1,000 live births versus 5.8. The rates for both groups had declined since the late 1980s, with the percentage point gap between the two narrowing somewhat in recent years (National Center for Health Statistics 2002, table 20). Certain Asian-origin groups report much lower than average infant mortality, while Hispanics as a group record infant mortality rates between those of whites and blacks. Native Americans and native Alaskans historically have recorded very high infant mortality rates.

Coping with discrimination can result in chronic levels of stress that have physical and mental health consequences. This discrimination-related stress is exacerbated, researchers have discovered, by empathizing with the discriminatory acts experienced by other members of their group. In one study, for example, researchers found elevations in blood pressure among black subjects when viewing videotaped vignettes of discriminatory acts toward blacks, such as poor service, verbal abuse, and police threats.

Similar disparities are found between racial and ethnic groups in the use of health services. To a limited extent, differences in utilization may be traced to differences in the types of health problems experienced. However, many of the differences reflect variations in lifestyle patterns and

---

Box 11-3

The Implications of Foreign Immigration for Healthcare

For over a century, immigrants to the United States have influenced the healthcare system through the importation of differing perceptions of health and healthcare and certain unconventional forms of medical treatment. In addition, they have introduced new health problems and reintroduced many conditions that had been essentially eliminated in America. During the last quarter of the 20th century the United States experienced a resurgence of immigration. The annual influx of legal immigrants reached a level not experienced since the 1930s. The large number of legal immigrants were thought to be matched during the 1980s and 1990s by the number of immigrants entering the United States illegally. For the first time since early in that century, immigration became a major issue for scholarly research and public policy debate.

This debate has not been inspired not so much by the renewed volume of immigration (although that certainly is an issue for some parts of the country) as by the nature of the immigrants. These "new" immigrants have for the most part originated in countries with cultures dissimilar to American culture. Unlike the well-educated, often professional immigrants to which the U.S. had grown accustomed, these new waves include large numbers of refugees from Southeast Asia, Latin America, and, now, the Middle East. They often arrive with only the clothes on their backs. Those coming from Asian cultures bring very "foreign" ways with them. Similarly, the estimated 4 to 8 million illegal aliens in the United States from Mexico, Central America, and the Caribbean often come from lower socioeconomic backgrounds.

This new immigration has many implications for health status and health care delivery. For those legally admitted immigrants in need of medical care—especially refugees—the problems are extreme. These immigrants often come from countries where healthcare delivery is poorly developed and/or disrupted by political conflict. These groups also present special problems in that the cultural distance between them and the U.S. system is great and they are typically impoverished. Some groups (e.g., Southeast Asians) have introduced new health problems that call for additional personnel and programs.

The burden imposed by illegal immigrants—to the extent that it can be documented—is several times more severe. In the late 1980s, the U.S.

---

cultural preferences. Perhaps more importantly, disparities in utilization often reflect differential treatment of members of various racial and ethnic groups by the healthcare system.

The hospital admission rate for whites tends to be around 20% lower than that for African Americans, despite the older age structure of the white population. Although whites generate a greater number of patient days per

Immigration and Naturalization Service estimated the annual cost of providing care for this population at over $93 million for each one million illegal immigrants. The problems are exacerbated due to the concentration of illegal immigrants in certain parts of the country. These areas include parts of Florida, Texas, and California, along with New York City. Since most of the health care provided is uncompensated, a severe strain is placed on the health care system. According to an article in *Hospitals* (April 5, 1986), one hospital in Miami lost $10 million the previous year caring for legal immigrants. Although the federal government has provided some financial assistance to health systems serving certain groups (e.g., Haitians, Nicaraguans, and Cubans), it has not begun to cover the costs of this care. Recent immigration reform that has "legitimized" large numbers of illegal aliens can be expected to further contribute to the demand for services.

Even as some hospitals are overwhelmed by the volume of medically indigent immigrants, fear and distrust keep many immigrants away from the healthcare system. Immigrants are likely to enter the system after considerable delay, and preventive measures such as prenatal care are rare. Problems associated with communications and cultural differences are multiplied for illegal immigrants who fear that any contact with an "official" can result in deportation. Members of some groups still utilize traditional health care techniques and, where possible, traditional healers.

Providers of healthcare have attempted to adapt to this new category of patient, even to the point of catering to those among them that can pay. Individual hospitals have modified their policies and practices in keeping with the concerns of ethnic patients, and some health systems have attempted to target ethnic patients. Some institutions are finding, contrary to the financial burden described above, that immigrants often pay out-of-pocket for services, making them relatively desirable customers. Some hospitals, in fact, have attempted to capitalize on their ethnic connections by encouraging the flow of more affluent foreigners into the United States for purposes of using the particular hospital's services. This has led to an unprecedented interest in "international medicine" among healthcare providers and planners.

As the U.S. becomes increasingly racially and ethnically diverse, the implications of immigration for the healthcare system can only grow. The system has been only moderately successful at adapting itself to the needs of these "different" types of patients, and this will be a growing challenge for the U.S. healthcare system in the 21st century.

1,000 population than African Americans, their average number of patient days per hospital episode is not that different from the figure for African Americans. As with admissions, there is no consistent pattern with regard to patient days and length of stay for other racial and ethnic groups. Whites are overrepresented among the nursing home population. African Americans and other racial and ethnic groups tend to be underrepresented, although Hispanics increasingly report a pattern similar to that of non-Hispanic whites.

In general, whites tend to utilize physicians at a higher rate than the rest of the population. Physician utilization rates, however, do not provide a complete picture of their healthcare utilization. There are certain differences in the types of tests and procedures performed on members of various racial and ethnic groups. It has been found, for example, that African Americans are likely to be subjected to more invasive forms of treatment than whites, all things being equal. At the same time, African Americans are less likely to receive major diagnostic and treatment procedures compared to whites with the same problem. This has been found for both physical and mental disorders. It is believed, however, that this is more a reflection of socioeconomic status and the conditions under which care is received than a function of racial differences (Harris et al. 1997).

One of the reasons for the differential treatment of members of racial and ethnic groups stems from the fact that non-whites have historically been left out of clinical trials (with the exception of the notorious Tuskegee experiments). The extent to which the needs of members of different racial groups vary is generally unknown due to their exclusion from research studies.

Given the middle-class white bias in the operation of the system, it is not surprising that clinicians often do not appreciate the perspective of the minority patient. The characteristics of non-whites often result in their being identified as "bad" patients. The failure of such patients to practice prevention, show up for appointments, follow doctors orders, etc., is often attributed to some character flaw rather than addressing the structural issues involved in creating the "bad" patient.

While racism involves majority attitudes toward racial minorities, ethnic disparagement is referred to as "cultural chauvinism". Cultural chauvinism is based on the notion that the majority culture is superior to the cultures characterizing ethnic subgroups or, more generally, that one culture is superior to another. While racial discrimination in the provision of healthcare based on race has been well documented and progress has been in addressing this issue, cultural chauvinism remains an important concern among students of healthcare. The historical emphasis of the system on white, middle class medicine has fostered the development of both class and ethnic biases. The system has operated as a one-size-fits-all system, and individuals were expected to conform to the mold regardless of their ethnic, religious or national background. If there was a mismatch between the delivery system and the patient, the fault, it was contended, lay with the patient, essentially blaming the victim.

Healthcare providers have exhibited a notorious insensitivity to the cultural precepts of ethnic groups. This has ranged from overt violations of rules regarding male/female relationships to failing to allow for linguistic differences to making assumptions about the social context of the individual without a knowledge of the culture.

The respective cultures of which the patient and medical practitioners are representatives may be sufficiently different to spawn numerous misunderstandings. Each cultural and subcultural group, by definition, brings its own set of beliefs, values, norms and culture-specific practices to the situation. These traits of group members cause them often to bring conflicting beliefs about the role of the supernatural in the disease etiology and treatment processes, the importance of health as a condition, and the appropriateness of human intervention in the disease management process. Ethnic minorities may have distinctive religious practices that may conflict with the norms of the health care system. The clash of standard medical protocol with the normative systems of various groups has the potential for negating any benefit to be derived from the operation of the health care system.

Many of the disparities noted may be due, at least in part, to problems that racial and ethnic minorities may have in accessing and effectively utilizing the health care system. A growing body of research shows differences in utilization levels across racial and ethnic groups and in the nature of the care that minority groups receive. Example after example can be found in which members of minority groups and subcultures do not receive comparable treatment to members of the majority. Sometimes this may be due to issues related to patient attitude, preferences, or perceptions. More often, however, the characteristics—real or perceived—of the patient contribute to differential treatment of the part of medical practitioners.

REFERENCES

Alliance for Aging Research (1998). *When Medicine Hurts Instead of Helps: Preventing Medication Problems in Older Persons*. Washington, DC: Alliance for Aging Research.

Benderly, Beryl Lieff (1997). *In Her Own Right: The Institute of Medicine's Guide to Women's Health Issues*. Washington, DC: National Institute of Medicine.

Benjamin, Lois (1991). *The Black Elite: Facing the Color Line in the Twilight of the Twentieth Century*. Chicago: Nelson-Hall.

Bogardus, Emory S. (1968). "Comparing racial distance in Ethiopia, South Africa and the United States," *Sociology and Social Research* 52:149–156.

Brook, Robert H., Kamberg, Caren J., Mayer-Oakes, Allison, Beers, Mark H., Raube, Kristiana, and Andrea Steiner (1991). *Appropriateness of Acute Medical Care for the Elderly: An Analysis of the Literature*. Santa Monica, CA: Rand Corporation.

Cockerham, William C. (1997). *This Aging Society*, 2nd ed. Upper Saddle River, NJ: Prentice Hall.

Dohrenwend, B.P. (1990). "Socioeconomic status (SES) and psychiatric disorders: Are the issues still compelling," *Social Psychiatry and Psychiatric Epidemiology* 25:41–47.

Lengermann, Patricia Madoo, and Ruth A. Wallace (1985). *Gender in America: Social Control and Social Change*. Englewood Cliffs, NJ: Prentice Hall.

National Center for Health Statistics (1998). *Health, United States, 1998*. Hyattsville, MD: National Center for Health Statistics.

Reed, Alyson (1999). *Civil Rights Journal*. Website URL: http://www.findarticles.com/cf_dls/m0HSP/1_4/66678569/p1/article.jhtml.

Ren, X.S., and B.C. Amick (1996). "Racial and ethnic disparities in self-assessed health status: Evidence from the national survey of families and households," *Ethnic Health* 1:293–303.

Rogers, Richard G., Robert A. Hummer, and Charles B. Nam (2000). *Living and Dying in the USA: Behavioral, Health, and Social Differentials in Mortality*. New York: Academic Press.

Schrijvers, C.T.M., K. Stronks, D. van de Mheen, and J.P. Mackenbach (1999). "Explaining educational differences in mortality: The role of behavioral and material factors," *American Journal of Public Health*, 89:535–540.

Smith, Tom W. (1996). "Research results reported in 'Anti-Semitism Decreases But Persists'," *Society* 33:2.

Wamala, S. P., M.A. Mittleman, K. Schenck-Gustafson, and K. Orth-Gomer (1999). "Potential explanations for the educational gradient in coronary heart disease: A population-based control study of Swedish women," *American Journal of Public Health*, 89:315–321.

ADDITIONAL RESOURCES

Auerback, Judith, and Anne Pigert (1995). "Women's health research: Public policy and sociology." *Journal of Health and Social Behavior*, extra issue:115–131.

Berkman, Lisa. F., and Ichiro Kawachi, editors (2000). *Social Epidemiology*. London: Oxford University Press.

INTERNET LINKS

Office of Minority Health (DHHS) homepage: www.omhrc.gov/omhhome.htm.

Chapter 12

Deviance and Control in Society and Healthcare

DEVIANCE AND SOCIAL ORDER

All societies maintain order through the operation of norms, whether they be informal customs and mores or formally enacted laws. Society members are socialized with regard to these rules of society, and the society's effective operation depends upon compliance with these rules. The institutions of society develop mechanisms to assure this compliance as they seek to achieve their goals. Of the various institutions, the political institution is most involved with the maintenance of social order. As will be seen, however, the healthcare institution also plays a role in maintaining social control.

Any violation of a social norm can be considered "deviance" and viewed negatively by the society in which it occurs. This violation could be as simple as bad manners (i.e., violating rules of etiquette), as serious as unethical professional behavior, or as legalistic as insurance fraud. All are forms of deviance because they represent deviations from accepted

277

social norms. All evoke some type of response from those in one's social environment and from society at large.

Most violations of norms involve momentary lapses on the part of the violator—neglecting to answer an elder respectfully, a single homosexual experience, or failing to see a stop sign while driving. However, in some cases the behavior becomes habitual to the point that a pattern emerges. A consistent pattern of norm violation would be considered "deviant behavior." Thus, the perpetually rude child, the lifelong homosexual, and the chronic traffic law violator are characterized by a pattern of deviance that goes beyond the occasional slip and could be defined as deviant behavior.

Although sociologists use the term "deviance" in their discussion of rule breaking, it is important to note that this does not represent a moral judgment (although some agents of social control would see it in those terms). Although some deviance may have a moral connotation, the rules are in place to assure "appropriate" behavior and not necessarily "right" or "good" behavior. Sociologists would argue, in fact, that there is no behavior that is inherently deviant. While it is true that all societies have rules forbidding murder, virtually all societies make exceptions to this rule under certain circumstances. Each society establishes it own set of norms, and behavior that is considered "normal" in one society may be considered abnormal in another. Each society sets the guidelines and determines the punishment in keeping with its particular view of the world. Thus, no act is inherently deviant, but must be defined as such by the social group.

Deviance arises within any social group and, indeed, as long as there are rules there will be deviance. The violation of norms occurs because the rules are not always clear, not every knows the rules, or there are individuals who can't (or won't) obey the rules. Indeed, *some* deviance is considered beneficial in society. No one likes a perfectionist and, besides, deviance serves a lot of useful social purposes. These include clarification of the rules, establishment of "bad examples", and providing a source of comparison for those who are not deviant.

The labeling of an attribute or action as deviant is a social process (Becker, 1963). What is defined as deviance is more a descriptor assigned by the social group that defines it than a quality of the individual considered deviant. Cultures vary widely, for example, in the extent to which they consider such bodily conditions as facial scars, obesity, shortness, and paleness as deviant (Freund and McGuire, 1999).

Some sociologists have raised the question as to why more people do not deviate from the rules. Surely there is ample opportunity in U.S. society. Part of the answer may rest with concerns over the reactions of others or even fear of the law. For the most part, though, it is felt that members of society abide by the rules because of the effective socialization that took place as they were developing as society members. Indeed, we typically comply with the rules without thinking. Most Americans follow the "rule" of brushing their teeth twice a day, and they do it without thinking about it. While driving, we reflexively stop for Stop signs even if there are no other cars for miles around. So it is with most of the rules of society.

Many people are considered deviant when it comes to their health behavior and the utilization of health services. There are certain subgroups (e.g., certain low-income minority populations) within U.S. society whose members do not follow healthy lifestyles and, in fact, are involved in risky health behavior. They do not obtain the necessary examinations and do not follow doctor's orders. They may use the hospital emergency room inappropriately, fail to return for followup care, and not pay their medical bills. Medical practitioners and the public in general tend to think of members of these groups as "bad patients" and attach a negative connotation to their deviant behavior.

This represents an excellent example of why some deviance will always be found in society. First, members of disadvantaged segments of society may not be aware of the rules that govern health behavior. How would they? We don't teach courses on appropriate health behavior, and the members of their social group are likely to know no more about appropriate responses in the face of health problems than they do. Unless one is plugged into the healthcare system, one doesn't know that regular checkups are important for a variety of reasons. Further, if one isn't enrolled in a health plan that encourages preventive behavior and regular checkups, how is one to know what is expected? U.S. society is quick to criticize misuse of the system by these populations, without realizing that society has failed to make them fully aware of the rules.

Neither has society provided the means for medical compliance on the part of these populations. Even if members of these groups were totally aware of the rules with regard to healthcare, they would be severely limited in their ability to comply with them. Given an appreciation of the need for regular checkups, how does one get around the facts that there is no physician in the community, there is no health insurance or other resources to cover the cost of the exam, or that it will take a full day of waiting (with lost income and babysitting costs) to obtain a 45-minute checkup?

This same line of reasoning could be applied to compliance with medical regimens and the pursuit of healthy lifestyles. The expectations of many subgroups, in fact, may dictate unhealthy lifestyles as the norm. True, there are some individuals who are not going to follow the rules of the healthcare system under any circumstances, but many are in a position where they cannot follow the rules even if they know them and are so inclined. To the sociologist, these do not represent flagrant examples of rule breaking but a reflection of the difficulty of complying with complex rules under circumstances of limited knowledge and resources.

While violations of customs may be thought to constitute bad taste and violations of mores thought to involve sin, violations of laws constitute crimes. Crime involves the violation of criminal laws enacted by a locality, state, or federal government. In healthcare, crime may take a variety of forms, from theft of drugs by hospital employees to insurance fraud to the performance of illegal abortions.

Many of the legal violations that occur within the healthcare institution involve white-collar crime. White-collar crimes do not involve violence and rarely bring police with drawn guns to the scene. Rather, white-collar criminals use their powerful occupational offices to enrich themselves or others illegally, often causing significant public harm in the process. Because of the nature of these crimes, these violations are sometimes referred to as "crime in the suites" rather than crime in the streets. The most common white-collar crimes are embezzlement, business fraud, bribery, and antitrust violations. While some white-collar crime causes limited harm, many such crimes—like the savings and loan scandal during the 1980s and the corporate scandals of the early twenty-first century—cause substantial loss to the public. The government program to bail out the savings and loan industry ended up costing the U.S. taxpayers $600 billion dollars or $2,500 apiece. Some of the most costly crimes—at least for taxpayers—involve Medicare and Medicaid fraud. Medicare fraud alone is estimated to cost the federal government (and American taxpayers) billions of dollars each year. (Box 12-1 presents and example of criminal deviance in healthcare.)

SOCIOLOGICAL EXPLANATIONS OF DEVIANCE

Sociologists go beyond merely describing deviance and seek explanations for its existence. The origins of deviance and its implications for the healthcare system are examined from different sociological perspectives.

The Structural-Functional Approach

From the structural-functional approach, the perspective accepted through most of this text, deviance is perceived as societal "dysfunction." As will be recalled, this approach would perceive normality and abnormality in terms of society members' ability to function in the performance of their socially assigned roles. The behavior of individuals who do not seek employment, fail their college exams, or cheat on their income tax returns is not defined as irresponsible or illegal from this perspective but as a failure to function normally. Similarly, individuals who practice risky health behavior, abuse the healthcare system or fail to comply with doctors' orders are found wanting due to their failure to carry out their roles pursuant to the efficient functioning of the healthcare system.

Such activities are interpreted from this perspective not with regard to their implications for the individual but for their implications for the functioning of society. Therefore, these behaviors represent dysfunctional factors in the operation of the social system. While the religious, government, social welfare and healthcare institutions may be used to try to ameliorate these problems, there is no place for "blame" within the structural-functional framework. These are all conditions that need to be corrected to restore efficient functioning to the social system.

Attempts to address dysfunctional aspects of the system may involve the elimination of the problems from the "critical path" of social system operation by incarcerating the nonfunctioning individuals in prisons or mental hospitals. However, the primary goal of attempts to restore system efficiency is to return individuals to productive roles within the various societal institutions. Thus, it is more important from this perspective that functioning be restored than for offenders to be punished. This places the healthcare institution in a pivotal role within the structural-functional framework.

The Symbolic-Interaction Approach

The symbolic-interaction paradigm explains how people define deviance in everyday situations. The central contribution of symbolic-interaction analysis is "labeling theory", the assertion that deviance and conformity result not so much from what people do, but from how others respond to these actions. Labeling theory stresses the relativity of deviance, noting that people may define the same behavior in any number of ways. Becker (1966) claims that deviance is, therefore, nothing more than certain behaviors that society members have labeled as deviant.

Examples of deviance from healthcare might include risky sexual behavior, medication noncompliance, and receiving a "kickback" for referring a patient to a medical facility. The response to and consequences of these actions depend on the circumstances and who is aware of the behavior. The social construction of deviance, then, is a highly variable process of detection, definition, and response.

Some of these conditions would be considered "primary deviance", provoking slight reaction from others and having little effect on a person's self-concept. On the other hand, other society members might take notice of someone's behavior and draw attention to it. If, for example, people begin to describe a young man as an "addict" and no longer welcome him into their social circle, he may become embittered, abuse drugs even more, and seek the company of those who approve of his behavior. Thus, the response to the primary deviance can set in motion secondary deviance, in which case a pattern of repeated norm violation is established and the individual

---

Box 12-1

Fraud in the Healthcare Industry

Fraud technically involves intentional misrepresentation on the part of an individual who knows that the misrepresentation could result in some unauthorized benefit to himself/herself or some other person. The most frequent kind of fraud in healthcare arises from a false statement or misrepresentation made to a third-party payer (e.g., Medicare) related to the provision of care. The violator may be a physician or other practitioner, a hospital or other institutional provider, a clinical laboratory or other supplier, an employee of any provider, a billing service, a beneficiary, a Medicare carrier employee, or any person in a position to file a claim for reimbursement for services.

Fraud schemes range from those perpetrated by individuals acting alone to broad-based activities by institutions or groups of individuals, sometimes employing sophisticated telemarketing and other promotional techniques to lure consumers into serving as the unwitting tools in the schemes. Some defraud several private and public sector victims simultaneously.

According to a 1993 survey by the Health Insurance Association of America of private insurers' healthcare fraud investigations, it was found that 43 percent of the offenses related to fraudulent diagnoses, 34 percent to billing for services not rendered, 21 percent for inappropriate waiver of patient deductibles or co-payments, and 2 percent for other offenses. In Medicare, the most common forms of fraud include:

- Billing for services not furnished
- Misrepresenting the diagnosis to justify payment
- Soliciting, offering, or receiving a kickback
- Unbundling or "exploding" charges
- Falsifying certificates of medical necessity, plans of treatment, and medical records to justify payment
- Billing for a service not furnished as billed; i.e., upcoding

No one really knows the extent of Medicare fraud. The U.S. General Accounting Office estimates that $1 out of every $7 spent on Medicare is lost to fraud and abuse. In 1999 alone, Medicare lost nearly $13.5 billion

---

begins to take on a deviant identity. The conversion of behavior from primary deviance to secondary deviance reflects the sociological maxim that if something is defined as "real", it becomes real in its consequences.

Secondary deviance represents a response to the reactions of society to primary deviance and marks the start of what has been called a "deviant career" (Goffman, 1963). As individuals develop a stronger commitment to

to fraudulent or unnecessary claims. An audit by the Center for Medicare and Medicaid Services (formerly the Health Care Financing Administration) revealed that "improper" Medicare payments topped $20 billion in fiscal 1997 for the second year in a row.

Of the $20.3 billion for fiscal year 1997, $5.9 billion—or slightly more than 29 percent of the total—was for physician services, which account for most of the 853 million Medicare claims paid annually. In analyzing the $5.9 billion in improper payments to doctors, the Office of the Inspector General (OIG) estimated that about $2.6 billion was attributable to insufficient or non-existent documentation. Another $560 million might be, but the OIG couldn't make that determination because it was prohibited from requesting the medical records of providers already under investigation. Other errors included incorrect coding ($1.7 billion), lack of medical necessity ($376 million), and non-covered/non-allowable services ($387 million).

In 1998 state officials in Florida reported that drug traffickers are changing professions because the money is bigger in healthcare fraud and the risk is less. Recent accounts show that Medicare has attracted its own class of organized criminals—persons who specialize in defrauding healthcare and health insurance systems. The GAO found the following about the criminal groups that had infiltrated the system: "These groups created as many as 160 sham medical entities . . . For the most part these entities only existed on paper. Once the structure was in place, subjects used a variety of schemes to submit claims to Medicare, Medicaid, or private insurance companies." According to OIG data, 1,700 healthcare cases are now under active investigation. Of these, slightly over 300 involve medical practices, approximately 80 percent of which have criminal fraud charges pending against them. Further, between January 1996 and June 1998, the OIG opened 2,977 cases involving medical practices, of which 1,631 were criminal investigations and 1,346 civil. During this same period, successful prosecutions of medical practices led to 49 criminal convictions and 54 civil judgments. A total of 1,156 doctors were excluded from Medicare participation.

Although most people who enter the healthcare field do so because of their interest in serving their fellow man, it is clear that numerous opportunities exist for illegal gain. Given the amount of money involved in the healthcare system, it is not surprising that opportunistic practitioners and administrators are tempted by prospect of "free money" and that unscrupulous operators target the healthcare industry for their illegal operations.

deviant behavior, they typically acquire a "stigma", a powerfully negative label that radically changes a person's self-concept and social identity. Stigma may convert the deviant condition into a master status, overshadowing other dimensions of identity so that a person is discredited in the minds of others and, consequently, becomes socially isolated. Sometimes an entire community stigmatizes an individual through what has been called a "degradation ceremony" (Garfinkel, 1956). A criminal prosecution is an example, operating much like a high school graduation in reverse: A person stands before the community to be labeled in a negative rather than a positive way (Macionis, 2000). A parallel in healthcare could be a competency hearing for an individual in which his or her deviant thought processes or behavior becomes officially labeled as mental illness.

Once society stigmatizes a person, society members may engage in retrospective labeling, or the reinterpretation of a person's past in the light of some present deviance (Scheff, 1984). For example, after discovering that a priest has sexually molested a child, others rethink his past. Or when it comes out that an acquaintance has been diagnosed with AIDS, associates are likely to recall that he seldom was seen in the company of women. Retrospective labeling distorts a person's biography by being highly selective, a process that can deepen a deviant identity.

The various symbolic-interaction theories all see deviance as a process. Labeling theory links deviance not to action but to the reaction of others. Thus, some people are defined as deviant while others who think or behave in the same way are not. The concepts of secondary deviance, deviant careers, and stigma demonstrate how being labeled as deviant can become a lasting self-concept.

Yet, labeling theory has several limitations. First, because it takes a highly relative view of deviance, labeling theory ignores the fact that some behavior—such as murder—is condemned in virtually every society. Labeling theory is thus most usefully applied to less serious deviance such as sexual promiscuity or mental illness.

Second, research on the consequences of deviant labeling is inconclusive (Smith and Gartin 1989; Sherman and Smith 1992). It is not clear whether the labeling produces further deviance or discourages it. Third, not everyone resists being labeled as deviant; some people actually seek it out. For example, people engage in civil disobedience (such as anti-abortion protests) leading to arrest in order to call attention to social injustice. A prime example of this from healthcare is the case of Jack Kervorkian, M.D.

The Social Conflict Approach

The social conflict paradigm sees deviance as a natural outgrowth of the conflict inherent in society due to the existence of social inequality. That is, who or what is considered "deviant" depends on which categories of people hold power in the society. Alexander Liazos (1972) points out that those perceived as deviant by society—i.e., "nuts, sluts, and 'perverts'"— all share the trait of powerlessness. Bag ladies (not corporate polluters) and unemployed men on street corners (not arms dealers) carry the stigma of deviance. Note that drug dealers—presumably trading with consenting adults who willing participate in the transaction—are often sentenced to life imprisonment, while financial managers who arguably destroy the economic "lives" (and, no doubt, in some cases, the physical lives) of thousands of people may serve a few months in prison if they are punished at all. A hospital administrator who looks the other way while his staff pads hospital bills or a physician who performs euthanasia on a suffering terminal patient is seldom considered a deviant—even if his behavior is unethical or even illegal. (See Box 12-2 for a discussion of society's treatment of deviants.)

Social-conflict theory explains this pattern in three ways. First, the norms—including the laws—of any society generally reflect the interests of the rich and powerful. People who threaten the wealthy are likely to evoke negative responses and be labeled as enemies of the social order by those in power. Social-conflict theorists argue that the law (and all social institutions) supports the interests of the rich and even speak of "capitalist justice" (Quinney 1977). Indeed, it is clear that political decisions are affected by the influence of major political contributors and lobbyists such as the American Medical Association, American Hospital association, the insurance industry and the pharmaceutical industry.

Second, even if their behavior is called into question, the powerful have the resources to resist deviant labels. Government officials or corporate executives who might order or condone the dumping of hazardous wastes are rarely held personally accountable. Similarly, those who promote inappropriate uses of a pharmaceutical—ultimately resulting in deadly side-effects—are seldom called to task for their behavior.

Third, the widespread belief that norms and laws are "natural" and beneficial masks their political character. For this reason, we may condemn the unequal application of the law but give little thought to whether the laws themselves are inherently fair (Quinney 1977). Critics have questioned the intent of laws and regulations governing welfare and Medicaid participation, and social conflict theorists would argue that they have the consequence—intended or unintended—of reinforcing social inequality.

SICKNESS AS DEVIANCE

The violation of a norm does not have to be deliberate, and this fact makes the discussion of deviance particularly important for the sociology of health and illness. "Illness" in its strict sense represents a violation of a biological norm—e.g., blood pressure above a specified threshold, HIV antibodies above a certain level, or the presence of an "abnormal" lump in a woman's breast. These biological deviations from established norms (established, by the way, through a process that is as much social as scientific) are significant

---
───── *Box 12-2* ─────

Images of Deviance: Nuts, Sluts, and Perverts

During the 1970s, some sociologists began to question the perception of deviance presented by their colleagues. The public's perception of deviance reflected reports in the media involving a preponderance of "street crime". While drug dealers, street gangs, and criminals account for some of the more sensational deviance, it could be argued that white-collar crime is much more prevalent and ultimately exacts a greater toll on society. Yet, the perception of an underclass of criminals dominates the public's concept of deviance.

As sociologists in the 1960s and 1970s embarked on the scientific study of deviance, they too focused on certain categories of deviants for their research. They did research, for example, on gang members, drug addicts, prostitutes and petty criminals. While the research involved an objective attempt at examining the conditions surrounding deviance and a well-intentioned effort to humanize the deviant, sociologists may have unwittingly helped perpetuate the stereotypical perception of the deviant.

This was the argument presented by Alexander Liazos and other critics of the dominant approach to the study of deviance. It was felt that by focusing on certain types of deviance (what Liazos termed "nuts, sluts and perverts") and not others, that the distorted perception of deviance in society was perpetuated. By concentrating attention on one segment of society to the exclusion of others, little attention was focused to the unethical, illegal and destructive actions of powerful individuals, groups and institutions in society.

The dominant approach led to the conclusion that deviance was concentrated among the lower classes of society and that an underclass of deviants

---

because a social connotation is almost invariably attached to them. These "deviants" come to be seen as different by those in their social circles from what they were before the diagnosis and, in certain cases—e.g., an HIV diagnosis—some level of stigma is likely to be attached. Through this process, "illness" is converted into "sickness." Sickness represents a threat to the social order and the meanings through which people make sense of their lives and organize the routines of their everyday existence.

Like crime, sickness is a form of deviance, or departure from group-established norms. Society typically imputes different kinds of responsibility for sickness than for crime. The way a society reacts to sickness and crime reaffirms its core values. Furthermore, the reaction of society to deviance (such as punishing the criminal or treating the sick person) reaffirm and revitalize the collective sentiments and maintain social solidarity. Thus, the treatment of the sick in all healthcare systems serves to reaffirm cultural norms and ideals for the sick and the well alike. (Violence as a form

existed that were qualitatively different from "normal" people. The drug dealer was thus presented as the typical representative of deviant behavior rather than the embezzling employee. It is no accident that those depicted as deviant tend to be the powerless in society and seldom the powerful.

Sociologists unwittingly contributed to this situation through the types of deviance they chose to study and by supporting an explanation of deviance that looked for etiology within the individual deviant rather than in the deviant's environment or social circumstances. In much the same way, health professionals of this period held individual patients to blame for not obtaining timely care, not returning for followup appointments, or failing to comply with medication orders. Even attempts at presenting deviants as different from normal people in minor ways inadvertently tends to emphasize the differences rather than the similarities. For example, researchers during this period tried to demonstrate that homosexuals were little different from those with other sexual orientations. Unfortunately, the minor differences became the focus of attention rather than the similarities.

The perception of deviance in U.S. society continues to be biased by the presentation of "nuts, sluts and perverts" as typical deviants. As Liazos and others have pointed out, this serves the purposes of other categories of deviants who may not perceive of themselves as deviant and certainly do not want others to do so. The more cynical would argue that this approach to deviance provides a smokescreen that obscures the more damaging activities of those in positions of power.

Source: Alexander Liazos (1972). "The Poverty of the Sociology of Deviance: Nuts, Sluts, and Perverts," *Social Problems, 20* (Summer): 103 120.

---

of deviance and its implications for the healthcare system are discussed in Box 12-3.)

MEDICINE AS A FORM OF SOCIAL CONTROL

"Social control" refers to the sanctioned, institutionalized means by which the agents of society's institutions preserve order. Social control is a process for maintaining social order through mechanisms that assure people's adherence to societal norms. Any social system strives to control people who don't fit into that system. The elderly, people with physical or mental disabilities, and alcohol and drug addicts represent a burden on society whose impact must be managed. Such people are subject to control by the criminal justice system, social welfare agencies and, increasingly, healthcare organizations.

———————— *Box 12-3* ————————

The Implications of Violence for Healthcare

Violence is the intentional use of force to harm a human being. Its outcome is injury—physical or psychological, fatal or nonfatal. In the U.S. injuries from all causes are the leading cause of death for persons under the age of 45, and 38 percent of all deaths from injury are the result of violence. Recent statistics further suggest that both the proportion and number of violent deaths are increasing. In 1988, for the first time, firearms killed more children than all other causes combined. These facts, it is argued, make violence a public health concern, as much as (or more than) a criminal problem.

Homicide is the leading cause of death among young black men and women in this country. Violence is endemic in some communities, a part of the culture of everyday life, creating a perpetual post-traumatic syndrome characterized by hyper-vigilance, defensiveness, assertiveness, and hostility. Comparing the experiences of inner-city kids today with his own adolescence in East Los Angeles, film actor, producer, and director Edward James Olmos fears that the act of killing, itself, has now become a form of addiction.

This paints a compelling picture of a social malady that appears to be getting worse. But how does this objective reality relate to the public's perception of violence as a social problem that warrants concern and action, among the many other issues that compete for our attention? Viewing violence only as a minority urban problem dangerously misconstrues the issue. The "post-crack, post-trauma" culture is not confined to the inner city. The language and voice of the inner city—with their recognized commercial potential—have been absorbed into the mainstream popular culture of youth, aided by the mass media.

The problem of "kids killing kids" and the deadly role of firearms in the escalating homicide rate are the most appropriate targets of public policy, and however heatedly Americans may disagree about all other aspects of gun use, surely everyone can agree that guns do not belong in the hands of children. Outside these limited circles, this issue is only beginning to emerge as a theme around which to rally and take action.

Violence is a major public health problem worldwide. Each year, millions of people die as the result of injuries due to violence. Many more survive their injuries, but live with a permanent disability. Violence is among the leading causes of death among people aged 15–44 years worldwide, accounting for 14% of deaths among males and 7% of deaths among females. In addition to death and disability, violence contributes to a variety of other health consequences. These include depression, alcohol and substance abuse, smoking, eating and sleeping disorders, and HIV and other sexually transmitted diseases.

Violence results from interplay of individual, relationship, community, and societal factors. Some of the factors associated with violence include a history of early aggression, impulsiveness, harsh punitive discipline, poor monitoring and supervision of children, associating with delinquent peers, witnessing violence, drug trafficking, access to firearms, gender and income inequality, and norms that support violence as a way to resolve conflict.

Public health officials have a very important role to play in reducing violence. Through their vision and leadership, much can be done to establish national plans and policies for violence prevention, to help facilitate the collection of data to document and respond to the problem, to build important partnerships with other sectors, and to ensure an adequate commitment of resources to prevention efforts.

In addition to the toll of human misery, violence puts a massive burden on national economies. For example, studies sponsored by the Inter-American Development Bank between 1996 and 1997 on the economic impact of violence in six Latin American countries calculated that expenditures on violence-associated health services alone amounted to 1.9% of the gross domestic product in Brazil, 5.0% in Colombia, 4.3% in El Salvador, 1.3% in Mexico, 1.5% in Peru and 0.3% in Venezuela. A 1992 study in the United States put the annual cost of treating gunshot wounds at $126 billion. Cutting and stab wounds cost an additional $51 billion.

The evidence shows that, as a general rule, victims of domestic or sexual violence have more health problems, significantly higher healthcare costs, and more frequent visits to hospital emergency departments throughout their lives than those without a history of abuse. The same is also true for victims of child abuse and neglect.

In calculating the costs of violence to a nation's economy, a wide range of factors need to be taken into consideration besides the direct costs of medical care and criminal justice. Indirect costs may include:

- The provision of shelter or other places of safety and associated care;
- Lost productivity as a result of premature death, injury, absenteeism, long-term disability and lost potential;
- Diminished quality of life and decreased ability to care for oneself or others;
- Life-long costs of maintenance for individuals disabled as a result of violence;
- Disruption of daily life as a result of fears for personal safety;
- Disincentives to investment and tourism that hamper economic development.

The implications of violence for the healthcare system has been given scant attention in the past. However, as more data on the direct and indirect costs of violence to the system have been generated, public and professional awareness of this issue has increased. The American Public Health Association has encouraged the defining of violence as a public health issue. Given that violence is an inherent part of American society, it clearly deserves to be a priority of the healthcare system.

The agents of social control may be law enforcement officers, social workers, or medical personnel, especially physicians and mental health professionals. These agents seek to secure adherence to social norms in an effort to eliminate or minimize deviant behavior. The significance of institutions of social control is not only that their agents sanction deviant behavior that occurs, but that they define what constitutes appropriate behavior in the first place.

In medicine, ideology and social control are closely related. When doctors transmit ideological messages that reinforce current social patterns, they help control behavior in ways that are defined as socially appropriate. When private hospitals divert indigent patients to other facilities, they are contributing to this process of control.

There are numerous classic examples of the use of medicine as a means of social control. Sometimes the approach is subtle, as in the case of variable criteria for physical fitness for military induction. Under the Soviet system, company physicians assessed the health status of workers and, remarkably, the level of sickness that was identified among workers dropped significantly during periods when the plant was behind quota. In the U.S., the mental health system has sometimes been utilized as a means of social control as individuals have been depicted as mentally ill to the gain of the accusing party. This was institutionalized within the Soviet Union through laws that stated that criticism of the government was an indisputable symptom of mental disorder, requiring that the offender be incarcerated indefinitely. Perhaps the most extensive application of medicine to social control was in the Prussian society of the nineteenth century where the stated purpose of the healthcare system was the assurance of a healthy society (and large numbers of battle-worthy males) for the furtherance of the goals of the state.

As an example of the operation of social control, it can be noted that the criminal justice system, social welfare, and healthcare blame individuals—not the system—for social problems. Low-income individuals who wait until they are gravely ill to seek care are considered "bad" patients, rather than victims of a system that denies them health insurance or convenient access to health services.

For socially powerful groups and institutions, diagnosis can be a tool for social control. The authority to diagnose deviance implies control, since giving a name to a condition has often been the starting point for the labeling process. Diagnosis reinforces parameters of normality and abnormality, demarcates the professional and institutional boundaries of the treatment system, and authorizes medicine to label and deal with people on behalf of society at large. This labeling is often the legal basis for provision of health services, welfare benefits, unemployment certification, workers' compensation claims, and legal testimony (Zola, 1972).

The healthcare system has extended its sphere to the point that a wide range of psychological, social, economic, and political problems have been "medicalized". Examples include sexuality and marital relations, dissatisfaction with work, problems related to birth, adolescence, aging and dying, learning disabilities and student psychological distress, and many other conditions. By addressing these conditions, practitioners often believe they are extending the caring function of the medical role while they are inadvertently expanding the control of medicine over society (Waitzkin, 1996). By focusing on individual troubles rather than on social issues, doctor-patient encounters may reinforce the social order as presently constituted.

Professional education and socialization contribute to the tendency toward medical social control. Lectures on social consciousness are not part of the medical school curriculum. To the contrary, professionals in training receive many lessons about individual pathophysiology and treatment. Within progressive medical schools, students may be exposed to information about emotional disturbances and social problems. But this training consistently emphasizes the importance of individual traits and individualized responses to the needs of the patient. Even in its more progressive and enlightened versions, professional education does not foster social criticism or social change as part of the medical mission (Waitzkin, 1996).

Situational constraints also place medical social control below the level of consciousness. When a client is in trouble, a professional usually feels that something should be done. Yet the professional also senses the limits of what he or she as an individual can do. For instance, when a patient's symptoms reflect stress at work, a doctor is likely to view a transformation of the workplace as beyond the responsibility or even the capability of the medical role. With rare exceptions, such as those involving physical abuse, disruption of familial relations is not an appropriate goal of medical intervention even when the pathology arises out of family dynamics.

These situational constraints contribute to the generally conservative influence of the healthcare system. On the one hand, medical discourse usually does not attend to institutional causes of suffering. This orientation leads health professionals to overlook social change as a possible therapeutic option. On the other hand, when doctors do consider institutional problems in their encounters with patients, this intervention frequently serves to support the status quo. When a professional encourages mechanisms of coping and adjustment, this communication conveys a subtle political content. By seeking limited modifications in social roles—at work and in the family, for instance—which preserve a particular institution's overall stability, the practitioner exerts a conservative political impact (Waitzkin, 1996).

THE MEDICALIZATION OF AMERICAN SOCIETY

Medicalization refers to the political and ideological process by which the medical profession increases its practical and ideological control over various aspects of society (Illich 1976). Medicalization is the process of legitimating medical control over an area of life, typically by asserting and establishing the primacy of a medical interpretation of that area. It refers to the increasing influence of medical institutions and the medical profession on aspects of life that previously had not been considered medical issues. For example, disruptive behavior by children is now more likely to be defined as attention deficit disorder, with drugs being prescribed for its treatment (Cockerham and Richey 1997).

The scientific objectivity of medicine passes no moral judgment, instead using clinical diagnoses such as "sick" and "healthy", rather than the "bad" or "good" of a moral assessment. Medicalization is also used to refer to the process by which the medical profession, as an agent of social control, gains control over the determinants of social problems and behaviors that are defined as sickness as opposed to badness.

With the medicalization of childbirth, aspects of women's reproductive lives that are not pathological were brought under the canopy definition of illness. Medical education during the emergence of the specialty of obstetrics and gynecology fostered the notion that the events of childbearing—pregnancy, labor and delivery, and puerperium—could best be understood in purely physical and pathological terms (Hahn, 1987). The medical profession ultimately persuaded the public and the regulators of healthcare that women needed doctors to manage their pregnancies and childbirth.

There is extensive evidence, however, that initial medicalization was linked more with doctors' professional interests than with the patients' well-being. Indeed, when medical control over childbirth was first consolidated, doctors and hospitals had abysmal records, especially for spreading infection to both mothers and babies (Oakley, 1984; Wertz and Wertz, 1979). More recently, impotency, fertility, and the process of conception have also become medicalized (Becker and Nachtigall, 1992; Tiefer, 1992, Sandelowski, 1991).

An illustration of the medicalization of a phenomenon is provided by the condition of "alcoholism." Until the middle of the twentieth century, most people viewed alcoholics as morally weak people easily tempted by the pleasure of drink. Gradually, however, medical specialists redefined alcoholism so that most people now consider it a disease, rendering individuals "sick" rather than "bad". Similarly, obesity, drug addiction, child abuse, promiscuity, and other behaviors that used to be moral matters are widely defined today as illnesses for which people need help rather than punishment.

According to Macionis (2000), whether we define deviance as a moral or medical issue has three consequences. First, it affects who responds to deviance. An offence against common morality typically provokes a reaction from members of the community or the police. Applying medical labels, however, transfers the situation to the control of clinical specialists, including counselors, psychiatrists, and physicians.

A second issue is how people respond to a deviant. A moral approach defines the deviant as an "offender" subject to punishment. From a medical, however, "patients" need treatment (for their own good, of course) and deserve sympathy. Therefore, while punishment is designed to fit the crime, treatment programs are tailored to the patient and may involve virtually any therapy that a specialist thinks might prevent future illness.

Third, and most important, the two labels differ on the issue of the personal competence of the deviant person. Morally speaking, whether the individual is right or wrong, at least the affected party is assigned responsibility for his behavior by society. Once defined as sick, however, we are seen as unable to control (or, if "mentally ill", even understand) our actions. People who are deemed incompetent are, in turn, often subject to treatment against their will (Macionis, 2000).

There is evidence that U.S. society is beginning to experience a certain amount of demedicalization. "Demedicalization" is the political and ideological process by which the medical profession loses influence over various aspects of society or, alternatively, the political and ideological process by which the medical profession, as an agent of social control, loses influence over which social problems and behaviors are defined as sickness as opposed to badness (Cockerham and Richey 1997). The medical profession is said to be threatened by deprofessionalization as other institutions challenge its authority on controversial issues. As physicians are forced to share power with a growing number of parties, the trend toward demedicalization is likely to continue.

To the extent that deviance (including sickness) becomes widespread, the possibility of the creation of what sociologists refer to as "social problems" arises. Box 12-4 discusses health as a social problem.

TRANSITION OF CONTROL: FROM CHURCH TO STATE TO HEALTHCARE

The relative influence of religious, government, and medical institutions in defining deviance has shifted in Western societies. As the Middle Ages waned and these three institutions became increasingly differentiated from each other, the religious institution still carried the greatest weight in defining deviance. This preeminence continued into the eighteenth

---

——————— *Box 12-4* ———————

Health Issues as Social Problems

When the level of a certain type of deviant behavior reaches a certain point, sociologists may define the behavior as a "social problem." For example, if the occasional jazz musician smoked marijuana and a few ghetto dwellers used heroin, this would represent scattered deviant behavior. However, if drug abuse becomes widespread to the point that it affects large portions of the population in one way or another and ties up the criminal justice system, then drug abuse becomes a social problem. Thus, sociologists define a "social problem" as a phenomenon that:

- Effects large numbers of individuals
- Represents a persistent pattern of deviance
- Adversely affects the individual and those around them
- Involves serious costs to society
- Is disruptive of society
- Must be addressed at the macro-level of society

Some observers have viewed healthcare in the U.S. in general as a social problem. Many aspects of health and healthcare have a social dimension as well as a medical dimension. Thus, if aspects of the healthcare system involve significant disruption of the operation of society, there may be reason to consider healthcare in this light.

There are a number of ways in which healthcare issues can be viewed as social problems. For example, there are large segments of the population

---

century, but in America and France (and later in other European countries) the emerging government institution began defining deviance. In America, the increasing preeminence of legal definitions was promoted by religious pluralism and the increasingly rational organization of the nation-state.

The significance of legal definitions of deviance diminished somewhat during the twentieth century, and medical definitions gained in importance. This shift in balance favoring medical definitions of deviance corresponds chronologically with a period of the rapid professionalization of medicine, when medical discoveries and technology proceeded quickly, and public faith in science and medicine was increasing. Compared to religious and legal definitions, medical definitions appear to be more rational and scientific, and are based on technical expertise rather than human judgment.

Medical control in defining deviance also engenders medical power in certifying deviance, which is another aspect of social control. The societal acceptance of medical definitions of deviance gives the medical profession unique power to certify individuals as sick or well.

that do not have access to healthcare because no facilities exist in their community or they have no insurance or other ability to pay for care. This means that many individuals access inappropriate sources of care or that their conditions worsen to the point that they show up with advanced states of illness. Large portions of the population do not know the basics of prevention or healthy living, resulting in an unacceptable level of ill health in the population. Some 70 percent of the deaths that occur each year are preventable. The infant mortality rate remains unacceptably high in the United States, despite more resources being devoted to neonatal care in the U.S. than in any other country.

Because so much of health-related behavior is social in nature, many aspects of healthcare can be viewed as social problems. For example, a whole range of behaviors tracked through the Behavioral Risk Factor Surveillance System (BRFSS) can be considered contributory to social problems. These include chronic smoking, chronic alcohol use, and unhealthy eating habits, among others. Certainly risky sexual behavior has emerged to the point of being qualified as a health-related social problem.

The impact of these health-related problems is not restricted to the individuals involved, and they all have implications for the wider society. They effect the functioning of other institutions and result in costs to other sectors of society. These are conditions that require a society-wide response for the most part, with individual treatment by the healthcare system likely to have limited effect on the overall problem. As the notion of what constitutes healthcare continues to be broadened, the notion of health-related issues as social problems is likely to gain attention.

The labeling of deviance involves an issue of legitimacy since the power to define sickness and to label someone as "sick" is also the power to discredit that person. If a person's mental health is called into question, than the rest of society does not have to take that person seriously.

If a back disorder is a legitimate basis for adopting the sick role (and thus be excused from work or to claim insurance), the physician is considered to be the appropriate agent for certifying a valid claim, thereby assuming the role of gatekeeper.

Physicians become the chief arbiters of claims for worker compensation for "repetitive strain" injuries; not surprisingly, company doctors selected by manufacturers or insurers typically are less likely to certify the injury or provide sympathetic care than are personal physicians. Similarly, from 1952 to 1979, when homosexuality was a legitimate basis for denying a person U.S. citizenship, psychiatrists were given the power to certify that a homosexual should be thus denied.

The mechanism for reintegrating the deviant individual into the social group is medical therapy, which for even relatively minor deviance involves a form of social control. Social control may seem more palatable or humane when the deviance is treated as sickness instead of crime or sin, but the potency of the control agencies is just as great. Even when the condition is considered medically "cured" or under control, stigma still adheres to such "illnesses" as alcoholism, drug abuse, mental disorders, syphilis, and cancer.

As the transition occurred from church to state to healthcare with regard to the management of deviance, the symbols involved changed. The cathedral was the symbol of the church, to be replaced by the courthouse for the state and, ultimately, the hospital for the healthcare system. These symbols were turned to by supplicants under the respective paradigms. The agent representing the controlling institution shifted from the priest to the judge to the physician. Interestingly, the hospital and the physician retain some of the attributes of the cathedral and the priest.

As the form of deviance shifted from sin to crime to sickness, the response changed from penance to incarceration to treatment and cure. Through each stage, the relationship between the deviant and the system remained unchanged. Whether confronted with a priest, a judge or a doctor, the deviant was at a power and knowledge disadvantage and forced to bend to the will of the institution in order to be made "whole".

When a person is certified as a deviant, the agency of social control must then deal with this offender. Religious responses to deviance include counseling, moral indignation, confession, repentance, penance, and forgiveness. Legal responses include parallel actions, such as legal allegations, confession, punishments, rehabilitation, and release with or without the stigma of a record. In the medical model, the responses entail the parallel mechanisms of diagnosis and therapy.

REFERENCES

Becker, Howard S. (1966). *Outsiders: Studies in the Sociology of Deviance*. New York: Free Press.

Becker, Gay, and Robert D. Nachtigall (1992). "Eager for medicalization: The social production of fertility as a disease," *Sociology of Health and Illness* 14:456–471.

Cockerham, William C., and Ferris J. Richey (1997). *The Dictionary of Medical Sociology*. Westport, CT: Greenwood.

Freund, Peter E.S., and Meredith B. McGuire (1999). *Health, Illness and the Social Body*, 3rd ed. Englewood Cliffs, NJ: Prentice Hall.

Garfinkel, Harold (1956). "Conditions of successful degradation ceremonies," *American Journal of Sociology* 61:420–424.

Goffman, Irving (1963). *Stigma: Notes on the Management of Spoiled Identity*. Englewood Cliffs, NJ: Prentice Hall.

Hahn, Robert A. (1987). "Division of labor: Obstetrician, woman, and society in *Williams Obstetrics*, 1903–1985," *Medical Anthropology Quarterly* 1(3):256–282.

Liazos, Alexander (1972). "The poverty of the sociology of deviance: Nuts, sluts and perverts," *Social Problems* 20:403–420.

Macionis, John (2000). *Society: The Basics*. Upper Saddle River, NJ: Prentice Hall.

Oakley, Ann (1984). *The Captured Womb: A History of the Medical Care of Pregnant Women*. Oxford: Basil Blackwell.

Quinney, Richard (1977). *Class, State and Crime: On the Theory and Practice of Criminal Justice*.

Scheff, Thomas J. (1984). *Being Mentally Ill: A Sociological Theory*, 2nd ed. New York: Aldine.

Sherman, Lawrence W., and Douglas A. Smith (1992). "Crime, punishment and stake in the community: Legal and informal control of domestic violence," *American Sociological Review* 57:680–690.

Smith, Douglas A., and Patricia R. Gartin (1989). "Specifying specific deterrence: The influence of arrest on future criminal activity," *American Sociological Review*, 54:94–105.

Tiefer, Leonore (1992). "In pursuit of the perfect penis: The medicalization of male sexuality," pp. 450–465 in M.S. Kimmel and M.A. Messner, eds., *Men's Lives*. New York: McMillan.

Sandelowski, Margarete (1991). "Compelled to try: The never-enough quality of conceptive technology," *Medical Anthropology Quarterly* 5:29–47.

Waitzkin, Howard (1996). "The politics of medical encounters," in Phil Brown (ed.), *Perspectives in Medical Sociology* (2nd edition). Prospect Heights, IL: Waveland Press.

Wertz Richard W., and Dorothy C. Wertz (1979). *Lying In: A History of Childbirth in America*. New York: Schocken.

Zola, Irving K. (1972). "Medicine as an institution of social control," *Sociological Review*, 20:487–504.

ADDITIONAL RESOURCES

Brown, Phil (1995). "Naming and framing: The social construction of diagnosis and illness." *Journal of Health and Social Behavior*, extra issue:34–52.

Chapter 13

The Sociology of Mental Illness

A SOCIOLOGICAL APPROACH TO MENTAL ILLNESS

Since mental illness is viewed as distinct from physical illness in the U.S. healthcare system, the topic requires special attention from medical sociologists. While the study of mental health and illness involves many of the same approaches utilized in the analysis of physical health and illness, there are some important differences. While the notion of sickness is considered to be a social construct, the typical physical condition does have some underlying biological abnormality associated with it. Thus, most, but by no means all, health conditions can be determined to have some clinically identifiable characteristics associated with them.

This is clearly not the case with most mental disorders. Conditions that involve abnormalities of mood, thought process, and/or behavior typically cannot be demonstrated to have an underlying pathological foundation. Thus, the very notion of mental illness, it could be argued, is a social construct. Society, or its agents in the form of mental health professionals, social workers, and law enforcement officers, identify certain characteristics as "abnormal" and group these symptoms into syndromes that are

---

Box 13-1

Some Misconceptions About Mental Illness

As we enter the 21st century, the American public continues to per-petuate many myths related to mental illness. These myths deter a rational consideration of the needs of the mentally ill and add to the stigma that peo-ple who suffer from mental disorders must bear. The following myths have been identified by various organizations serving the mentally ill:

The mentally ill are violent and dangerous. People with mental illness are no more violent than the general population. In fact, people with mental illness are more often the victims of violence than perpetrators of violent acts. Isolated acts of violence by those with severe mental disorders tend to receive inordinate attention, and the mentally ill are unfairly portrayed as unpredictable or sinister in dramatic presentations on television, and in movies, magazines, and novels.

Mental illness is contagious. It is not contagious, since there is typically no "pathogen" to transmit. While there may be a higher risk of developing symptoms of mental illness if a past or present family member is so affected, this may be due to many factors.

The mentally ill have low IQs and usually live in poverty. Many studies have shown that most mentally ill individuals have average or above average intelligence. Mental illness affects individuals at all economic levels. Many mental patients end up in poverty due to the stigma attached to being labeled mentally ill, making it difficult for them to enter or re-enter the work force.

---

subsequently determined to constitute "mental disorders". The existence of this process clearly distinguishes mental illness from physical illness. (There are many misconceptions held concerning mental illness and these are discussed in Box 13-1).

DEFINING MENTAL ILLNESS

The approach used in defining physical illness can be used in defining mental health and illness. From a *medical model* perspective, mental health would be thought of as simply the absence of symptoms of mental illness. From this perspective, mental illness refers collectively to all diagnosable mental disorders or health conditions that are characterized by alterations in thinking, mood, or behavior (or some combination thereof) associated

Most people with mental health problems require hospitalization. Most people affected by mental disorders can best be helped by community-based mental health services. Community-based services include: prevention education; crisis stabilization; outpatient counseling; medication; service coordination; community residences; job training; and family, friendship, self-help, and recreational support services.

Most people do not recover from mental illnesses. Most mental illnesses are temporary, although—like other illnesses—some can be disabling. A previously well-adjusted person may have an episode of mental illness lasting weeks or months, and then go for years—even a lifetime—without further difficulties. To continue to label such a recovered person "abnormal" is inaccurate. Some people have bouts of disturbances. Between episodes they can be perfectly well. When they are well they understandably resent being treated as other than normal.

People who have recovered from a mental illness, cannot work successfully at a job. People who experience mental illnesses are all different. As such, their career potentials depend on their particular talents, abilities, experience, and motivation—as well as their current state of physical and mental health. Well-known political leaders, artists, and many others have achieved greatness despite the handicap of a mental illness. With modern treatment and support, people who have had mental illnesses can reasonably expect to work at responsible jobs and continue to contribute to society.

with distress and/or impaired functioning. Proponents of the medical model often view mental disorders as having physiological/anatomical foundations and prescribe physiological/anatomical treatment. While the medical model is not a very comfortable fit with most notions of mental health and illness, this model has continued to exert significant influence due to the role of psychiatrists whose approval is typically required for treatment, hospital admission or discharge, and drug prescription.

From the perspective of the *functional model*, mental health can be defined as a state of successful mental functioning, resulting in productive activities, fulfilling relationships, and the ability to adapt to change and cope with adversity. Conversely, mental illness would refer to conditions of thought, mood or behavior that prevent successful functioning and interfere with relationships and the individual's ability to cope. Many conditions that might be better described as "mental health problems" as opposed to diagnosable mental disorders might fall into this category. Almost everyone has experienced mental health problems in which the manifest distress matches some of the signs and symptoms of mental disorders. From this perspective, an individual who is adequately performing his social roles, despite the existence of symptoms that could be interpreted as mental illness, is considered healthy.

Due to the nature of mental illness, the *psychological model* is seldom applied in defining mental health and illness. This model assumes that the individual can make a rational decision as to whether he is sick or well. This assumption does not hold when dealing with individuals with conditions that might cause them to have a distorted notion of their ability to function. As will be seen later, the stress-related aspects of this model have important implications for the onset and progression of mental disorders and should not be ignored.

A model that relates specifically to mental illness is the *societal reaction model*. Proponents of this perspective contend that there is no such thing as mental illness in a scientific sense. Mental illness is a concept constructed by society as a means of controlling residual deviant behavior—i.e., behavior that doesn't fit nicely into the sin or crime categories but is nevertheless found to be objectionable. Thus, the behaviors or attributes that society (or powerful interests in society) reacts negatively to become labeled as mental illness. It is no surprise that those who are typically labeled as mentally ill are those who are on the margins of society and relatively powerless.

The societal reaction approach argues that certain behaviors of certain categories of people are selectively chosen for labeling as mental illness. For example, middle-class therapists may label certain "normal" behaviors of lower-class patients as symptoms of mental disorder although they are common to all members of this category. Further, the fact that most of the behavior patterns of symptomatic individuals are normal in no way detracts from the mental illness label.

Once the label is applied, the affected individual is seen in a new light by society and by himself. The individual begins to act in keeping with the label—i.e., in response to societal expectations. Permanent stigmatization may result and continue to be attached to the individual regardless of the outcome of the episode.

Finally, the *legal model* has more application with regard to mental illness than physical illness. All states have laws that afford the authorities the ability to ascertain the competency of individuals to manage their affairs, stand trial and otherwise act competently. Although input from the mental health system is required, the standard is ultimately a legal one. Thus, individuals may be legally adjudged too sick to manage their affairs, stand trial, or make decisions with regard to their own treatment. The most common application of the medical model relates to involuntary mental hospitalization, wherein an individual is found to be incompetent in terms of his life situation or a danger to himself or others.

TYPES OF MENTAL DISORDERS

Mental health professionals identify over 300 different "mental disorders" and typically categorize them as either mild or severe disorders. They may also be categorized based on the etiology of the condition. In the U.S., mental disorders are diagnosed based on the *Diagnostic and Statistical Manual of Mental Disorders, fourth edition (DSM-IV)*.

Mild Mental Disorders

Many mild mental disorders are a consequence of anxiety on the part of the affected individuals. Anxiety is one of the most widespread and easily understood of the major symptoms of mental disorders. Each of us encounters anxiety in many forms throughout the course of our routine activities. It may often take the concrete form of intense fear experienced in response to an immediately threatening experience, such as narrowly avoiding a traffic accident, and is aroused most intensely by immediate threats to one's safety. It also occurs commonly in response to dangers that are relatively remote or abstract. Intense anxiety may also result from situations that one can only vaguely imagine or anticipate.

Anxiety has evolved as a vitally important physiological response to dangerous situations that prepares a person for confronting or evading a threat in the environment. The appropriate regulation of anxiety is critical to the survival of virtually every higher organism in every environment. However, the mechanisms that regulate anxiety may break down in a wide variety of circumstances, leading to excessive or inappropriate expression of anxiety. Specific examples include phobias, panic attacks, and generalized anxiety. In phobias, high-level anxiety is aroused by specific situations or objects that may range from concrete entities such as snakes, to complex circumstances such as social interactions or public speaking. Panic attacks are brief but intense episodes of anxiety that often occur without a precipitating event or stimulus.

Generalized anxiety represents a more diffuse and nonspecific kind of anxiety that is most often experienced as excessive worrying, restlessness, and tension occurring with a chronic and sustained pattern. In each case, an anxiety disorder may be said to exist if the anxiety experienced is disproportionate to the circumstance, is difficult for the individual to control, or interferes with normal functioning. Anxiety disorders were originally referred to as neuroses and were thought to represent milder forms of severe psychiatric disorders (psychoses).

Severe Mental Disorders

Persons suffering from any of the severe mental disorders present with a variety of symptoms that may include inappropriate anxiety, disturbances of thought and perception, dysregulation of mood, and cognitive dysfunction. Disturbances of thought and perception are most commonly associated with schizophrenia. Similarly, severe disturbances in expression of affect and regulation of mood are most commonly seen in depression and bipolar disorder. Symptoms associated with mood, anxiety, thought process, or cognition may occur in any patient at some point during his or her illness.

Disturbances of perception and thought process fall into a broad category of symptoms referred to as psychosis. The threshold for determining whether thought is impaired varies somewhat with the cultural context. Like anxiety, psychotic symptoms may occur in a wide variety of mental disorders. They are most characteristically associated with schizophrenia, but psychotic symptoms can also occur in severe mood disorders.

One of the most common groups of symptoms that result from disordered processing and interpretation of sensory information are hallucinations. Hallucinations may be auditory, olfactory, gustatory, kinesthetic, tactile, or visual. For example, auditory hallucinations frequently involve the impression that one is hearing a voice. In each case, the sensory impression is falsely experienced as real.

Disturbances of mood characteristically manifest themselves as a sustained feeling of sadness or sustained elevation of mood. As with anxiety and psychosis, disturbances of mood may occur in a variety of patterns associated with different mental disorders. The disorder most closely associated with persistent sadness is major depression, while that associated with sustained elevation or fluctuation of mood is bipolar disorder. Along with the prevailing feelings of sadness or elation, disorders of mood are associated with a host of related symptoms that include disturbances in appetite, sleep patterns, energy level, concentration, and memory.

Cognitive function refers to the general ability to organize, process, and recall information. Disturbances of cognitive function may occur in a variety of disorders. Progressive deterioration of cognitive function is referred to as dementia. Dementia may be caused by a number of specific conditions including Alzheimer's disease. Impairment of cognitive function may also occur in other mental disorders such as depression. It is not uncommon to find profound disturbances of cognition in patients suffering from severe mood disturbances. Cognitive impairment often occurs in a host of chemical, metabolic, and infectious diseases that exert an impact on the brain.

During the last half of the twentieth century, mental health professionals identified numerous "new" mental disorders and/or redefined existing conditions as mental disorders. Eating disorders were identified as one of the conditions of the 1980s and three main types of eating disorders—anorexia nervosa, bulimia nervosa, and binge-eating disorder—were identified. Attention deficit hyperactivity disorder (ADHD) was defined in children and this has now become one of the most common mental disorders diagnosed, in children and adolescents, affecting an estimated 4.1 percent of youths ages 9 to 17. Autism was also identified as a condition during this period, with autism thought to affect an estimated 1 to 2 per 1,000 population. Alzheimer's disease was identified as a more precise diagnosis for what in the past was generalized as senile dementia. Alzheimer's disease is the most common cause of dementia among people age 65 and older, affecting an estimated four million Americans.

MENTAL DISORDERS IN AMERICA

The burden of mental illness on health and productivity in the United States and throughout the world has long been profoundly underestimated. Data developed by the massive Global Burden of Disease study, conducted by the World Health Organization, the World Bank, and Harvard University, reveal that mental illness, including suicide, ranks second in the burden of disease in established market economies, such as the United States.

Major depression alone ranked second only to ischemic heart disease in magnitude of disease burden. Schizophrenia, bipolar disorder, obsessive-compulsive disorder, panic disorder, and post-traumatic stress disorder also contributed significantly to the burden represented by mental illness. Mental disorders impose an enormous emotional and financial burden on ill individuals and their families. These disorders are also costly to society in reduced or lost productivity (indirect costs) and in medical resources used for care, treatment, and rehabilitation (direct costs).

The costs of mental illness to U.S. society are substantial. A recently completed NIMH study found that, in 1992, mental disorders cost the U.S. $94 billion in indirect costs and $66.8 billion in direct costs (under managed care) for a total of $160.8 billion. The direct costs of mental health services in the United States in 1996 totaled $69.0 billion. This figure represents 7.3 percent of total health spending. An additional $17.7 billion was spent on Alzheimer's disease and $12.6 billion on substance abuse treatment. Direct costs correspond to spending for treatment and rehabilitation nationwide.

Indirect costs—measured in terms of lost productivity at the workplace, school, and home—were estimated in 1990 at $78.6 billion (Rice & Miller, 1996). More than 80 percent of these costs stemmed from disability rather than death because mortality from mental disorders is relatively low.

An estimated 22.1 percent of Americans ages 18 and older—about 1 in 5 adults—suffer from a diagnosable mental disorder in a given year. When applied to the 2000 U.S. Census residential population estimate, this figure translates to over 63 million people. In addition, 4 of the 10 leading causes of disability in the U.S. and other developed countries are mental disorders. These include major depression, bipolar disorder, schizophrenia, and obsessive-compulsive disorder. Many people suffer from more than one mental disorder at a given time. In a given year 11 percent of the adult population will seek mental health treatment and $150 billion per year are spent on treatment. About 28 to 30 percent of the population has either a mental or addictive disorder (Regier et al. 1993; Kessler et al. 1994).

The epidemiology of mental disorders is made somewhat problematic by the difficulty of identifying a mental illness "case". Diagnosis of mental disorders is a problem, since it is not always possible to establish a threshold for a mental disorder, particularly in light of how common symptoms of mental distress are and the lack of objective, physical symptoms. Therefore, current epidemiological estimates cannot definitively identify those who are in need of treatment. Some individuals with mental disorders are in treatment and others are not; some are seen in primary care settings and others in specialty care. In the absence of valid measures of need, rates of disorder estimated in epidemiological surveys serve as an imperfect proxy for the need for care and treatment.

Epidemiological estimates have shifted over time because of changes in the definitions and diagnosis of mental health and mental illness. In the early 1950s, the rates of mental illness estimated by epidemiologists were far higher than those of today. One study, for example, found 81.5 percent of the population of Manhattan, New York, to have had signs and symptoms of mental distress (Srole, 1962). This led the authors of the study to conclude that mental illness was widespread.

Other studies began to find lower rates when they used more restrictive definitions that reflected contemporary depictions of mental illness. Instead of classifying anyone with signs and symptoms as being mentally ill, this more recent line of epidemiological research only identified people as mentally ill if they had a cluster of signs and symptoms that, when taken together, impaired people's ability to function (Pasamanick, 1959; Weissman et al. 1978). By 1978, the President's Commission on Mental Health (1978) concluded conservatively that the annual prevalence of specific mental disorders in the United States was about 15 percent. Current prevalence estimates comes from two epidemiologic surveys: the Epidemiologic Catchment Area (ECA) study of the early 1980s and the National Comorbidity Survey (NCS) of the early 1990s. A subpopulation of 5.4 percent of adults is considered to have a "serious" mental illness (SMI) (Kessler et al. 1996). About half of those with a "serious mental illness" (SMI) as defined by federal regulations (or 2.6 percent of all adults) were identified as being even more seriously affected, that is, by having "severe and persistent" mental illness (SPMI) (Kessler et al. 1996). This category includes schizophrenia, bipolar disorder, other severe forms of depression, panic disorder, and obsessive-compulsive disorder.

About 20 percent of children are estimated to have mental disorders with at least mild functional impairment. Federal regulations also define a sub-population of children and adolescents with more severe functional limitations, known as "serious emotional disturbance" (SED). Children and adolescents with SED number approximately 5 to 9 percent of children ages 9 to 17 (Friedman et al. 1996b).

Estimates generated from the ECA survey indicate that 19.8 percent of the older adult population has a diagnosable mental disorder during a one-year period. Almost four percent of older adults have SMI, and just under one percent has SPMI (Kessler et al. 1996).

SOCIAL FACTORS IN MENTAL HEALTH AND ILLNESS

Anthropological and cross-cultural studies show that cultural beliefs about the nature of mental illness influence the community's view of its course and treatment. These views may affect, in turn, the actual duration of the illness. It has long been thought that major mental illness is almost inevitably chronic and incurable. Research now shows that schizophrenia and many other severe forms of mental illness (such as manic-depressive illness and depression) have extremely diverse courses, ranging from complete recovery through patterns of waxing and waning, to nearly complete disability.

Another line of research shows that diagnoses of mental illness differ across cultures and subcultures. For example, among psychiatric inpatients in the United States, African Americans are more likely than white Americans to be diagnosed with schizophrenia and less likely to be diagnosed with affective disorder. Mexican Americans in the Los Angeles area tend to view people with symptoms of schizophrenia as vulnerable and ill, but they explain those symptoms as resulting from "nerves" and from being "sensitive" and assume that recovery is possible. In contrast, Anglo Americans in the same area are more likely to categorize the same people as "crazy," with little or no hope of recovery.

Culturally based variations in diagnosis also occur because current diagnostic categories are derived largely from research among majority populations, particularly those in hospitals or specialty psychiatric clinics. Such studies tend to support the impression that the observed expressions of illness are universal. The patterns of onset and duration and even the nature and clustering of specific symptoms vary widely across cultures. These findings have many practical as well as theoretical implications. For example, at present, the vast majority of medically trained clinicians in our healthcare system come from the white majority, while a sizable proportion of their clients, especially in public facilities, are members of racial or ethnic minorities.

As with physical illness, both mental health status and sickness behavior are correlated with a variety of sociocultural variables. The major correlates of mental illness are described below.

Age and Mental Illness

There is a well-documented relationship between the prevalence of mental illness and age, although the nature of the relationship has undergone substantial modification in recent years. Until the 1970s, it was believed that aging had a cumulative effect on mental health just as it was thought to have on physical health (Warheit et al. 1975), with the prevalence of mental illness thought to increase with advancing age. However, many observers argued that this pattern reflected selectivity in terms of the mental disorders measured, use of statistics for institutionalized patients, and the tendency to attribute many symptoms of old age to mental illness.

A more contemporary depiction suggests a nonmonotonic and much more irregular relationship. This change in perceived relationship between age and mental illness is a function not so much of actual changes in the distribution of mental illness within the population as of a revision in terms of the conditions classified as mental disorders. The inclusion of alcoholism, drug abuse, and suicide under the heading of mental illness has created a "bulge" in the 15–25 age cohort. Further, the advent of adolescent treatment centers has meant that many more adolescents are being defined as mentally disturbed than in the past. At the same time, attributing many symptoms of aging to Alzheimer's disease has reduced the perceived prevalence of mental illness among the elderly.

As was the case with physical illness, the quantity and type of mental health services utilized vary dramatically with age. The very young utilize few such services, while the utilization rates for other cohorts vary widely. In terms of inpatient care for the mentally ill, the elderly have historically been overrepresented, although this may be a reflection of selective data.

By the 1970s, young adults had become overrepresented among psychiatric inpatients. This shift reflects changes in institutionalization policies and the redefinition of certain behaviors (e.g., alcohol and drug abuse) as mental illness. In 2000, the highest inpatient admission rates to all facilities were for the 15-to-44 cohort. By far the lowest rates were for the 15-and-under cohort (National Center for Health Statistics 2002, table 3).

For outpatient care overall, the 15-to-35 age cohort appears to dominate utilization. However, this pattern is probably more a function of help-seeking by females in these age cohorts than of mental problems in this age group overall. The picture is further complicated when the source of treatment is considered. Those utilizing community mental health centers, which have become the most common settings for care, tend to have demographic attributes different from those utilizing psychiatrists or psychoanalysts. Further, those utilizing medical doctors or clergymen for mental health counseling are also characterized by differing demographic characteristics.

Sex and Mental Illness

The relationship between sex and mental health status is fairly well documented, although the conclusions are not without controversy. As noted earlier with regard to physical health, females appear to be characterized by a higher level of psychiatric morbidity. This assertion is based on reported symptoms, clinical evaluations by community researchers, and frequency of presenting themselves for mental healthcare (Cockerham 1997). Even this must be qualified, however. While women exhibit higher scores on indices (MMPI-2) of depression, hysteria and paranoia, men have higher scores for antisocial behavior, problems with authority, and type A behavior (Gumbiner and Flowers 1997).

Many observers suggest that females are not, in fact, "crazier," but that differences in identified prevalence rates are a function of other factors. These factors include a tendency for females to perceive symptoms as emotional rather than physical, a greater tendency for females to admit to symptoms of either physical or mental character, and the willingness of society to interpret females' characteristics as emotional rather than physical.

Males and females tend to be characterized by quite different psychiatric disorders. Females tend to be characterized by milder, more common anxiety disorders. Males, on the other hand, tend to predominate with regard to the less common but more serious psychoses such as schizophrenia and personality disorders. A major exception is found in the case of depression, for which women report a rate twice as high as men (Cockerham 1997). As with physical illness, it appears that females are characterized by a greater occurrence of symptoms while males are afflicted with more extreme conditions.

Females tend to be much heavier users of mental health services than males. This predominance, however, primarily reflects use of outpatient services; when inpatient mental healthcare is examined, males appear to be heavier utilizers of these services. In 2000, for example, the rate of discharge from general hospitals for patients with mental disorders was 81.2 per 10,000 population for males and 73.2 for females (Hall, 2002, table 6).

A preponderance of males among the institutionalized population is explained to a certain extent by contemporary patterns of mental hospitalization. The conditions most likely to warrant institutionalization are the extreme psychotic conditions such as schizophrenia and manic-depression. Males tend to have higher rates of the former, and females of the latter. However, depressed patients are much more likely to be admitted to general hospital psychiatric wards than they are to mental hospitals. Women, therefore, turn up less often in the mental hospitalization statistics. The various types of substance abuse tend to be much more common among males than females. For both inpatient and outpatient mental health treatment, females are overrepresented among those voluntarily seeking care and males among those involuntarily receiving care.

Females exhibit higher levels of utilization regardless of the type of therapist. For psychiatrists, clinical psychologists, social workers, and even general practitioners and clergymen, females constitute the majority of the patients/clients.

Race and Ethnicity and Mental Illness

The distribution of mental illness with regard to race and ethnicity has been of great interest to researchers and health professionals. This interest has been sparked in part by the controversial nature of the relationship, especially as it relates to racial comparisons. Since the development of modern concepts of mental illness in the nineteenth century, attempts have been made to profile the mental health status of various racial and ethnic groups. In its most malevolent form, this effort has been subverted in an attempt to portray certain groups as mentally inferior.

Race and ethnicity are major risk factors for mental illness and psychosocial dysfunction. African Americans and Hispanics are at higher risk for many mental disorders. Some of this increased risk is due to the lower average socioeconomic status of most racial and ethnic minorities and their concentration in more hazardous urban environments. However, race and ethnicity have health consequences simply not accounted for by socioeconomic status and place of residence.

After several decades of research, it is now believed by many that the impression of higher rates of mental disorder among blacks and certain other racial and/or ethnic groups is a function of at least three factors. These include: (a) collection of data historically from public mental institutions; (b) a middle-class bias in the diagnosis of mental disorders; and (c) a failure to consider important intervening variables such as social class. Recent studies, in fact, have found little support for significant differences between blacks and whites in terms of the prevalence of mental disorders. However, Hispanics have been found in these same studies to have higher than average rates, while Asian-Americans record lower than average prevalence rates. Differences in education and occupational status, for example, may account for some of the variation. More importantly, social class is often pointed to as the major contributing factor to prevalence differentials.

The relationship between mental disorder and ethnicity is even cloudier, given the wide variation in the types of ethnic groups in U.S. society. Some groups, such as Mexican-Americans, appear to be characterized by higher than average rates of disorder (Kessler 1994). Others, such as Japanese- and Chinese-Americans, appear to be relatively "disease-free" (Kuo 1984).

Once again, the observed differences may reflect differentials in types of disorders rather than overall prevalence. These differentials in turn may be a function of social class or other socioeconomic differences, or even migration status. In any case, it is extremely difficult to compare subgroups of the population in terms of either prevalence or types of disorder, due to numerous possible intervening variables.

The rate of institutionalization for psychiatric treatment is much lower for whites than for non-whites. This is true whether the site of institutionalization is the government mental institution, a private psychiatric facility, or the psychiatric ward of a general hospital (National Center for Health Statistics 1998, table 97). This is true for the second largest racial/ethnic group—Hispanics—as well. It should be noted that African Americans face a greater likelihood of involuntary commitment, and this accounts for some of the difference in hospital utilization.

Marital Status, Living Arrangements, and Mental Illness

The preponderance of research now indicates that the different marital statuses—never married, married, divorced, and widowed—are at varying risks of mental illness. The consensus is that the married are much better off overall in terms of mental health than are those in any of the other marital categories. There is less consensus concerning the category at greatest risk;

different studies have variously identified the never married, the divorced, and the widowed. Changes in marital status are also contributors to higher levels of morbidity, with divorce being a contributor to the onset of major depression for both men and women. The impact of such changes, however, is clearly greater for women (Bruce and Kim 1992).

As for many of the variables discussed, the relationship may not be as direct as it appears. There are those that argue for marital status-specific disorders and others that contend that reliance on marital categories overlooks important differences between the sexes. Another school of thought suggests that it is not marital status per se that correlates with risk of mental disorder but living arrangements. For example, those living alone (regardless of marital status) have been found to be at greater risk of mental disorder (Hughes and Gove 1981). Until the complexities of these relationships can be unraveled, it appears that marital status will be retained as a reasonable predictor of the prevalence of mental disorder.

Socioeconomic Status and Mental Illness

Early on in the study of the social epidemiology of mental disorder, it was asserted that the lower classes were more prone to psychiatric pathology than the affluent (Hollingshead and Redlich 1958). However, more recent studies have failed to consistently demonstrate a clear relationship between income and the prevalence of mental illness. What has been demonstrated is the fact that the relative prevalence of mental illness by social class depends heavily on the type of disorder examined. Even so, the apparent correlations between mental illness and certain other variables (e.g., race and age) are essentially eliminated when socioeconomic status is controlled (Warheit et al. 1975).

For the American population, the highest rates of diagnosable mental disorder have been found among the groups with the lowest socioeconomic status. For example, people with less than a high school education or less than in $20,000 annual income experienced psychiatric disorders at almost four times the rate found among those with a college education or an annual income of $70,000 or more.

Recent research on schizophrenia suggests that, while poverty does not cause the disorder, it is powerfully related to the experience of those suffering from it, their resources for coping with it, and perhaps their likelihood of recovery. Socioeconomic or other psychosocial deprivations and stresses do seem to play a causal role in both the onset and course of depressive, substance abuse, and antisocial disorders. Further, researchers now know that virtually all major psychosocial risk factors for mental illness are more prevalent at lower socioeconomic levels. Alleviating acute socioeconomic deprivation can often lessen the more serious long-term psychological consequences of these disorders.

The relationship between educational level and mental illness, like that for physical illness, appears to be fairly clear-cut. In fact, some researchers have suggested that the social class differentials noted above are a function of differing levels of education. As the level of education increases, there appears to be an increase in the prevalence, but a decrease in the severity, of disorders. The better educated appear to be more characterized by anxiety disorders, while the less educated appear to be more frequently psychotic. Gallo et al. (1993) found a clear relationship between educational level and the likelihood of depression onset in older adults. Ironically, the rate of suicide is much higher among the better educated, but this is generally attributed to the differing means of coping characterizing various educational levels.

Religion and Mental Illness

Associations between either religious affiliation or degree of religiosity and sickness behavior are among the most idiosyncratic of the relationships discussed. These relationships have been subjected to limited research so that clear patters are difficult to discern. Further, in the U.S. at the beginning of the twenty-first century, religious affiliation and participation appear to be associated with so many other variables that it is difficult to tease out the influences of those variables per se.

The findings on the correlation between religion and mental illness are not particularly clear-cut. For one measure of mental disorder at least—feelings of nervous breakdown—it has been found that the highest rates were among members of fundamentalist denominations, followed by Baptist and Jews (Gurin et al. 1960). In terms of religiosity, it has been found that the more religious are characterized by lower levels of psychiatric morbidity (Stark, 1971).

There appears to be little difference in the rate of mental hospitalization for the major religious groups in the United States. There are some patterns specific to particular religions. Jews, for example are found to have higher rates of psychiatric care, particularly outpatient care, than other religious groups.

Many psychiatric inpatients indicate that spiritual/religious beliefs and practices help them to cope. Lindgren and Coursey (1995) reported 83% of psychiatric patients felt that spiritual belief had a positive impact on their illness through the comfort it provided and the feelings of being cared for and not being alone it engendered. Religious/spiritual commitment may enhance recovery from depression, serious mental or physical illness, and substance abuse, help curtail suicide, and reduce health risks.

THE TREATMENT OF MENTAL DISORDERS

While scant attention was paid to the treatment of physical illnesses, there is ample reason to consider therapeutic issues when mental illness is being considered. Many aspects of the diagnosis and treatment of mental illness are controversial and often reflect the operation of social factors. Over the past three decades, the complex patchwork of mental health services in the United States has become so fragmented that it is referred to as the *de facto mental health system* (Regier et al. 1993). Its shape has been determined by many heterogeneous factors rather than by a single guiding set of organizing principles. The de facto system has been characterized as having distinct sectors, financing, duration of care, and settings.

The four sectors of the system are the specialty mental health sector, the general medical/primary care sector, the human services sector, and the voluntary support network sector. Specialty mental health services include services provided by specialized mental health professionals (e.g., psychologists, psychiatric nurses, psychiatrists, and psychiatric social workers) and the specialized offices, facilities, and agencies in which they work. Specialty services have been designed expressly for the provision of mental health services.

The general medical/primary care sector consists of health care professionals (e.g., family physicians, nurse practitioners, internists, pediatricians, etc.) and the settings (i.e., offices, clinics, and hospitals) in which they work. These settings were designed for the full range of health care services, including the delivery of mental health services. The human services sector consists of social welfare, criminal justice, educational, religious, and charitable services. The voluntary support network refers to self-help groups and organizations. These are groups devoted to education, communication, and support, all of which extend beyond formal treatment.

In terms of financing, the system is divided into a public (i.e., government) and a private sector. The term "public sector" refers both to services directly operated by government agencies (e.g., state and county mental hospitals) and to services financed with government resources (e.g., Medicaid and Medicare). Private sector financing involves payments through insurance plans and by individuals.

Care is divided between services for the treatment of short-term acute conditions and those devoted to the long-term care of chronic (i.e., severe and persistent) conditions, such as schizophrenia, bipolar disorder, and Alzheimer's disease. The former, provided in psychiatric hospitals, psychiatric units in general hospitals, and in beds "scattered" in general hospital wards, includes brief treatment-oriented services. Long-term care includes residential care as well as some treatment services. Residential care is often referred to as "custodial," when supervised living predominates over active treatment. Non-institutional settings for care include physicians offices and other medical clinics, non-physician therapists' offices, community mental health centers, and the home. In today's environment, most of the diagnosis and treatment of mental disorders takes place in such non-institutional settings.

According to recent national surveys (Regier et al. 1993; Kessler et al. 1996), approximately 15 percent of the U.S. adult population use mental health services in any given year. Eleven percent receive their services from either the general medical care sector or the specialty mental health sector, in roughly equal proportions. In addition, about five percent receive care from the human services sector, and about three percent receive care from the voluntary support network.

Slightly more than half of the 15 percent of the adult population that use mental health services have a diagnosable mental or addictive disorder (8%), while the remaining portion has a mental health problem (7%). Bearing in mind that 28 percent of the population has a diagnosable mental or substance abuse disorder, only about one-third with a diagnosable mental disorder receives treatment in any year. Thus, the *majority* of those with a diagnosable mental disorder are not receiving treatment.

One of the major developments in the treatment of mental disorder in the second half of the twentieth century was the deinstitutionalization movement. "Deinstitutionalization" refers to the shift in the setting of care for mental disorders from large state hospitals to federally supported community mental health centers and community-based clinics. This movement to outpatient services began in the 1950s as new medications allowed many mentally ill individuals to function normally for extended periods of time. The failure of both local and federal governments to adequately fund the mental treatment of the uninsured and underinsured has resulted in many chronically mentally ill patients becoming homeless. As a consequence, the term deinstitutionalization has become synonymous with "dumping people on the streets".

CRITICAL PERSPECTIVES OF MENTAL ILLNESS

Many medical sociologists, psychiatrists, and other mental health professionals have found much to be critical about with regard to the field of mental health and illness. Detractors have questioned the very concept of mental disorder as a "real" health condition. Others, perhaps conceding that such disorders might exist beyond being social constructs, point out the fallacies involved in the defining and categorizing of mental disorders.

Critics raise issues with regard to the diagnosis process and question many of the forms of treatment that are utilized.

The sociological concept of "labeling" has experienced its most extensive application in the area of mental illness. From this perspective, a diagnosis of "mental illness" represents a label. This label contributes to behavior that could be viewed as evidence of mental illness. Thus, from this viewpoint mental illness is the result of a role imposed upon individuals by others. If someone is labeled as mentally ill this label may become a self-fulfilling prophecy. Such labeling, Szasz (1961) claims, simply enforces conformity to the standards of people powerful enough to impose their will on others.

Some renegade psychiatrists contend that there is no such thing as mental illness and refer to mental illness as a myth. They argue that what we label as mental illness is simply behavior and ways of thinking that are not accepted by society. They are not necessarily rooted in the physiology of individuals and therefore should not be referred to as illnesses. Much of what is called mental illness is not a disease like cancer or pneumonia and should not be viewed using a medical model. Thus, from this perspective, the only conditions that should be called mental illness are those linked, without question, to physiological processes and anatomical structure.

This view argues that the myth of mental illness is maintained by psychiatrists and clinical psychologists who profit from the view that mental illness is a medical problem. From a broader perspective, the mental illness label may be used as a way of controlling problem populations who are threats to society but are not criminal. This perspective would argue for extremely blurred lines between the sane and insane. (Box 13-2 deals with being sane in insane places.)

SOCIAL STRESS AND ITS CONSEQUENCES

One phenomenon related to mental health that has been extensively studied by medical sociologists and others is social stress. "Stress" involves a heightened mind-body reaction to stimuli inducing fear or anxiety in the individual (Cockerham and Richey 1997). Stress in this sense is the response to a stressor in the environment or a stressful life event. Stress typically starts with a situation that a person finds threatening or burdensome. The individual responds to stress through various physical and mental reactions.

Most threats individuals face in modern society are symbolic, not physical, and seldom require a physical response. Indeed, such traditional physical responses as fighting are discouraged in contemporary society.

Thus, the human organism is often left with no course of action, perhaps not even verbal insults. This inability to respond externally leaves the body physiologically mobilized for action that never comes, creating a situation that can result in damage to the body (Cockerham, 2001).

A number of studies have shown that the human organism's inability to manage stress can lead to the development of cardiovascular complications and hypertension, peptic ulcers, muscular pain, compulsive vomiting, asthma, migraine headaches, and other health problems. Research has demonstrated the effects of stress on the cardiovascular system and shown how the failure to cope with job-related stressors promotes heart disease.

David Mechanic (1962, 1978) explains the stress experience from the standpoint of both society and the individual, suggesting that the meaning of the crisis lies not in the situation, but rather in the interaction between the situation and the person's ability to cope with it. The impact of a crisis depends on the ability of the person to manage it.

Extending this concept of stress from the individual to societal components, Mechanic states that a person's ability to cope with problems is influenced by a society's preparatory institutions, such as schools and the family. A person's emotional control and ability to cope are also related to society's incentive systems—that is, society's rewards (or punishments) for those who do (or do not) control their behavior in accordance with social norms (Cockerham, 2001).

Hence, the extent of physiological damage or change within an individual depends on: 1) the stimulus situation and the individual's interpretation of it; 2) the individual's capacity to deal with the stimulus situation; 3) the individual's preparation by society to meet problems; and 4) the influence of society's approved modes of behavior. Mechanic (1962:8) emphasizes the contribution of society toward an individual's adaptation to stress, noting that the extent to which an individual experiences stress is a function of the means—mostly learned—that the individual has available for dealing with the situation.

Sociologists have found that the group context influences the individual's ability to manage stress. Moss (1973) illustrates the significance of group membership in helping individuals cope with information they find stressful. He suggests that stress and physiological change are likely to occur when people experience information that goes against their beliefs or desires. The social support provided through group membership affords protection for the individual. Subjective feelings of belonging, being accepted, and being needed have consistently shown themselves to be crucial in the relieving of symptoms of stress.

Social interaction with family, friends, and acquaintances often plays an important part in the decision to seek help for psychiatric symptoms.

Box 13-2

On Being Sane in Insane Places

During the 1970s questions began being raised by individuals inside and outside of psychiatry as to the appropriateness of the process used to diagnose the mentally ill. The 1960s and 70s had become the "golden age" of psychiatry, as new therapies were introduced, psychotropic drugs were brought to market, and the general public developed a fascination with psychotherapy. The assumption was made that mental health professionals could definitively distinguish between the "sane" and the "insane", and this process was codified in the *Diagnostics and Statistical Manual* produced by the American Psychiatric Association.

Many critics of psychiatry raised questions concerning the appropriateness of the standard diagnostic process and raised questions concerning the ability of mental health professionals to distinguish between the sane and insane. After all, they argued, most mentally disordered individuals were normal with regard to most aspects of their lives and, conversely, most normal people displayed certain behaviors that could be considered abnormal at least some of the time. How, then, was it possible to definitively draw the line between the sane and the insane?

In the early 1970s, psychologist David L. Rosenhan devised an experiment to test the ability of mental health professionals to distinguish between the sane and the insane. He identified 8 individuals from various walks of life who were "prepped" to become patients at a dozen mental hospitals. The patients were to present themselves with a certain set of symptoms (e.g., hearing voices, feeling of emptiness) in an attempt to obtain admission to

---

For example, a poor person might be motivated to seek help after a friend's description of some serious disease that could possibly be related to her symptoms, symptoms that were formerly not worrisome but now became significant, even though she had experienced no change in the symptoms themselves. Similar factors may be involved in the decision to seek nonmedical forms of help. Thus, the motivation to do something about a health problem often results from social interaction that heightens the significance imputed to the symptoms.

One dimension of response to stress involves "coping behavior"—that is how individuals respond to stressful situations in order to make them more manageable. However, this is typically not an individualistic response to stress, but a socially induced one resulting from the sociocultural context of the individual and the group influences that are exerted. Sociologists view the coping process in terms of social resources, the intervention of other individuals, and the availability of structural and

one or more of the hospitals. The mental hospitals represented the full range of facilities, from impoverished public hospitals to expensive private hospitals. Once admitted, these pseudopatients were instructed to eliminate any of the admitting symptoms and act "normal"—that is, to behave in the same manner they would if they were outside the hospital. However, they were told that they would have to find their own way out of the hospital.

None of the pseudopatients had any problem being admitted to any of the facilities where they presented themselves. They were typically diagnosed with some form of schizophrenia. One admitted they began to carry on in a normal fashion as instructed. The only thing that might have been considered out of the ordinary was their responsibility for taking notes on their experiences within the various mental institutions. The length of the hospital stay ranged from two days to 52 days, with an average of 19 days.

The combination of 8 pseudopatients and 12 hospitals resulted in a large number of episodes of institutionalization. However, none of the pseudopatients was ever identified as "sane" by staff at any of the institutions in the study. While notes from the patients charts often included positive comments (e.g., "friendly", "cooperative"), no clinician ever suggested that the patient may actually be sane and not in need of treatment. The fact that they were present in the institution was *a priori* proof that they were insane.

On the contrary, their behavior was interpreted as symptomatic of the mental condition of the patient rather than the normal behavior it was. For example, the clinical notes for one patient described the not unusual situation of being closer to his mother and some point in his life and closer to his father at some other point. The pseudopatient also indicated that he had lost touch with some of his friends and had made new ones in the interim. These seemingly normal situations were interpreted as symptomatic of the

(*continued*)

community resources that may potentially moderate or buffer the effects of stressors. Informal social resources include the quantity and quality of social contacts and networks. Formal social resources include knowledge of, and physical and financial access to, treatment, preventive and assistance services, such as professional counselors (Cockerham and Richey, 1997).

Within some segments of society, coping behavior may involve prayer and the seeking of religious counsel. In others, it may involve the use of alcohol or drugs. The way people in society react to stressful situations, then, is more a function of their group affiliation than of any individual traits.

A "social stressor" is a factor found in the social environment that induces stress in individuals. These include both significant life events and chronic strains (Pearlin, 1989). Life events that induce stress include divorce, marriage, or job loss. (Note that both positive and negative events can induce stress.) Chronic strains are relatively enduring conflicts,

schizophrenia characterizing the individual, in that he had ambivalent feelings toward his parents and was unable to maintain stable relationships with family and friends.

Because of their fear of being discovered as "frauds", the pseudopatients initially took their notes in secret. However, when they discovered that none of the staff cared what they were doing, they opening took notes. In some cases, this behavior reinforced the perception of insanity held by the staff; the behavior was described as "writing behavior" and recorded as a symptom associated with their disorders.

While the sanity of the pseudopatients went undetected by the staff, this was not the case with their fellow "inmates". In every case, a significant portion of other patients saw through the pretense. They would often tell the pseudopatients that they weren't "crazy" and accuse them of being a journalist or a professor—someone who was studying or investigating the hospital.

Ultimately, all of the pseudopatients were discharged from the various institutions with the universal discharge diagnosis of "schizophrenia in remission". Note that none of them was cured of their condition (in fact they received virtually no treatments) yet each was still considered to be mentally ill although in a state of remission.

Among the many conclusions drawn from the study were the following. Mental health professionals could not definitively distinguish between

problems, and threats that many people face on a daily basis. Chronic strain may reflect role overload, conflict within role sets, inter-role conflict, role capacity in which a person is "trapped" in an unpleasant role, or role restructuring in which a person changes relationships within roles. Role strain can have serious effects on individuals because the roles themselves are important, especially when they involve jobs, marriage, and parenthood (Cockerham, 2001).

One of the attempts to quantify life stress has been the Holmes and Rahe (1967) "Social Readjusment Rating Scale." This tool allows individuals to indicate the number of events (both positive and negative) that have occurred to them during the past year and then calculate a stress score. Research has found that those with higher scores are more likely to have suffered illness during the period in question. (See Table 13–1 for an updated version of the original social readjustment rating scale.)

Although the Holmes and Rahe scale is found to measure stress and life events reasonably there are some criticisms of it. For example, the scale does not adequately account for differences in the relative importance of various life events among ethnic and culture subgroups. Also, some events, such as divorce, can be regarded as a consequence of stress instead of a cause.

the sane and the insane. The labeling of certain behaviors as psychotic was more a function of the non-clinical characteristics of the diagnostician and the individual being diagnosed and the environment in which the behavior occurred. Further, once an individual was labeled as mentally ill, there was no further questioning of his condition on the part of mental health professionals. In fact, any subsequent behavior was interpreted in the light of the patient's diagnosis rather than the reverse.

Finally, it was concluded that much of the behavior of institutionalized patients was not a function of their disorder but represented a means of accommodation to the situation. That is, staff holds certain notions of the behavior that is appropriate for mental patients and they "reward" the patients for behaving in keeping with their expectations. While they may have been labeled as mentally ill, most mental patients are not stupid and can appreciate the importance of behaving in keeping with the expectations of those who maintain absolute control over their existence. Thus, to behave as a "normal" person was likely to attract unfavorable attention to the patient; in order to remain in the good graces of the hospital staff, mental patients found it expedient to act "crazy".

Source: David L. Rosenhan (1973). "On Being Sane in Insane Places," *Science* 179:250–258.

PSYCHOSOCIAL CONTRIBUTIONS TO ILLNESS

The notion of a relationship between the mental condition of an individual and his health status is not new. Classical philosopher/physicians and primitive healers alike realized that there was a mind-body connection. There has been a historical flirtation in medical science with the notion of "psychosomatic" conditions. However, the emergence of the medical model as the dominant explanatory framework at the end of the nineteenth century pushed the importance of psychosocial factors to the background, and it was well into the twentieth century before psychosomatic illness was rediscovered. This time, however, there was a growing body of empirical evidence supporting the existence of a mind-body connection, supported even by biochemical and neurologic evidence.

A "psychosomatic" illness is a physical disorder related to or resulting from an underlying emotional or psychological state. The assumption is held that specific attitudes or psychological states are correlated with particular physiological changes of a disease-like nature. For example, unexplained feelings of anger and hostility can be translated into disorders such as high blood pressure and irregular heartbeat. It is not clear exactly

Table 13–1. The Life Event Assessment Scale

The Life Event Assessment Scale is used to measure the amount of stress in an individual's life. Respondents indicate the stressors to which they were exposed in the past 12 months and calculate the their scores based on these stressors. A total score of anywhere from about 250 to 500 or would be considered a moderate amount of stress. Individuals who score higher than that may face an increased risk of illness.

Life event	Points
Health	
An injury or illness which:	
Kept you in bed for a week or more, or sent you to the hospital	74
Was less serious than that	44
Major dental work	26
Major change in eating habits	27
Major change in sleeping habits	26
Major change in usual type/amount of recreation	28
Work	
Change to a new type of work	51
Change in your work hours or conditions	35
Change in your responsibilities at work:	
More responsibilities	29
Fewer responsibilities	21
Promotion	31
Demotion	42
Transfer	32
Troubles at work:	
With your boss	29
With co-workers	35
With persons under your supervision	35
Other work troubles	28
Major business adjustment	60
Retirement	52
Loss of job:	
Laid off from work	68
Fired from work	79
Correspondence course to help you in your work	18
Home and family	
Major change in living conditions	42
Change in residence:	
Move within the same town or city	25
Move to a different town, city or state	47
Change in family get-togethers	25
Major change in health of a family member	55
Marriage	50

Table 13–2.   (*Cont.*)

Life event	Points
Pregnancy	67
Miscarriage or abortion	65
Gain of a new family member:	
Birth of a child	66
Adoption of a child	65
A relative moving in with you	59
Spouse beginning or ending work	46
Child leaving home	
To attend college	41
Due to marriage	41
For other reasons	45
Change in arguments with spouse	50
In-law problems	38
Change in the marital status of your parents:	
Divorce	59
Remarriage	50
Separation from spouse:	
Due to work	53
Due to marital problems	76
Divorce	96
Birth of a grandchild	43
Death of spouse	119
Death of other family member:	
Child	123
Brother or sister	102
Parent	100
Personal and social	
Change in personal habits	26
Beginning of ending school or college	35
Change in school or college	35
Change in political beliefs	24
Change in religious beliefs	29
Change in social activities	27
Vacation trip	24
New, close, personal relationship	37
Engagement to marry	45
Girlfriend or boyfriend problems	39
Sexual difficulties	44
"Falling out" of close personal relationship	47
An accident	48
Minor violation of the law	20
Being held in jail	75
Death of a close friend	70
Major decision about your immediate future	51
Major personal achievement	36

(*continued*)

Table 13–2. (*Cont.*)

Life event	Points
Financial	
Major change in finances	
Increased income	38
Decreased income	60
Investment or credit difficulties	56
Loss or damage of personal property	43
Moderate purchase	30
Major purchase	37
Foreclosure on a mortgage or loan	58
TOTAL SCORE	

SOURCE: M.A. Miller and R. H. Rahe (1997). "Life Changes Scaling for the 1990s." *Journal of Psychosomatic Research*, 43: 279–292.

how these states affect one's physical condition, but recent biochemical research indicates that a strong positive (or negative) attitude is reflected within every cell of the person's body. The diseases that result from these psychological states appear to be a complex mix of physical, psychological and social conditions. Some, in fact, actually reflect the expectations of the social group (as indicated by wide variations in the response of the affected individual to menstruation and pregnancy).

Researchers have identified seven "classic" psychosomatic disorders—ones that have long been associated with negative emotional or psychological state, along with several newly identified conditions. The classic disorders are: hypertension, hyperthyroidism, neurodermatitis, rheumatoid arthritis, peptic ulcer, ulcerative colitis, and asthma. The list of newly identified psychosomatic conditions is lengthy and includes: hypoglycemia, migraine headaches, vertigo, narcolepsy, most endocrinal problems, many pediatric problems, pelvic pain, menstrual irregularity, frigidity and impotence. There is also evidence that certain cancers may be linked to specific mental states.

A number of factors have contributed to the identification of psychosocial factors as a legitimate contributor to health conditions. The influence of psychoanalysis and the scientific study of the role of psychological factors in a variety of situations attracted attention to the possibility of psychologically initiated illnesses. Further, the demonstration of the placebo effect provided evidence of the role the mind played in a patient's illness progression. These realizations were occurring at a time when the diminishing importance of biological agents in the etiology of illness caused researchers to look elsewhere for explanations.

At the same time, some surprising statistics were being generated by the research that took place during the last quarter of the twentieth century. It was found, for example, that 30 percent of a primary care practice was devoted to emotional and psychological conditions rather than physical problems. Thus, marital problems, depression, hypochondriasis, alcoholism and anxiety were taking as much of the physician's time as colds, viruses, and hypertension. Further, 30–60 percent of patients (depending on the study) claiming a physical problem actually suffer from a psychosomatic or psychoneurotic problem. In fact, as much as 50 percent of the population may suffer from some type of psychosomatic problem.

The issue of psychosomatic illnesses has been problematic for a number of reasons. Clinicians know less about these types of conditions than many others due to a lack of research funding on the topic. Further, physicians in general have limited training in the management of psychosomatic problems. They feel uncomfortable dealing with such disorders and are often less sympathetic toward this type of patient. These conditions do not fit the medical model mold and are not responsive to the primary tools of the physician (i.e., surgery and drugs).

Like virtually every health condition that we have considered, psychosomatic illnesses are not randomly spread throughout the population. Instead, they tend to affect some groups more than others. Among those in U.S. society more likely to be affected by psychosomatic conditions are: nonwhites, females, the poor, the elderly, the widowed, separated or divorces, and the unemployed, retired or disabled. Thus, populations that are often considered "vulnerable" when it comes to physical illnesses are the ones most affected by psychosomatic disorders.

REFERENCES

Bruce, M.L., and K.M. Kim (1992). "Differences in the effects of divorce on major depression in men and women," *American Journal of Psychiatry*, 149:914–917.

Cockerham, William C. (1997). *The Sociology of Mental Disorder*. Englewood Cliffs, NJ: Prentice Hall.

Cockerham, William C., and Ferris J. Richey (1997). *The Dictionary of Medical Sociology*. Westport, CT: Greenwood.

Cockerham, William C., (2001). *Medical Sociology* 8th ed. Upper Saddle Creek, NJ: Prentice Hall.

Friedman, R.M., J.W. Katz-Levey, R.W. Manderschied, and D.L. Sondheimer (1996). "Prevalence of serious emotional disturbance in children and adolescent." In R.W. Manderscheid and M.A. Sonnenschein (Eds.), *Mental Health, United States, 1996* (pp. 71–88). Rockville, MD: Center for Mental Health Services.

Gallo, J.J., D.R. Royall, and J.C. Anthony (1993). "Risk factors for the onset of depression in middle age and later life," *Social Psychiatry and Psychiatric Epidemiology*, 28:101–108.

Gartner J, D.B. Larson, G. Allen (1991), Religious commitment and mental health: a review of the empirical literature. *Journal of Psychology and Theology*, 19(1):6–25.

Gumbiner, J., and J. Flowers (1997). "Sex differences in MMPI-1 and MMPI-2," *Psychological Reports*, 81:479–482.

Gurin, G., J. Veroff, and S. Feld (1960). *Americans View Their Mental Health*. New York: Basic Books.

Hall, Margaret, and Maria F. Owings (2002). "2000 National Hospital Discharge Survey," *Advance Data* No. 329.

Hollingshead, August B., and Frederick C. Redlich (1958). *Social Class and Mental Illness: A Community Study*. New York: John Wiley.

Holmes, T.H., and R.H. Rahe (1967). "The social readjustment rating scale." *Journal of Psychosomatic Research*, 11:213–225.

Hughes, Michael D., and Walter R. Gove (1981). "Living alone, social integration, and mental health," *American Journal of Sociology*, 87:48–74.

Kessler, R.C., K.A. McGonagle, S. Zhao, C.B. Nelson, M. Hughes, S. Eshleman, H.U. Wittchen, and K.S. Kendler (1994). "Lifetime and 12-month prevalence of DSM-III-R psychiatric disorders in the United States. Results from the National Comorbidity Survey." *Archives of General Psychiatry*, 51:8–19.

Kessler, Ronald C., Katherine A. McGonagle, Shanyang Zhao, Christopher B. Nelson, Michael Hughes, Suzann Eshleman, Hans-Ulrich Wittchen, and Kenneth S. Kendler (1994). "Lifetime and 12-month prevalence of DSM-III-R psychiatric disorders in the United States," *Archives of General Psychiatry*, 51:8–19.

Kessler, R.C., P.A. Berglund, S. Zhao, P.J. Leaf, A.C. Kouzis, M.L. Bruce, R.M. Friedman, R.C. Grossier, C. Kennedy, W.E. Narrow, T.G. Kuehnel, E.M. Laska, R.W. Manderscheid, R.A. Rosenheck, T.W. Santoni, and M. Schneier (1996). "The 12-month prevalence and correlates of serious mental illness", in Manderscheid, R.W. and Sonnenschein, M.A. (Eds.), *Mental Health, United States, 1996* (DHHS Publication No. (SMA) 96-3098, pp. 59–70). Washington, DC: U.S. Government Printing Office.

Kuo, W.H. (1984). "Prevalence of depression among Asian-Americans," *Journal of Nervous and Mental Disease*, 161:449–457.

Mechanic, David (1962). "The concept of illness behavior." *Journal of Chronic Illness*, 15:189–194.

Mechanic, David (1978). *Medical Sociology*. New York: The Free Press.

Moss, Gordon E. (1973). *Illness, Immunity, and Social Interaction*. New York: John Wiley.

National Center for Health Statistics (1998). *Health, United States, 1998*. Hyattsville, MD: National Center for Health Statistics.

National Center for Health Statistics (2002). *Health, United States, 2002*. Hyattsville, MD: National Center for Health Statistics.

Pasamanick, B.A. (1959). *The epidemiology of mental disorder*. Washington, DC: American Association for the Advancement of Science.

Regier, D.A., M.E. Farmer, D.S. Rae, J.K. Myers, M. Kramer, L.N. Robins, L.K. George, M. Karno, and B.Z. Locke (1993). "One-month prevalence of mental disorders in the United States and sociodemographic characteristics: The Epidemiologic Catchment Area study." *Acta Psychiatrica Scandinavica*, 88:35–47.

Rice, D.P., and L.S. Miller (1996). "The economic burden of schizophrenia: Conceptual and methodological issues, and cost estimates." in M. Moscarelli, A. Rupp, and N. Sartorious (Eds.), *Handbook of mental health economics and health policy. Vol. 1: Schizophrenia* (pp. 321–324). New York: John Wiley and Sons.

Srole, L. (1962). *Mental Health in the Metropolis: The Midtown Manhattan Study*. New York: McGraw-Hill.

Stark, Rodney (1971). "Psychopathology and religious commitment," *Review of Religious Research*, 12:165–176.

Szasz, Thomas S. (1961). *The Manufacture of Madness: A Comparative Study of the Inquisition and the Mental Health Movement*. New York: Dell.

Warheit, G., C.E. Holzer III, and J.J. Schwab (1975). "An analysis of social and racial differences in depressive symptomatology," *Journal of Health and Social Behavior*, 14:291–299.

Weissman, M.M., J.K. Myers, and P.S. Harding (1978). "Psychiatric disorders in a U.S. urban community: 1975–1976." *American Journal of Psychiatry*, 135:459–462.

ADDITIONAL RESOURCES

American Psychiatric Association. *Diagnostic and Statistical Manual for Mental Disorders, fourth edition (DSM-IV)*. Washington, DC: American Psychiatric Press, 1994.

Center for Mental Health Services (1998). *Mental Health, United States, 1998*. Washington, DC: U.S. Government Printing Office.

Dohrenwend, Barbara S., and Bruce P. Dohrenwend (1981). *Stressful Life Events and Their Contexts*. New York: Prodist.

Kessler, Ronald C., Katherine A. McGonagle, Shanyang Zhao, Christopher B. Nelson (1994). "Lifetime and 12-month Prevalence of DMS-III-R Psychiatric Disorders in the United States." *Archives of General Psychiatry*, 51:8–19.

Lin, Nan, Mary W. Woelfel, and Stephen C. Light (1985). "The buffering effect of social support subsequent to an important life event." *Journal of Health and Social Behavior*, 26:247–263.

Murray C.J.L., and A.D. Lopez (editors) (1996). *Summary: The global burden of disease: a comprehensive assessment of mortality and disability from diseases, injuries, and risk factors in 1990 and projected to 2020*. Cambridge, MA: Harvard University Press.

Robins L.N., and D.A. Regier, eds. (1991). *Psychiatric Disorders in America: The Epidemiologic Catchment Area Study*. New York: The Free Press.

Schumaker, J.F., ed. (1992). *Religion and Mental Health*. New York: Oxford University Press.

Stewart, Miriam J. (1989). "Social support: Diverse theoretical perspectives," *Social Science and Medicine*, 28:1275–1282.

Thoits, Peggy A. (1995). "Stress, coping, and social support processes: Where are we? What next?" *Journal of Health and Social Behavior*, extra issue:53–79.

Turner, R. Jay, and Donald A. Lloyd (1995). "Life-time traumas and mental health: The significance of cumulative adversity," *Journal of Health and Social Behavior*, 40:374–404.

Turner, R. Jay, Blair Wheaton, and Donald A. Lloyd (1995). "The epidemiology of social stress," *American Sociological Review*, 60:125–140.

Williams, David R., David T. Takeuchi, and Russell K. Adair (1992). "Socioeconomic status and psychiatric disorder among blacks and whites," *Social Forces*, 71:179–194.

INTERNET LINKS

World Health Organization (Burden of disease) site: http://www.who.int/msa/mnh/ems/dalys/intro.htm.

National Institute of Mental Health (NIMH) homepage: www.nimh.nih.gov.

Chapter 14

Social Change, Technology, and Healthcare

THE NATURE OF SOCIAL AND CULTURAL CHANGE

A certain amount of social change is inevitable in every society. The change may be subtle and virtually unnoticed by those who are actually "living it." Or it may be cataclysmic and have a dramatic impact on the entire population. Although the change that occurs in isolated traditional societies may go almost unnoticed, change always occurs. On the other hand, social change is glaringly obvious in modern societies and particularly in the United States. Everywhere we turn Americans find changes in the physical environment, the social environment, and the lifestyles of society members. In fact, it could be argued that "change" itself has become a value in American culture. The society's emphasis on "progress" and technological advancement make a certain amount of change inevitable. This is perhaps epitomized by the hawker's favorite phrase: New and Improved! The rate at which Americans change jobs, residences, and even lifestyles reinforces the notion that change has become a national value.

Change is ubiquitous in the healthcare arena, and substantial energy and resources go into initiatives seeking to introduce innovations into healthcare and, by extension, society. There is always the prospect of the breakthrough drug or procedure that will revolutionize medical care. Billions of dollars are expended for research on products and procedures that could eventually engender significant changes in the delivery of care.

Ironically, this emphasis on change as it relates to healthcare runs counter to the basically conservative nature of the institution. The benefits of any new approach must be scientifically demonstrated before its adoption by clinicians and, even then, there may be substantial resistance to its acceptance. Healthcare provides a clear example of the tension that results from society's quest for improvement and an institution's inherent urge to maintain the status quo. Healthcare also clearly illustrates the concept of "cultural lag", in which technological developments far outpace social and ethical concepts.

There are a number of reasons—both internal and external—why change is inevitable in society. Internally, every society undergoes constant turnover in personnel. Each generation is somewhat different from the previous one if only in subtle ways. Even in traditional societies, alternating periods of famine and plenty may affect the physical characteristics of the population and cause more children to survive in one generation than in another. Changes in a society's values may occur (often influenced by external forces). For example, a warlike society may concede that the toll exacted from constant warfare is too costly and begin to minimize military values. Changes in technology within the society are likely to occur as well. Some of these may be introduced from the outside but, even left to their own devices, societies will make discoveries and invent new tools or techniques. Imagine the social implications of the discovery of a permanent water supply by a hunting and gathering society that for generations had spent most of its time migrating in search of water.

External forces for change exist as well. Changes occur in the environment over time and more dramatic changes might be brought about by the forces of nature. Indeed, the history of man on earth has been one of constant adaptation to a changing environment. Another major external force for change is acculturation. "Acculturation" refers to the process of borrowing traits from other cultures and, thus, involves changes in the social environment rather that the physical environment. As long as societies are in contact with each other they will borrow objects, techniques and ideas from one another. Anthropologists offer countless examples of situations in which the culture of a society was significantly changed through even limited contact with another society.

With regard to internal forces for change, social conflict theorists would argue that tension and conflict within a society inevitably produce change. Social conflict arising from inequality (involving race and gender as well as class) can force change in every society, including the U.S. The struggle between the "haves" and "have nots" results in conflict and the resolution of this conflict is likely to result in social change. From this perspective, society is in a constant state of disequilibrium, rather than equilibrium, as it goes through cycle after cycle of organization, disorganization and reorganization. As the character of the haves and have nots is modified over time, change in the nature of society is inevitable.

Migration within and among societies is another social process that promotes change. Between 1870 and 1930, tens of millions of immigrants entered the industrial cities of the United States, now joined by other millions during the 1990s. Millions more from rural areas of the United States joined the rush to the city. As a result, farm communities declined, cities expanded into metropolises, and the United States became a predominantly urban nation. Similar changes are taking place today as people move from the Snowbelt to the Sunbelt and mix with new immigrants from Latin America and Asia.

One of the major forces for social change involves the modification of the ideals and values of society and the associated behavior patterns. The importance of the healthcare institution today owes a lot to changes in the value system that occurred in the second half of the twentieth century. While societies seldom totally forsake a value, they often demonstrate a shift in relative importance over time. Earlier note has been made of the value shifts from an emphasis on the family and religion to an emphasis on economic success, educational achievement and the quest for health. A shift away from self-sufficiency as a value to reliance on formal institutions contributed to the rise of healthcare, as did the growing value placed on technological advances.

Change in one dimension of a cultural system usually sparks changes in others, although not necessarily in the same way or at the same pace. For example, the increased participation of women in the labor force is linked to changing family patterns, including later age of first marriage and a high divorce rate. At the same time, the growing numbers of women physicians has had a significant impact on the medical profession and the delivery of care. Such connections illustrate the close relationship among various elements of a cultural system.

In a given society, some elements of the cultural system change faster than others. Ogburn (1964) introduced the concept of cultural lag, contending that material culture invariably changes at a faster pace than nonmaterial culture. New surgical techniques are routinely developed and often outpace the ability of the system to adapt to them. Even more dramatic examples are found in the cases of genetic engineering and human cloning. These changes in technology raise numerous social concerns and, given that we still struggle with issues like abortion and euthanasia, these issues defy resolution. Cultural lag theory contends that society will ultimately "catch up" to changes in material culture as changing knowledge and technology make old forms of organization obsolete and call for innovation. Even so, social resistance to such changes causes lags in the adoption of new technologies and organizational structures. As Cockerham and Richey (1997) point out, cultural lag is a useful concept for examining how social disorder and ethical dilemmas result from variable rates of social and cultural change within the larger social milieu.

Medical technology that makes it possible to prolong life has developed more rapidly than our ethical standards for deciding when and how to use it. The same is true for virtually any medical innovation. For instance, a less invasive surgical technique may eliminate the need for long hospital stays, but because of delays in acceptance by physicians and resistance from insurance companies with regard to reimbursement, years may pass before the technique is made available to patients. Cultural lag is especially apparent in the ethical controversies created by changing medical technology, such as the moral and legal controversy surrounding the termination of life support for terminally ill patients (Cockerham and Richey 1997).

Social change is set in motion in at least three ways. The first is through invention, or the process of creating new cultural elements. This is clearly a factor affecting the healthcare system. Billions of dollars are spent on research, with the intent of "inventing" a new surgical technique or drug. The process of invention goes on constantly, as indicated by the thousands of applications submitted annually to the U.S. Patent Office.

Discovery, a second cause of change, involves recognizing and or understanding something already in existence. Discovery is also a common development in healthcare, from the serendipitous discovery of penicillin to the painstaking process of unraveling the genetic code.

The third cause of social change is diffusion, or the spread of objects or ideas within a particular society or from one society to another. The ability of new information technology to send information around the world in seconds means that the level of cultural diffusion has never been greater than it is today. The process involved in the diffusion of medical innovations has been thoroughly researched and, at the consumer level, the ability to diffuse vast amounts of information via the Internet has served to dramatically expand access to valuable information.

THE CULTURAL FRAMEWORK FOR HEALTHCARE

Social change in the United States could not have occurred at the pace at which it has without substantial change in underlying cultural traits.

The restructuring of U.S. institutions in the twentieth century was accompanied by a cultural revolution resulting in extensive value reorientation within American society. The values associated with traditional societies that emphasized kinship, community, authority, and primary relationships became overshadowed by the values of modern industrialized societies. "Health" came to be recognized as a distinct value in American society, with the quest for health coming to dominate much of the activity of the American population.

The "modern" values that emerged within the United States after World War II supported the development of a healthcare system that is unique among the world's healthcare systems. The values that emerged in the twentieth century and serve to color the nature of American society today place emphasis on economic success, educational achievement, and scientific and technological advancement. These emergent values supported the ascendancy of healthcare as a dominant institution during the last half of the twentieth century.

The extent to which societal values influence the nature of the healthcare system cannot be overemphasized. The emphasis Americans place on economic success led to the establishment of the world's most profit-oriented healthcare system. The emphasis placed on education assured a premium for the long training period required for medical personnel. The value placed on technology clearly influenced the direction of the healthcare system, resulting in by far the world's most high-tech system. Most important, perhaps, is an emphasis on "activism" in that it called for a healthcare system that featured an instrumental orientation that demanded direct, aggressive action in the face of health problems.

These shifts in value orientation, to a great extent, reflect the demographic transformation of U.S. society in the twentieth century. While it is true that the development of modern scientific medicine required the formulation of germ theory as its foundation, the evolution of contemporary U.S. healthcare corresponded substantially with the demographic changes characterizing the first half of the twentieth century. It is one thing to develop the capacity for inoculating against various disease organisms—this is readily done in developing countries—but it is quite another to establish a value system that fosters a mammoth, highly specialized industry that not only accounts for a disproportionate share of the gross national product but also exerts a tremendous influence over the everyday lives of U.S. citizens.

The cumulative effect of the demographic and epidemiologic transitions of the 20th century and shifting American values contributed to the nature of the healthcare system that is in place as we enter the 21st century. There is no reason to believe that social, economic and political change will not continue to play a more important role in determining the future of healthcare than developments within healthcare itself.

IMPLICATIONS OF SOCIAL CHANGE

A great deal of research has been focused on the implications of social change for a society. Social change is sometimes intentional but often unplanned. Industrial societies actively promote many kinds of change. Scientists, for example, seek more efficient forms of energy, and advertisers try to convince us that life is incomplete without this or that new gadget. People often band together to form social movements, organized efforts to encourage or oppose some dimension of change. Our nation's history is the story of all kinds of social movements, from the colonial drive for independence to today's organizations supporting or opposing abortion, gay rights, and the death penalty. Ironically, while U.S. society places great value on change, it is loathe to formally institute society-wide change through government action. Thus, while all welcome innovations in healthcare, few support planning efforts that would contribute to orderly change within the institution.

Rarely can anyone envision all the social consequences that technological changes set in motion. No one could foresee, for example, how much the mobility provided by the automobile would alter life in the United States, scattering family members, threatening the environment, reshaping cities and creating suburbs and ultimately gutting the medical centers of many central cities. Neither could automotive pioneers have predicted the 50,000 deaths caused by car accidents each year in the United States alone or the fact that automobile accidents would become the leading cause of accidental deaths and result in accidents becoming one of the five leading causes of death in U.S. society. At the same time, such developments as the introduction of safe drinking water and smoking bans have implications for social behavior and health status. For this reason, researchers often speak in terms of the unintended consequences of social change.

An important example of this phenomenon drawn from healthcare involves the technological advances that have allowed the healthcare system to save severely low-birth weight babies and to save the lives of those suffering severe trauma and burns. The life-saving technology that was developed during the last half of the twentieth century has resulted in a substantial increase in the number (and proportion) of individuals in U.S. society who suffer from significant disabilities. These survivors may suffer from severe physical and/or mental handicaps and be forced to rely upon society for a lifetime of continued (and often expensive) support services. Clearly, no one involved in the desperate fight to save a premature baby has gives much thought to the long-term consequences of the application of this technology. Nevertheless, the creation of large numbers of disabled individuals within society has clearly been an unintended consequence of these well-intentioned activities.

Social change can have both "good" and "bad" consequences and much of the meaning attached to social change depends on one's perspective. One group's benefit may be another's liability as demonstrated by the case of surgical technology. The introduction of new, non-invasive surgical techniques may be seen as a boon for consumers, insurers, and those who master the new techniques. On the other hand, this breakthrough may be seen as a setback for hospitals that stand to lose inpatient admissions and for established surgeons whose livelihood depends on the performance of invasive surgery. Similarly, the increase in the proportion of female physicians may be seen as a positive development by some parties and a negative one by others.

An example of this situation involves the introduction of the Internet into the healthcare arena. Certainly the World Wide Web was not designed as a means of transmitting health-related information. Yet, during the 1990s the Internet as a source of health-related information began to surpass all other sources, including the physician and the health plan. By the end of the decade there were more sites devoted to health-related topics than any other subject, and healthcare consumers were eagerly surfing the Internet in search of everything from disease information to drug side effects to the location of a specialist.

Healthcare consumers were becoming as current as healthcare providers with regard to therapeutic procedures, drug dispensing, and disease symptomology. As a result, patients began showing up at the doctor's office armed with extensive information, some of which the physician may not have had access to. Granted, not all of the health-related information on the Internet is accurate but, accurate or not, the fact that a better-informed patient was showing up at the doctor's office has had significant implications for the doctor-patient relationship.

This relationship has also been changed due to the ability of doctors and patients to interact directly with each other via the Internet. Although slow in coming, by 2000 a significant number of physicians had begun contacting their patients through this medium. While this may be thought to detract from personal contact between doctor and patient, more likely it has increased the ability of the physician to interact with a larger number of patients. The use of the Internet by medical practices to provide test results, monitor patient compliance, and otherwise maintain contact has changed the dynamics of healthcare delivery. The ability of patients to make appointments, obtain test results, and review their medical record has further changed the dynamics of healthcare delivery, far beyond the expectations of early pioneers of the Internet.

LEVELS OF SOCIAL CHANGE

Social change can take place of a number of different levels in society. Broad societal trends affect the various institutions and, like the others, healthcare was swept up in these trends characterizing the twentieth century. Changes in the U.S. social structure and value system created an environment in which a large and powerful healthcare system could develop. The declining role of the family and church in the provision of healthcare and the growing involvement of governments at all levels in the healthcare system resulted in dramatic changes. The establishment of the Medicare and Medicaid programs in the 1960s were political developments that had profound implications for the healthcare institution. Demographic changes established the baby boomers as the dominant cohort in society and this group has influenced numerous society-wide changes in the institution.

The organizational level or the level at which healthcare is delivered is another level at which change can occur. In fact, for most Americans this is the area of greatest personal impact. During the last 20 years of the twentieth century Americans experienced a major transformation in the delivery and financing of care. A new generation of therapeutic techniques was introduced along with a new generation of pharmaceuticals, the delivery of care shifted from primarily an inpatient setting to an outpatient setting, and the manner of financing care was modified as managed care became a dominant feature of the healthcare landscape and tens of millions of Americans ended up without health insurance.

At the same time, the healthcare institution experienced shifting power relationships as the unfettered influence of the physician was challenged by other competing providers, and third-party payors began to increasingly set the parameters for reimbursement and, hence, the delivery of care. Employers, who were bearing most of the cost of private insurance, began to play a more active role, bringing about numerous changes in the delivery of care. Many of these developments reflected the shift from an emphasis on medical care to an emphasis on healthcare described earlier in the text.

At the lowest level of social structure, change occurred with regard to statuses and role relationships. The status of the physician came into question during the last years of the twentieth century, as evidence on the fallibility and limitations of physicians became more abundant. The introduction of increasing numbers of women and foreign-trained physicians into the physician ranks also led to a changing image of the physician. Baby boomers, now armed with information from the Internet, influenced the shift way from the dependent patient to an aggressive consumer-patient demanding a role in the therapeutic process. These developments have had a significant impact on the doctor-patient relationship and on the manner in which care is delivered.

TECHNOLOGY, SOCIAL CHANGE, AND HEALTHCARE

Every society exhibits some level of technology. It can range from the rudimentary and unobtrusive to the complex and intrusive. The influence of technology on life in the United States is something Americans take for granted, and society members seldom consider the subtle implications of technology for their lives.

A society's technology reflects underlying cultural values. Industrial technology raises living standards and extends lives. High levels of education become the rule because industrial and post-industrial jobs demand a literate and skilled work force. Further, industrial societies extend political rights and have the potential to reduce economic inequality. While advanced technology gives us work-saving machines and miraculous forms of medical treatment, it also contributes to unhealthy levels of stress and has created weapons of mass destruction.

The value that American culture places on technology has led to the establishment of a "technological imperative", a prevalent idea in most Western societies (especially the United States) which argues that, if we have the technological capability to do something, then we should do it. The technological imperative implies that action in the form of the use of an available technology is always preferable to inaction.

The notion of a technological imperative was first forced on the American consciousness during the Viet Nam war when a technology far beyond the demands of the situation was brought to bear—essentially because it was available. Although the application of technology to healthcare is certainly considered more benign than that for warfare, once a technology becomes available, its use becomes inexorably routinized and considered standard. The failure to apply a new standard of care—no matter how inappropriate for the individual patient—would be considered unacceptable (Koenig, 1988).

The technological imperative has become deeply ingrained in many institutional responses to health crises. For example, most hospitals have created (and thus need to use) several high-technology wards, such as coronary and neonatal intensive care units, deliberately equipped and staffed to provide maximum multiple technological responses to patients' conditions. Similarly, much health insurance gives priority to high-tech medicine (such as treatment in a coronary care unit) over low-tech or nontechnological responses (such as home care).

According to Freund and McGuire (1999), there are also serious ethical questions about the use of medical responses that themselves cause pain or other suffering. For example, under what conditions should a patient or a patient's family be allowed to refuse a prescribed treatment, such as chemotherapy or surgery? The technological imperative has considerable legal support in many states; patients and their families must go to court to assert (and sometimes lose) the right to decide to refuse treatment or life supports.

Considerations such as these make decisions related to the use of technology appropriate for the entire society as well as individual practitioners, patients, and families to consider. Indeed, many issues such as cloning, genetic engineering, and stem cell research are being debated in the halls of Congress. These issues are difficult for the courts, in part because the courts have historically deferred to the medical profession as the proper authority on matters such as these.

The technological imperative has important policy implications that society at large must address. The unbridled use of technology has meant that 5–6 percent of Medicare enrollees account for 25–35 percent of all Medicare expenditures, with these incurred mostly during the last year of life. It allows thousands of low-birth weight and premature babies to be kept alive at tremendous expense and with a high risk of permanent disabilities. It means that individuals can receive expensive organ transplants, even those who have "deliberately" destroyed their livers through alcohol addiction.

Ultimately, society must weigh the costs incurred as a result of the technological imperative against the benefits derived from expending these resources in some other manner. By the end of the twentieth century such issues were being raised with increasing frequency, but the proponents of high-tech medicine are strongly entrenched and can claim strong societal support. It will be interesting to see the impact that the shift to a biopsychosocial approach to care and the growing emphasis on holistic, more low-tech treatment will have on the technological imperative. (Box 14-1 considers the possible end of the medical imperative in healthcare.)

SOCIAL MOVEMENTS AND HEALTHCARE

Like all institutions in society, healthcare is influenced by the social movements that occur within society. Some of these movements take place in the larger society and outside of healthcare. Others occur squarely within the healthcare institution. Regardless of the site of the movement, sociologists contend that these movements take two forms: valued-oriented movements and norm-oriented movements.

The drive for equality for women in U.S. society can be viewed as a value-oriented movement. This movement initially focused on the workplace and called for the equal treatment of women by employers. Demands for fair pay and equal opportunity were joined by demands for more women-friendly, employer-sponsored insurance provisions. This movement was ultimately extended to the healthcare arena and, joined with feminist supporters from other arenas, resulted in a demand for fairer treatment of women by the healthcare system. This involved more sensitivity to the needs of women on the part of providers, an end to the medical exploitation of women, and more representation in clinical research, among other issues. The crux of the movement was the value placed on women and their needs, and this movement was successful at identifying inequities that required redress.

An example of a norm-oriented movement would be the campaign in support of legalized abortion. While this movement was tied to a certain extent to the more value-oriented women's equality movement, the focus was less on a value and more on a norm. Ultimately, it did not matter whether legislators and policy makers changed their value orientation toward women's rights or a woman's right to control her own body. What mattered is that legislation was passed that permitted the performance of abortions. Ultimately, many beneficiaries of the legal provision of abortion had little affinity for the broader women's equality movement. Their primary concern was having access to safe, legal abortion services.

Like the women's equality movement, many social movements that originated outside of healthcare ultimately had important implications for the institution. The women's equality movement could be seen as part of a broader movement usually referred to as the "feminist movement." This movement went well beyond the workplace in its scope and called for equality for women in all aspects of society. The movement challenged, for example, male-only organizations and male-only sports teams. One of its areas of greatest impact, however, was in the healthcare arena. The movement pointed up the attitude held toward women in the healthcare system and the subsequent treatment of women by healthcare providers. The movement admonished women to retake control of their health and become knowledgeable, active participants in their own healthcare. The problems highlighted by this movement in the 1970s and 1980s had a significant influence on women's health issues.

Another example of a social movement that originated outside of healthcare is the "War on Poverty" of the 1960s. During this period of raised social consciousness, poverty in America was rediscovered. Social observers pointed out the pervasive existence of hidden poverty in America's urban and rural areas and bemoaned the paradox of poverty amid an increasingly affluent society. One of the by-products of this process was the discovery of the unfavorable health status characterizing the poor and their lack of access to services to address their health issues. The circumstances of poverty contributed to poor health status and prevented individuals in these circumstances from having the resources to address these health problems. Further, a "culture of poverty" was discovered that led to generational transfer of poor health through the persistent lack of health knowledge and through a tradition of distrust of and/or misuse of the healthcare delivery system.

Box 14-1

The End of the Technological Imperative in Healthcare?

The healthcare delivery system in the United States was increasingly characterized by its technological component during the second half of the 20th century. As a society we became obsessed with biotechnology and increasingly put our trust in equipment. The emphasis on technology was such that many observers noted the existence of a "technological imperative" or the tendency to utilize technology because it existed rather than because it was a better approach. The U.S. system became known as a high tech/low touch system in which the human side of medicine was subordinated to the technical side and the cost of providing care increased commensurate with increases in the use of technology.

By the end of the 20th century, there was evidence of a backlash against the technological imperative, with a number of factors contributing to this development. On the practical side, hospitals and other healthcare providers were finding the cost of keeping technologically current to be increasingly prohibitively expensive. By the 1990s, hospital administrators were resisting demands from their medical staffs for new technology, demands that would have been routinely approved a decade earlier. Not only were budgets too tight to afford expensive technology, but third-party payers were discouraging the use of excessive technology and ratcheting down reimbursement in cases where its use was considered appropriate. Medicare and other

---

This movement that was intended to reduce poverty in the U.S. included a strong healthcare component. It was argued that it was impossible for sick people to go to school or to hold jobs. As long as they were sick, there was no way out of the situation. Thus, major healthcare initiatives were established to address these needs. A community health center initiative was launched, and programs were developed to encourage practitioners to serve in underserved areas. The most important result of this movement, however, was the establishment of the Medicaid program to provide government-subsidized healthcare to the deserving poor. Through a federal/state program funds were provided to reimburse providers for treating Medicaid enrollees. This was clearly a political response to a healthcare dilemma, and the program served to provide healthcare to tens of millions of Americans who otherwise would have had no access to care.

Other social movements have originated within the healthcare arena, initiated by healthcare providers, consumers, or other entities within or related to the healthcare institution. An example of this is the consumerism movement that has periodically emerged to have an impact on the healthcare delivery system. The consumer movement in healthcare was first

third-party payors were increasingly reluctant to approve reimbursement for new technology on the grounds, rightly or wrongly, that it was "experimental" technology.

Another source of resistance to technological imperialism came from consumers who were reacting to the impersonality of the system and to the high cost of care. The growing emphasis on healthcare (as opposed to medical care) and the increasing popularity of holistic approaches tempered the obsession with technology that characterized earlier decades. These consumers were joined by a new generation of physicians who were more interested in "whole person" healthcare and, despite growing up in the computer age, less enamored with high-tech medicine. Managed care plans even got into the act by insisting that an "appropriate" level of care be provided, and this often meant providing less technology than clinicians might desire.

Evidence was also developed that pointed to both the unfavorable cost-benefit ratio of some advanced technology and the failure of expensive advanced technology to provide much more diagnostic bang for the buck than some traditional technologies. These findings have generated a healthy skepticism even among some parties who had been strong advocates of advanced technology.

Obviously, technology is not going to disappear from U.S. healthcare and, indeed, we will continue to be the most high-tech system in the world. Current developments, however, suggest that the role of technology in the future healthcare system may be quite different than it was at the end of the 20th century.

documented during the 1970s and 1980s as patients began to react to some of the less favorable characteristics of the system. There was a growing resistance to the god-like status of the physician and an emergent desire to take a more active role in one's own therapy. The knowledge and capabilities of physicians were questioned, and the motives and practices of hospitals brought under fire for the first time. Insurance practices were also questioned, and various initiatives launched to make more information available to patients about physicians, hospitals, and health plans.

Just as consumerism was taking hold in healthcare, managed care came to dominate the organization and financing of care. Consumers who had begun to play a role in decision making were now told that decisions with regard to their care would be made by the managed care plan. The trend toward consumer choice was quickly snuffed out as restrictions were placed on access to care for plan enrollees.

By the mid-1990s, however, a significant backlash had developed among consumers with regard to managed care. A new generation of healthcare consumers, led by the baby boom cohort, chaffed under the restrictions imposed by managed care plans. These new consumer/patients

Insisted on playing a role in their care and had the resources to influence the operation of the system. As this huge cohort began to flex its muscles, managed care plans began backing away from many of their restrictions on access to care. Concepts central to managed care—but detrimental to the consumer—such as gatekeepers and capitated payments were deemphasized in favor of arrangements that allowed more consumer choice. Indeed, many futurists see consumer choice as the major characteristic of the healthcare system for the first decade of the twenty-first century.

Numerous other movements can be cited within healthcare. These include the holistic health movement, campaigns to legalize marijuana for medicinal purposes, the physician-assisted suicide movement, and others. Quite often these movements have less to do with the technical provision of care and more to do with the social, political and ethical aspects of care. As such, their implications range far beyond the healthcare arena into the larger society.

FUTURE SOCIOCULTURAL CHANGE IN THE U.S.

As illustrated above, the healthcare institution is as much influenced by the sociocultural changes that occur in society as it is by developments within healthcare itself. While it is hard to predict what developments might occur in healthcare over the next several years, we can foresee certain developments within the broader society that will have an impact on the healthcare institution. Some of the more important developments are discussed in the sections that follow.

Demographic Trends

Today, perhaps more than at any time in the past, demographic trends are shaping the demand for health services, both at the national and local level. The shifts that have occurred in value orientation in this century, to a great extent, reflect the demographic transformation of U.S. society. Beginning with the demographic transition that commenced with the beginning of the twentieth century through the epidemiological transition that started mid-century to the dramatic demographic shifts of the last third of the century, changes in the nature of the American population were to have significant implications for the healthcare system.

Changing Age Structure

The age distribution is perhaps the single most important demographic predictor of the demand for health services. The aging of America has obviously been one of the most publicized demographic trends in history.

Its implications for health services demand have been well-documented along with the likely impact of this trend on other aspects of society. The overall aging of the population is not nearly as directly significant for changing healthcare demand as is the "internal" restructuring of age distribution.

The development with the most implications for future healthcare demand is the movement of the huge baby boom cohort into the "middle ages". There are 77 million baby boomers who are used to having things their way. When they have to contend with the onset of chronic disease and the natural deterioration that comes with aging the healthcare system will be impacted significantly.

An automatic accompaniment to the aging of America has been the feminization of the U.S. population. The changing age distribution has important implications for the population's sex distribution. Generally speaking, the older the population, the greater the "excess" of females. Except for the very youngest ages, females outnumber males in every age cohort. Now, by the time we are considered "elderly", females outnumber males two to one, and, at the oldest ages, there may be four times as many women as men. For the older age cohorts (65 and older) the sex ratio is less than 70, compared to 95 for the total population. In the mid-1990s, the "excess" number of females over males approximated eight million. This means that women will constitute an ever-growing proportion of those that seek healthcare.

Racial and Ethnic Diversity

Another demographic trend that characterizes the American population is increasing racial and ethnic diversity. After a mid-century phase of homogeneity, America has once again become a nation of immigrants, with the numbers of newcomers from foreign lands equaling historic highs. Long-established ethnic and racial minorities are growing at faster rates than are native-born whites. As a result, the visibility of non-Hispanic whites in the U.S. population is decreasing.

Non-Hispanic whites accounted for 80 percent of the U.S. population in 1980, 76 percent in 1990 and 69 percent in 2000. In fact, most of the population growth during the next two decades will be accounted for by immigration. By 2000 nearly half of all American children will be members of minority groups, and by 2025 or so, minorities will be in the numerical majority.

Changing Household and Family Structure

Another demographic development that should be noted is the changing household and family structure. This trend is no surprise to demographers, although it has seldom been linked to health issues. For decades, the family has been undergoing change. First it was high divorce rates, then it was less people marrying (and those who did marry married at a later age); then it was less people having children (and those that did have children had fewer of them and at a later age).

This has meant that the "traditional" American family (with two parents and x number of children) has become a rarity, accounting for only 26 percent of the households in 2000. Today, married couple (without children) households have become the most common household form, but this type of household accounts for less than 30% of total households. Non-traditional households are becoming the norm. The fastest growing household types are single-parent households. Father-only or mother-only families (children present in both) are projected to grow by over 34 percent over the next 20 years. The absolute increase in mother-only families will be over two million.

Consumer Trends

Although patterns of consumer attitudes in U.S. society tend to be complex, it is clear that a new orientation is occurring with regard to healthcare. For the most part, today's consumer is much more knowledgeable about the healthcare system, much more open to innovative approaches, and much more intent on playing an active role in the diagnostic, therapeutic and health maintenance processes. This is in stark contrast to the traditional healthcare consumer during the Golden Age of medicine in the 1950–1960s when physicians and hospitals were regarded with something akin to reverence and patients had complete faith in the healthcare system.

These new attitudes are concentrated among the under-50 population and among certain demographically-distinct populations. The movement toward gaining control of one's own healthcare is spearheaded by the baby boom cohort that is now beginning to face the chronic conditions associated with "middle age". This is the population that has been responsible for the success of health maintenance organizations, urgent care centers, and birthing centers. This is the group that has been influential in limiting the discretion and control of physicians and hospitals.

The approach to healthcare characterizing this population is much more patient centered and emphasizes the non-medical aspects of healthcare. It is much less trusting of professionals and institutions and is control-oriented to the point of stubbornness. This cohort is much more self-reliant than previous generations and emphasizes self-care and home care. It is both outcomes oriented and cost sensitive. It is a generation that prides itself in getting results and extracting value for its expenditures. While this cohort influenced changes by "voting with its feet" during the 1980s, its members will increasingly be in the positions of power that will allow its members to start reshaping the healthcare landscape. This cohort has also provided the impetus for the rise of "alternative therapy" as a competitor with mainstream allopathic medicine.

To a certain extent, these changed attitudes toward healthcare reflect the rise of consumerism related to all segments of society. *Consumers* (as opposed to *patients*) demand healthcare information, insist on participating in healthcare decisions that directly affect them, and expect that the healthcare they receive will be of the highest possible quality. Consumers want to receive their healthcare close to their homes, with minimal interruption to their family life and work schedules. They also wish to maximize their healthcare dollars, especially when chronic illness quickly depletes their lifetime maximum insurance benefits.

REFERENCES

Cockerham, William C., and Ferris J. Richey (1997). *The Dictionary of Medical Sociology*. Westport, CT: Greenwood.

Freund, Peter E.S., and Meredith B. McGuire (1999). *Health, Illness and the Social Body*, 3rd ed. Englewood Cliffs, NJ: Prentice Hall.

Koenig, Barbara (1988). "The technological imperative in medical practice: The social creation of a 'routine' treatment," pp. 465–496 in M. Lock and D.R. Gordon, eds., *Biomedicine Examined*. Dordrecht, Netherlands: Kluwer.

Ogburn, William F. (1964). *On Culture and Social Change*. Chicago: University of Chicago Press.

ADDITIONAL RESOURCES

Coile, Russell C., Jr., (2002). *Futurescan 2002: A Forecast of Healthcare Trends 2002–2006*. Chicago: Health Administration Press.

Gallagher, Eugene B. (1988). "Modernization and medical care." *Sociological Perspectives*, 31:59–87.

Hardey, Michael (1999). "Doctor in the house: The Internet as a source of lay health knowledge and the challenge to expertise." *Sociology of Health and Illness*, 21:820–835.

Link, Bruce G., and Jo Phelan (1995). "Social conditions as fundamental causes of diseases." *Journal of Health and Social Behavior*, extra issue:80–94.

Nathanson, Constance A. (1996). "Disease prevention as social change: Toward a theory of public health," *Population and Development* 22:609–637.

Glossary

Absolute poverty: The poverty level of individuals and populations measured in absolute (rather than relative) terms; a level of deprivation that could be considered life threatening.

Access: The ability of individuals or groups to obtain health services. Access may be it influenced by service availability, as well as access to transportation, insurance and other factors.

Achieved status: A social position that a person assumes voluntarily and reflects the individuals abilities; status based on achievement ideally discounts inherent traits (such as gender and race).

Activities of daily living (ADL): The tasks that individuals must perform in order to take care of themselves (e.g., dressing, toilet use). The level of disability characterizing an individual is often determined by the number of ADLs he can or cannot perform.

Acute condition: A health condition characterized by rapid onset, usually short duration, and a clear-cut disposition (e.g., cure, death), typical of developing countries and younger populations.

Admission: The formal placement of an individual into a hospital or other inpatient facility, typically limited to episodes of care involving an overnight stay. The number of admissions is a commonly used measure of hospital utilization.

Age-sex pyramid: *See* Population Pyramid.

Age-specific rate: The level of occurrence (per 1,000, 10,000, 100,000 population) of a phenomenon for a specific age cohort.

Ageism: Prejudice and/or discrimination directed toward the elderly in society.

Agency for Healthcare Research and Quality (AHRQ): A federally-funded research institute under the auspices of the Department of Health and Human Services that supports studies on the utilization of health services and the efficacy of various treatment modalities.

Alienation: A situation in which an individual is dissociated from his culture and/or social milieu, resulting in a state of isolation and powerlessness.

Alternative therapy: An umbrella term that refers to a variety of therapeutic modalities (e.g., homeopathy, acupuncture, nutritional therapy) utilized by patients as alternatives to mainstream allopathic medicine. Increasingly referred to as complementary therapies.

Ambulatory care: Any type of treatment that is provided to an "ambulatory" patient that does not require an overnight hospital stay. Also referred to as outpatient care.

American Hospital Association (AHA): The primary professional association for hospitals and certain other healthcare organizations in the U.S.; the major spokesperson for the hospital industry.

American Medical Association (AMA): The primary professional association for physicians in the U.S.; the major spokesperson for the medical profession.

Anomie: A condition in which the individual is alienated from social norms, thereby lacking the moral guidance that society typically provides; normlessness.

Anticipatory socialization: Social "training" that prepares an individual for an anticipated future role (such as parent or medical student).

Anxiety disorder: An emotional condition characterized by fear, nervousness or other disquieting characteristics; a mild form of mental illness.

Ascribed status: A social position conferred on an individual (often at birth) based on inherent characteristics (such as sex and race); ascribed statuses are generally acquired involuntarily.

Assimilation: The process through which members of minority populations gradually adopt patterns of the dominant culture.

Assisted living facility: A residential facility that provides a controlled environment for individuals who require assistance with activities of daily living but do not require intensive medical care.

Attitude: An individual's cognitive evaluations, feelings, or action tendencies toward some person, object, or idea.

Authority: Power conferred on individuals through legitimate means.

Average length of stay (ALOS): The number of days on average patients remain in a hospital or other institution, calculated as the number of patient days during a period (usually a year) divided by the number of admissions during that period.

Avoidance: The process of deliberately attempting to remain ignorant of one's physical or mental condition.

Baby Boomers: The segment of the U.S. population (born between 1946 and 1964) that constitutes the largest cohort in the age distribution.

Behavioral health: An approach to the management of mental illness that emphasizes the behavioral component of the individual's condition.

Belief: A tenet that society members hold to be true, although it cannot be independently verified.

Blue-collar occupation: Lower prestige job that typically involves manual labor.

Bureaucracy: An organizational model involving a rational approach to effective task performance.

Capitalism: An economic system in which the means of producing goods are privately owned.

Capitation: An arrangement whereby providers are paid a predetermined per capita fee for providing a specified range of services to a specified population.

Case analysis: A technique used by epidemiologists to identify the incidence of specific health conditions within a population and track the progression of these conditions over time.

Case-mix: The combination of diagnoses that make up the distribution of cases treated by a particular provider (e.g., the proportion of cases that are obstetrical, cardiac, etc.). Alternatively, the overall characteristics (e.g., age, sex) of a group of enrollees for which a case manager is responsible.

Caste system: A closed social stratification system based primarily on ascription, with one's social status assigned at birth.

Cause-and-effect: A relationship in which a change in an independent variable causes a change in a dependent variable.

Cause of death: The reason for the death of an individual provided on the standard death certificate and used in mortality analyses.

Census Bureau: The federal agency within the U.S. Department of Commerce with responsibility for conducting the decennial census and a variety of other censuses and survey activities.

Center for Medicare and Medicaid Services (CMS): The federal agency within the U.S. Department of Health and Human Services that manages the Medicare and Medicaid programs; formerly the Health Care Financing Administration (HCFA).

Centers for Disease Control and Prevention (CDC): The CDC is the federal agency responsible for monitoring various infectious diseases and tracking the course of any epidemic condition. The CDC is an important source of epidemiological data.

Chronic condition: A health condition characterized by slow onset, lengthy progression, and a usually indefinite disposition, typical of modern, industrial societies, and older populations.

Cohort: A segment of the population that is distinguished by exposure to a particular condition—e.g., all people born in the United States between 1946 and 1951 or all American soldiers exposed to Agent Orange in Viet Nam.

Commercial insurer: A category of for-profit insurance plan that typically reimburses providers on a fee-for-service basis. Commercial insurers represented the major category of non-government insurance until the emergence of managed care.

Condition, health: A departure from a state of physical or mental well-being.

Consumer: Any individual in the community that is a potential user of an organization's products or services.

Continuum of care: A range of clinical services provided during a sickness episode that represent a continuous process of care from initial diagnosis to ultimate disposition of the case.

Crude birth rate (CBR): A simple measure of the level of fertility of a population based on the number of births per 1,000 population; the birth rate may be misleading since the denominator includes the total population and not just the population at risk.

Crude death rate (CMR): A simple measure of the level of mortality of a population based on the number of deaths per 1,000 population; the crude death rate may be misleading since there are significant variations in death rate by age.

Cultural conflict: A situation in which the norms of two cultures or subcultures are incompatible and create conflict for the individuals involved; a situation in which an individual is confronted with cultural patterns that are in conflict with his internalized patterns.

Cultural integration: A situation in which the components of a cultural system are in harmony.

Cultural lag: A social condition that results when some cultural elements change at a faster rate than others, thereby causing the development of some components of the culture to lag behind others.

Cultural relativism: The practice of evaluating a culture according to that culture's standards and not those of the evaluator; the opposite of ethnocentrism.

Cultural universals: Traits that are part of every known culture.

Culture: The set of intangible traits (beliefs, values and norms) and tangible artifacts that characterize a particular society; a people's way of life.

Culture shock: The personal disorientation that accompanies exposure to an unfamiliar way of life.

Current Procedural Terminology (CPT): A coding system used by physicians to code procedures performed. This code is tied to the fees charged.

Custodial care: Refers to non-medical care provided to individuals, typically in long-term care facilities, who cannot take care of themselves. There is no intent to cure, thus the term "custodial". Also referred to as "personal care".

Custom: The most basic type of social norm in society; an informal rule for guiding social behavior; a folkway.

Death role: The pattern of role obligations and privileges associated with the status of being terminally ill; an extension of the sick role.

Deinstitutionalization: A process through which institutionalized patients (typically the mentally ill) are discharged from inpatient facilities with the assumption that supportive services and treatment will be provided within the community.

Demand (for health services): The combined healthcare needs and wants of a population that constitutes the volume and type of health services "demanded" by the population (which may or may not approximate utilization).

Demographic transition: The process by which a population reduces it death rate as a result of health measures associated with modernization, contributing to an unprecedented surge in population growth followed by a decline in fertility due to higher standards of living. The process ends when fertility levels fall to essentially match mortality levels thereby creating a stable population.

Demographics: The set of biosocial and sociocultural characteristics of a population that determine its demographic composition.

Department of Health and Human Services (DHHS): The principal agency within the U.S. government for the coordination of the health-related responsibilities of the federal government.

Depression: A mental condition characterized by depressed mood and a lack of interest in social interaction; a form of psychosis.

Deviance: Any act or behavior that violates societal norms.

Deviant behavior: A pattern of social norm violation that becomes habitual and persistent.

Diagnosis Related Groups (DRGs): A system of classifying diagnoses and/or procedures for grouping hospital inpatients into categories based on relative resource utilization and used as a basis for prospective reimbursement by the Medicare program.

Diagnostic and Statistical Manual (DSM): A coding system patterned on the International Classification of Disease utilized for classifying mental disorders.

Disability: The level of incapacity within a population as measured by the number of cases of physically and/or mentally handicapped individuals, or by the level of restricted activity (e.g., school-loss days or work-loss days); a condition resulting in incapacity.

Discharge: The official release of a patient after an episode of care at a hospital or other inpatient facility involving at least one night in the hospital. The number of discharges is a frequently used indicator of the utilization level for a hospital.

Discrimination: The differential treatment of various categories of people based on some societally recognized trait (e.g., race, ethnicity).

Disease: A term used in a number of different ways but generally referring to a state of pathology within an individual organism.

Doctor-patient relationship: The on-going two-way interaction between a doctor and a patient.

Durable medical equipment (DME): Biomedical and assistive equipment utilized in the provision of care for institutionalized, homebound or ambulatory patients. Wheelchairs and hospital-type beds are examples of durable medical equipment.

Elasticity: The tendency for the demand for health services to rise or fall in response to non-clinical factors (e.g., insurance coverage, consumer preferences).

Elective procedure: A procedure that is not covered by insurance typically because it is not considered medically necessary (e.g., cosmetic surgery). A consumer may "elect" to have such a procedure performed if he is willing to pay out of pocket for the service.

Emergency care: Medical care provided for a serious medical condition resulting from injury, illness, or mental disorder that arises suddenly and requires immediate attention.

Encounter: Refers to one patient visit to a provider, usually regardless of the number of procedures performed.

Endemic: A situation in which a pathological condition is common to a large portion of a population, to the extent that its presence might be considered "normal".

Epidemic: A situation in which a health condition appears in a population in the form of an "outbreak"; generally refers to a condition that is contagious or communicable.

Epidemiological analysis: An approach to the study of health phenomena that involves the relationship between individuals and their social environment and the distribution of health problems among various segments of the population.

Epidemiological transition: Process occurring during the 20th century in most of the world's countries whereby the aging of the population resulted in a shift from a predominance of acute health conditions to a predominance of chronic health conditions.

Episodic care: The traditional approach to the provision of health services in which each physician visit for each reason is considered a separate episode unrelated to any other episodes of care for that episode. This is in contrast managed care that focuses on the total and continuous management of the condition or the patient.

Estimate, population: A calculated estimation of the population for a particular area or population category for some current or past time period.

Ethnic group: A subgroup within society recognized by virtue of its shared cultural heritage and (usually) its minority status.

Ethnicity: Referring to the shared cultural heritage characterizing an ethnic group.

Ethnocentrism: The practice of judging another culture by the standards of one's own culture; the opposite of cultural relativism.

Etiology: The factor or factors that cause a particular health condition.

Euthanasia: The act of assisting in the death of a person suffering from a terminal condition; mercy killing.

Extended family: A family unit including other relatives in addition to the nuclear family (parents and their children), typically involving three or more generations.

Fee-for-service: The traditional means of paying for health care in the United States whereby insurers or patients pay a separate fee for each service that a physician, hospital or other provider performs. This is in contrast to managed care in which the provider receives a specified amount of reimbursement for managing a range of services.

Feminism: The advocacy of social equality for men and women.

Fertility: The reproduction experience of a population, most often expressed in terms of total births and/or birth rates.

Folk medicine: A treatment model based on herbal remedies and a reliance on natural cures; a precursor of modern Western medicine.

Folkway: The most basic of social norms involving informal rules for everyday behavior; a custom.

Formal organization: A large secondary group that is organized for the efficient achievement of goals.

Functionalist theory: See Structural-Functional Paradigm.

Gatekeeper: The person or organization that controls a consumer's access to health services. Traditionally, the physician served as an informal gatekeeper, and formal gatekeepers such as health plan authorization personnel and discharge planners play an important role in managing utilization in today's healthcare environment.

Gender: The significance that a culture attaches to being male or females; the social distinction between males and females.

Gender role: The attitudes and behaviors that a culture associates with males and females; sex role.

Genocide: A systematic process for destroying a specific population.

Geographic information system (GIS): Computerized application for performing spatial analysis and generating maps reflecting the analysis.

Germ theory (of disease): Theoretical framework that contends that every disease has a specific pathogenic cause the treatment for which can be accomplished by removing or controlling that cause; the basic for the medical model used in modern allopathic medicine.

Gerontology: The study of aging and the elderly.

Group: Two or more individuals who interact with each other on an ongoing basis and develop shared social understandings.

Health: A state of wellness whose definition depends on one s perspective. In the narrowest sense, health has been defined as the absence of disease and disability. In its broadest sense, it has been defined as a state of complete physical, social, mental and spiritual well-being.

Health belief model: A social psychological model of health behavior that attempts to explain the motivation of people to avoid the threat of illness.

Healthcare: Any formal or informal action taken in an attempt to restore, maintain or enhance health status.

Health demography: A subdiscipline of demography that deals with the interaction of a population's demographics, its health status and its healthcare system.

Health maintenance organization: An organization of healthcare providers that provides a comprehensive range of services to an enrolled population for a fixed, prepaid sum.

Health plan: A generic term that applies to any type of insurer that provides coverage for health services, including companies that self-insure their employees.

Health Plan Employer Data and Information Set (HEDIS): An attempt to standardize health plan performance in terms of quality, access, satisfaction, utilization, and finance for use in comparing various health plans; the survey instrument used to gather HEDIS data.

Health Professions Shortage Area (HPSA): Areas designated by the U.S. Public Health Service that have shortages of various categories of health care providers.

Health promotion: Any activity or system that is designed to proactively maintain, improve, or enhance the health status of individuals or populations. Health promotion generally includes both preventive care and lifestyle-related health behavior. This is in contrast to the traditional approach of addressing health problems reactively after they have developed.

Health service area: The geographic area served by a healthcare provider; a formal service area designated by the federally government or some other entity.

Health status indicator: A measure of the relative health condition of a person or population, usually in the form of an index score generated through self-reports or from statistics on the population in question.

Holism: An approach to healthcare that involves a holistic perspective on the diagnosis and treatment of health problems. This approach involves an emphasis on the whole person rather than a specific disease or organ and takes into consideration non-clinical factors related to the patient and his environment in managing an individual's health.

Home health care: Medical care delivered in the home rather than in a clinic or hospital setting; the limited range of services that can be provided by home health agencies.

Hospice: A healthcare organization that provides personal care and palliative treatment for terminally ill patients.

Ideology: The set of doctrines that support a particular political, economic or social system.

Illness: A state of suffering as a result of a disease; a state of ill-health. Social scientists distinguish between illness and sickness, with illness referring to the personal (as opposed to social) aspect of the condition.

Incidence: The number of new cases of a disease, disability, or other health-related phenomenon recorded during a specified period of time.

Incidence rate: The calculation of the amount of new cases of disease or disability within a population, usually expressed in terms of the number of newly diagnosed cases per 100, 1,000, 10,000 or 100,000 persons.

Indemnity insurance: The traditional form of health insurance in the United States in which the insured pays the cost for each service after it has been provided (assuming it is covered by the benefits package). This is in contrast to a managed care approach that involves prepayment for a package of services that are covered under the health plan.

Index: A composite "score" derived from the combination of individual factors thought to be related; the index score can then be compared to other respondents or populations.

Indigent care: Health services provided at no cost to individuals who are considered "medically indigent"—i.e., they are not covered under any type of insurance plan or do not otherwise have the resources to pay for care.

Infant mortality rate (IMR): The number of deaths to infants under one year of age per 1,000 live births during a specific time period (usually one year).

In-group: A social group commanding its members' esteem and loyalty; a privileged group.

Immigration: The relocation of individuals from one country to another country.

In-migration: The process of moving into a geographic area with the intent of establishing residence.

Inpatient: Technically, any patient that spends at least one night (or 24 hours) in an institution such as a hospital or residential treatment program.

Institution: A component of the social system involving patterns of behavior directed to the accomplishment of a specific societal goal.

Institutional discrimination: Biased actions inherent in the operation of a formal organization.

International Classification of Disease (ICD): The standard classification system utilized to categorize the universe of diagnoses and procedures utilized in contemporary medical science.

Intergenerational social mobility: The upward or downward social mobility of society members in relation to their parents' social status.

Intervention: Any action taken in an attempt to remedy a health condition.

Intragenerational social mobility: A change in social status occurring during a person's lifetime.

Labeling theory: A theory that asserts that deviance and conformity reside not so much from what people do, but from how others respond to their actions.

Language: A system of symbols that allows people to communicate with one another and serves as the basis for cultural transmission.

Latent function: The indirect and often unintended consequences of a particular cultural pattern.

Lay referral system: The network of family, friends and associates that helps to interpret the individual's condition and direct him toward a source of care.

Length of stay: The number of days an individual remains in a hospital or other healthcare facility. The length of stay is in an important consideration in utilization management and the average length of stay is used as an indicator of utilization for a hospital.

Life event: An occurrence in an individual's life that is likely to induce stress (e.g., loss of job, birth of child, death of spouse).

Life expectancy: The average number of years members of a population can be expected to live.

Lifestyle: The set of attitudes, values, preferences and behavior patterns that distinguish subsets of the population from each other; often used interchangeably with "psychographic characteristics".

Lifestyle analysis: An analytical approach that analyzes a population on the basis of the lifestyle characteristics associated with various subsets within the population; often used interchangeably with "psychographic analysis".

Limitation of activity: A measure of disability that involves a determination of the ability of an individual to carry out various activities. Usually presented in terms of bed-restricted days, school-loss days, work-loss days, etc.

Living arrangement: Used to describe the nature of household relationships as a supplement to marital status. Includes such categories as married without children, married with children, living alone, cohabitation, and unrelated individuals living together.

Long term care (LTC): Refers to any type of care for the elderly and/or disabled that involves on-going, usually institutionalized management of the patient whether or not medical care is necessary. Nursing homes are the traditional form of long term care but various other types of long term care facilities have become common.

Malinger: To pretend to be suffering from a non-existent or no longer active disorder in order to obtain sympathy or avoid responsibilities.

Managed care: A planned and coordinated approach involving positive and negative incentives for both enrollees and providers for "managing" the services received by a population enrolled in a particular health plan.

Manifest function: The recognized and intended function of a social pattern.

Marital status: The official status of individuals in terms of marriage, typically including the categories of never married, married, divorced, widowed and, sometimes, separated.

Market: Any geographic area or population grouping that can be conceptualized as potential customers.

Market area: The targeted geographic area in which the primary market potential for a health care organization is located; often used interchangeably with "service area".

Market research: A multi-step process involving the systematic gathering and analysis of market data that assists an organization in developing strategies and making decisions.

Market segment: A specific subset of a population that differs from other subsets in a way significant to their use of health services.

Master status: One of a person's social positions that overshadows other statuses; the status of patient becomes one's master status in the case of a serious health condition.

Median age: An indicator of the average age of a population, whereby the median age represents that age at which half of the population falls below and half falls above.

Medicaid: The federally sponsored and state-administered government health insurance program for the low-income population in the United States.

Medicalization: Of deviance, the redefining of moral or legal deviance and medical deviance; of society, the expansion of the healthcare institution to the point that it exerts an inordinate influence over the other institutions of society.

Medically indigent: Individuals who for whatever reason do not have access to health insurance and or not able to pay for health service out of pocket. The medically indigent may not be poverty-stricken but are "insurance poor."

Medically necessary: A characteristic of a procedure or service provided under an insurance plan that reflects a clear medical need for the procedure or service. This is in contrast to elective procedures (e.g., cosmetic surgery) that may be performed in the absence of medical necessity.

Medicare: The federally-sponsored insurance program that covers the elderly population in the United States. All elderly citizens are eligible for basic coverage, with certain additional coverage optional.

Meritocracy: A system in which social position is based on personal merit and/or credentials.

Metropolitan statistical area (MSA): An official designation for a large concentration of population that includes a central city, a county and its surrounding counties.

Migration: The physical movement of individuals or groups from one location to another, typically with the intent of a permanent change of residence.

Minority: Any category of people defined by physical or cultural differences that is accorded inferior status in a society.

Modernization: The process, usually initiated by industrialization, through which a society transitions from a traditional society to a modern society.

Monopoly: The domination of a market by a single organization or group of organizations.

Morbidity: The level of sickness and disability within a population.

Mortality: The level of death characterizing a population, usually expressed in terms of the number of deaths and/or death rates.

Mores: A type of social norm that controls behavior that society places significance on, such as ethics, sexual relations, and other moral issues.

National Center for Health Statistics (NCHS): The federal agency responsible for the collection, management and dissemination of most national data on health and healthcare

Need: In this context, need refers to the actual need for health services within a population as measured by the prevalence of clinically identifiable health problems. This is in contrast to the wants and desires for health services that might characterize a population. Need should represent the baseline level of health problems affecting a population.

Network: A web of weak social ties.

Nonverbal communication: Communication involving body movements, gestures and facial expressions rather than speech.

Norms: Rules and expectations with which a society guides the behavior of its members.

Notifiable disease: A disease whose presence must be reported to public health officials. Typically an infectious disease, notifiable conditions are generally first reported to local health departments and this information is compiled nationally by the Centers for Disease Control and Prevention (CDC).

Nuclear family: A family composed of one or two adults and their children; a one- or two-generation family unit.

Nursing home: An inpatient facility that provides around-the-clock care for incapacitated individuals; typically limited nursing care is provided with personal, custodial care the dominant means of managing nursing home residents.

Occupancy rate: The percent of the beds in a hospital or other inpatient facility that are occupied by patients during a particular time period. The occupancy rate is an indicator of the level of utilization of a hospital, with occupancy for licensed beds versus operational beds often calculated separately.

Office visit: The standard measure for use of physician services and the typical "encounter" that is recorded to measure utilization of physicians and other services.

Oligopoly: The domination of a market by a small number of organizations; the provision of healthcare is often referred to as a monopoly but it more accurately involves an oligopoly.

Out-of-pocket payment: Reimbursement for health services made by patients who are not covered by insurance or for whom the particular service is not covered.

Outcome: The eventual result of a healthcare episode.

Outcome measurement: A formal process for assessing the effectiveness of treatment and patient satisfaction with treatment results.

Outgroup: A social group that one is not a part of and toward which one feels competition or opposition.

Out-migration: The flow of residents out of a geographic area.

Outpatient: An individual who receives any type of health service that does not require an overnight stay in a hospital or other inpatient facility. Similar to an ambulatory patient, although homebound patients would be considered outpatients but not ambulatory patients.

Over-the-counter drug (OTC): A drug that can be purchased from a pharmacy without a prescription written by a physician.

Paradigm: An explanatory framework; a worldview.

Patient: Any individual who receives "formal" health services from a licensed healthcare provider; the official designation necessary for an individual to enter the sick role.

Panel survey: A sample of respondents who have agreed to provide information for a research project over an extended period of time.

Patient origin: The source of patients for a health service based on place of residence (usually identified by ZIP code).

Payer: An agency, insurer or health plan that is responsible for payment for health services provided to designated enrollees or other beneficiaries.

Peer group: A social group whose members have interests, social position, and/or age in common.

Personality: The consistent patterns of acting, thinking and feeling characteristic of a particular individual.

Physician: A person who has successfully completed a prescribed course of studies in medicine at a qualified institution and has the requisite credentials for practicing medicine.

Physician-assisted suicide: Euthanasia; acts of omission or commission on the part of a physician or someone under the physician's supervision that results in the death of a terminally ill patient.

Placebo: An inert substance provided in place of a drug as part of a clinical trial; the effect created in a patient who believes he has received an actual treatment.

Pluralism: A situation in which racial and ethnic groups maintain their distinctiveness but enjoy social parity.

Population at risk: The total number of persons within a population that are at risk of a particular condition. E.g., the number of persons at risk of childbirth would equal the number of fertile child-bearing age women within the population.

Population-based health care: An approach to the provision health services that focuses on the needs of the total population rather than the needs of individuals. Actions focus more on groups than on individuals and outcomes are measured in terms of improvement in overall health status rather than individual clinical successes.

Population pyramid: A stacked bar graph visually depicting the age and sex composition of a specific population.

Post-industrial society: A society based on an economic system that emphasizes service work and high technology rather than manufacturing.

Power: The ability to achieve desired ends despite opposition; control based on force rather than authority.

Preferred provider organization (PPO): A form of health plan that encourages the use of a specified network of providers in exchange for lower rates for plan enrollees. The PPO typically negotiates discounted rates with providers in the network, with the intent of passing these discounts to consumers in the form of lower premiums.

Prejudice: A rigid and irrational generalization about a particular subgroup within society.

Prevalence: The total number of cases of a disease or disability within a population at a specific point in time.

Prevalence rate: The calculation of the amount of disease or disability within a population, usually expressed in terms of the number of existing cases per 100, 1,000, 10,000 or 100,000 persons.

Preventive care: Any activity intended to prevent disease and/or improve health status carried out prior to the onset of a health problem. Preventive care includes health education, screening, and various health behaviors (e.g., tooth brushing) that protect the individual from the onset of health conditions.

Price: The dollar amount that a provider charges for a service provided, typically referred to as a "fee" in health care. This is distinguished from "cost" which refers to the provider's cost of providing the service.

Primary care: The provision of basic, routine health services including preventive services. The physicians typically involved in primary care are general and family practitioners, general internists, obstetricians, and pediatricians, although other types of providers (e.g., behavioral health therapists) may be thought to provide "primary" care.

Primary group: A small social group whose members share personal and enduring relationships.

Product line: A business development approach common in other industries that has been tried with limited success in healthcare. Product line development involves the identification of a vertical set of services (e.g., cardiac care) and the subsequent operation and marketing of the set of services as a business line. In healthcare, it is often referred to as a service line.

Profession: A prestigious, white-collar occupation that requires extensive formal education.

Projection, population: A calculated figure indicating the size of the population for a particular area or population category for some point in the future.

Provider: An individual or organization that is licensed to provide health services, products and/or equipment.

Provider network: A group of providers that have been formally contracted to provide services to enrollees in a particular health plan; in many plans, enrollees are restricted to providers that belong to the network.

Psychographics: Subjective information reported by people regarding their beliefs, feelings, attitudes and behavior patterns; also referred to as lifestyles and utilized as a basis for predicting health behavior.

Public health: The set of activities designated for public health agencies that include disease surveillance, health status monitoring, air and water monitoring, food inspection, the registration of vital events, and the control of infectious conditions.

Purchaser (of health services): Any organization or individual that pays for health services. In common usage, purchaser has come to refer to "group purchasers" such as large employers and business coalitions that represent large numbers of covered lives and can negotiate with providers due to their purchasing power.

Race: A category of people defined based on physical characteristics considered significant by society; non-scientific distinctions made between populations based on physical characteristics.

Racism: The belief that one racial category is innately superior or inferior to another.

Rate: The level of occurrence of a phenomenon per a specified number of persons—e.g., per 100, 1,000, 10,000 or 100,000.

Ratio: The proportion of a characteristic in relation to another characteristic. E.g., a sex ratio of 95 means there are 95 males per 100 females.

Reference group: A social group that serves as a point of reference to an individual and as an example of desirable behavior.

Region, geographic: Generally a geographic area that extends beyond any one political jurisdiction to create an internally consistent region of some type (e.g., Appalachia). Also, refers to officially designated census regions into which the United States is divided by the federal government.

Registry: The systematic recording and reporting of events or situations characterizing a population—e.g., a tumor registry containing all reported cases of cancer within a specified area.

Rehabilitation: Treatment provided after an acute care episode to assist patients in regaining the physical or mental abilities lost due to injury or illness.

Relative deprivation: A perceived social or economic disadvantage relative to some standard of comparison.

Relative poverty: The state of having less economic resources than others in society, regardless of the absolute level of economic resources available.

Relative risk: The probability of the occurrence of a particular health condition within a population relative to the risk for some other population.

Religiosity: The importance of religion in an individual's life; the extent of participation in religious activities.

Risk: The exposure that individuals or population groups experience with regard to various health problems. The risk of contracting AIDS, for example, varies with the types of behaviors in which an individual participates.

Role: The set of rights and responsibilities associated with a particular status or social position.

Role conflict: The tension that occurs when an individual occupies two or more statuses whose roles are incompatible.

Role set: The group of roles that characterize an individual based on the set of statuses characterizing the individual.

Rural area: An area designated by the Census Bureau for data collection purposes that does not meet the minimum standards for an urban area.

Sample survey: A survey in which a subset of the population has been selected for participation in a study. The intent is to draw conclusions concerning the total population based on the sample of respondents that have been interviewed.

Satisfaction survey: A survey that attempts to measure the level of satisfaction with regard to health services or health plans on the part of patients, family members, plan enrollees, or other categories of customers.

Secondary care: A level of health services that involves moderate intensity care and a moderate level of resources and skill levels. Secondary care is more complex than routine care but less intensive than specialized tertiary services.

Secondary group: A large and impersonal social grouping whose members pursue a particular goal or activity.

Secularization: The process through which the significance of the religious institution is displaced by an emphasis on more secular institutions.

Segmentation, benefit: The grouping of individuals into market segments based on the benefits sought from a product—e.g., convenience, service.

Segmentation, demographic: The grouping of individuals into market segments based on such demographic characteristics as age, sex, income, and race.

Segmentation, geographic: The grouping of individuals into market segments based on location of residence or work.

Segmentation, psychographic: The grouping of individuals into market segments based on lifestyle and attitudinal characteristics.

Segmentation, usage: The grouping of individuals into market segments based on their level of utilization of a product or service. Segments may initially be identified as users and non-users, with the users broken down into subcategories based on their level of usage.

Self-administered questionnaire: Survey forms that are completed by the respondents with little or no input from survey administrators.

Service area: The geographic area from which a health care organization draws the majority of its customers; often used interchangeably with "market area".

Sex: The biological distinction between males and females.

Sex ratio: An indicator of the relative proportions of males and females within a population. Typically calculated in terms of the number of males per 100 females.

Sexism: The belief that one sex is innately superior or inferior to another.

Sick role: The set of rights and obligations associated with the social position of patient.

Sickness: A social state involving an impaired social role; the public manifestation of illness.

Sign: A manifestation of ill-health identified through clinical tests.

Significance, statistical: The determination that a research finding reflects a statistical association and not simply a chance correlation.

Social: Of or related to a society or group.

Social change: The transformation of culture and social institutions over time.

Social-conflict paradigm: A theoretical framework that holds that society is constantly in a state of conflict due to the inherent inequalities that exist; conflict rather than order is seen as the natural state of affairs.

Social construction of reality: The process by which individuals shape reality through social interaction.

Social control: Organized attempts by society to regulate society members' thoughts and behavior.

Social dysfunction: Undesirable consequences resulting from a particular social pattern.

Social interaction: The process through which individuals act and react in relation to others.

Social mobility: The process through which an individual or group changes it position in society relative to other positions.

Social movement: An organized effort to encourage or oppose some dimension of change.

Social stratification: The division of society into a hierarchy based on societally determined characteristics and involving inequality in terms of socioeconomic status.

Social structure: Any relatively stable pattern of social behavior.

Socialization: The process through which an individual is exposed to the social patterns of society; the informal or informal training one receives prior to adopting a social position.

Socialized medicine: A system of healthcare in which the government owns most facilities and employs most medical practitioners.

Society: A social system; the interrelated set of components that comprise a distinct social system.

Socioeconomic status: An indicator of an individual or group's position in the social structure based on such measures as income, occupation, and/or education.

Stakeholder: Any individual, organization or constituency that has a stake in the operation of an organization or a healthcare system.

Standardization: A process through which dissimilar populations are statistically adjusted to allow for meaningful comparisons.

Status: A recognized social position that an individual occupies.

Status consistency: The degree of consistency in an individual's social standing across various dimensions of stratification.

Status set: The group of statuses that an individual occupies at a given point in time.

Stereotype: An exaggerated depiction of a group that is applied to all people in that category of persons.

Stigma: An attribute of an individual that evokes a negative response from society members.

Stress: The tension faced by an organism when confronted with a real or perceived threat.

Stressor: Anything in an individual's environment that can induce stress.

Structural-functional paradigm: A theoretical framework that sees society as a complex system whose parts work together to promote solidarity and stability; order rather than disorder is seen as the natural state of affairs.

Subculture: Cultural patterns held by a subgroup of society (typically based on religion, ethnicity, lifestyle or other cultural feature) that distinguish members of the group from the dominant society; the group that is characterized by the patterns.

Survey instrument: Questionnaires used in survey research.

Symbol: Any object or idea that carries symbolic meaning for individuals who share a common culture.

Symbolic-interaction paradigm: A theoretical framework that sees society as a product of the everyday interaction of members of society; a view of society based on interpersonal relationships and interaction rather than social institutions.

Symptom: A manifestation of a health condition that is experienced by the affected individual; a characteristic of the condition known only to the individual.

Syndicated research: A form of contract survey research in which a professional research firm conducts a survey and sells the results to interested parties in the area or, alternatively, the research firm enlists the front-end participation of area healthcare organizations in the development of the survey.

Synthetic data: Population estimates and projections that are generated using statistical techniques and models. Synthetic data are distinguished from actual data collected by means of censuses and surveys.

Tertiary care: Specialized health services for the treatment of serious health conditions that require specialized clinicians, sophisticated equipment and facilities, and substantial support services.

Third-party payer: Any agency or organization that is responsible for reimbursing the cost of health services provided on the part of an insured individual. The provider provides the service to the patient, with the insurer being the "third party" that pays for the care.

Total institution: A setting in which individuals are isolated from the rest of society and manipulated by administrative staff; a social organization that develops beliefs, values and norms in isolation from the dominant society.

Tradition: Beliefs, values and social patterns passed from one generation to another.

Uncompensated care: Health services provided to medically indigent populations that have no ability to pay for care. Uncompensated care is sometimes informally used to refer to any shortfall between charges and reimbursement for services.

Underinsured: Individuals or groups in a population who are technically covered under some health insurance plan but have such limited benefits or unfavorable copay or deductible provisions that they do not have adequate coverage.

Uninsured: Individuals or groups in a population who are not covered under any health insurance plan.

Universal coverage: Situation in which an entire population is covered by a form of medical insurance.

Urbanization: The process of establishing cities as the dominant community type; the way of life that results from the establishment of cities.

Utilization (of health services): The amount and type of health services actually used by a particular population, as opposed to the demand for services.

Wellness: A healthcare process that fosters awareness of healthy lifestyles to allow individuals to achieve optimum physical and mental health.

White-collar crime: Crime committed by individuals of high social position in the course of their occupations.

White-collar occupation: Higher-prestige work that involves mostly mental activity.

Value: Any idea or object that a society places value on; a guiding principle of a culture.

Vital statistics: Data collected by government agencies related to "vital events"—e.g., births, deaths, marriages, divorces, and abortions.

Vulnerable population: Any population segment within a society that is placed at inordinate risk of health problems due to health status, environmental factors, lack of insurance, marginality, and any number of other factors.

Years of potential life lost: A measure of disability and premature death that is calculated in terms of the number of years that an individual would have expected to live (or to have quality of life) had it not been for disability or death. This is sometimes transformed into "productive" years of life lost.

Index